ATLAS *of* COLORECTAL SURGERY

With contributions by

SUSAN GALANDIUK, M.D.

Associate Professor
Department of Surgery
University of Louisville School of Medicine
Louisville, Kentucky

HEIDI NELSON, M.D.

Associate Professor
Department of Surgery
Mayo Medical School
Consultant
Department of Surgery
Mayo Clinic and Mayo Foundation
Rochester, Minnesota

With illustrations by

GILLIAN LEE, F.M.M.A, F.I.M.I., A.M.I

DIANE KINTON, B.A. (HONS)

SANDIE HILL, B.A. (HONS)

ATLAS *of* COLORECTAL SURGERY

MICHAEL R. B. KEIGHLEY, M.S., F.R.C.S.

Barling Professor of Surgery and Head
Department of Surgery
The University of Birmingham
The Medical School
Professor of Surgery
Queen Elizabeth Hospital
Edgbaston
Birmingham, United Kingdom

VICTOR W. FAZIO, M.D., F.R.A.C.S., F.A.C.S.

Professor
Department of Surgery
Ohio State University College of Medicine
Health Sciences Center at Cleveland Clinic
Rupert B. Turnbull Chairman
Department of Colorectal Surgery
The Cleveland Clinic Foundation
Cleveland, Ohio

JOHN H. PEMBERTON, M.D.

Professor of Surgery
Division of Colon and Rectal Surgery
Department of General Surgery
Mayo Medical School
Mayo Graduate School of Medicine
Consultant
Colon and Rectal Surgery
Mayo Clinic and Mayo Foundation
Rochester, Minnesota

ROLLAND PARC, M.D.

Chairman
Department of Surgery
University of Paris
Professor of Surgery
Centre de Chirurgie Digestive
Hopital Saint-Antoine
Paris, France

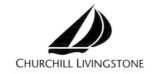

CHURCHILL LIVINGSTONE

New York, Edinburgh, London, Madrid, Melbourne, San Francisco, Tokyo

Library of Congress Cataloging-in-Publication Data

Atlas of colorectal surgery / Michael R.B. Keighley . . . [et al.] ;
   with illustrations by Gillian Lee ; with contributions by Susan
   Galandiuk, Heidi Nelson.
       p. cm.
   Includes bibliographical references and index.
   ISBN 0–443–07570–0
   1. Colon (Anatomy)—Surgery—Atlases. 2. Rectum—Surgery—
  Atlases. I. Keighley, M. R. B.
   [DNLM: 1. Colon—surgery—atlases. 2. Rectum—surgery—atlases.
  3. Colonic Diseases—surgery—atlases. 4. Rectal Diseases—surgery—
  atlases. WI 17 A876 1996]
  RD544.A85 1996
  617.5′ 547—dc20
  DNLM/DLC
  for Library of Congress   96–16863
                                    CIP

Distributed in the United Kingdom by Churchill Livingstone, Robert Stevenson House, 1–3 Baxter's Place, Leith Walk, Edinburgh EH1 3AF, and by associated companies, branches, and representatives throughout the world.

Accurate indications, adverse reactions, and dosage schedules for drugs are provided in this book, but it is possible that they may change. The reader is urged to review the package information data of the manufacturers of the medications mentioned.

The Publishers have made every effort to trace the copyright holders for borrowed material. If they have inadvertently overlooked any, they will be pleased to make the necessary arrangements at the first opportunity.

Acquisitions Editor: *Miranda Bromage*
Assistant Editor: *Ann Ruzycka*
Production Editor: *Robert Carmenini*
Production Supervisor: *Sharon Tuder*
Desktop Coordinator: *Jo-Ann Demas*
Cover Design: *Jeannette Jacobs*

Printed in the United States of America

First published in 1996   7 6 5 4 3 2 1

To Margaret, my wife, whom I owe everything for allowing me to pusue my surgical and academic interests

Michael R.B. Keighley

To Elise, whose patience is infinite, whose sense of humor has survived twenty years intact (mostly), and whose single-minded devotion to Johnny, Jeffrey, Lauren, and Margaret is unshakable, allowing me the privilege and luxury to pursue tasks such as this—all my love.

John H. Pemberton

This book is dedicated to a gracious woman, my mother, Kathleen Eleanor Hills Fazio . . . whose sacrifices enabled me to become a doctor.

Victor W. Fazio

Preface

The contribution of *The Atlas of Colorectal Surgery* to colorectal surgery is not to be yet another textbook! Our objective is to provide a clear, concise account of surgical technique and procedure in coloproctology. This book is aimed at coloproctologists and general surgeons and for those in training.

We have deliberately avoided descriptions of indications or outcome. This is a book devoted to "how it is done." The four authors of this atlas are experts with extensive experience in North American and European practice. Inevitably, we express individual views, and for this reason commentaries are provided by each of us on the subjects presented.

We have spared no expense on artwork in order to provide a comprehensive visual impact of how it is done. To avoid duplication, certain common issues, such as anastomotic technique, are dealt with at the start of the text and are cross-referenced for the reader so as to create a slim volume that avoids repetition. Thus, general surgical technique, the use of stomas, and the overall conduct of operative procedures in our field are dealt with as separate items.

We have made no attempt to provide a comprehensive bibliography. This is not a textbook, but a manual of operative surgery that we hope will sit on the shelves of every general surgeon and become a household volume for those in training.

Michael R. B. Keighley, M.S., F.R.C.S.
John H. Pemberton, M.D.
Victor W. Fazio, M.D., F.R.A.C.S., F.A.C.S.
Rolland Parc, M.D.

Contents

1

Approaches

John H. Pemberton

Positioning

Positioning of the patient on the operating room table may seem to be an unimportant detail, but most surgeons can recall having to complete an abdominoperineal resection in a patient whose perineum has slid away. A few tricks and a moment or two spent before preparing and draping are often repaid generously.

Combined Position

The Lloyd-Davies position (Figs. 1-1 and 1-2) has been modified to include the use of Allen stirrups, but the principle remains the same: The patient's perineum hangs off the end of the table. In order to prevent intense low back pain postoperatively, the sacrum should be supported with a pillow, as illustrated. If the buttocks are correctly positioned, then the patient will not slide forward when the table is placed in steep Trendelenburg for the pelvic dissection portion of an abdominal approach. Alternatively, a well-padded shoulder rest will prevent the patient from moving on the table.

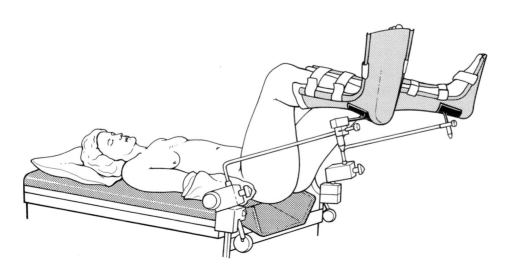

Figure 1-1.

1

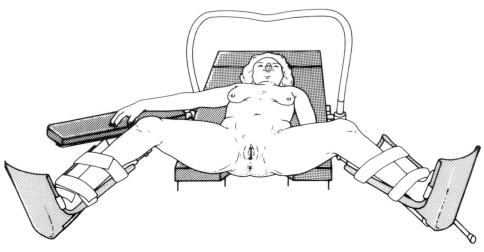

Figure 1-2.

The Allen stirrups are positioned such that the peroneal (lateral popliteal) nerve, which is easily injured using other types of stirrups, is not subject to any pressure. After placing the heel securely in the footrest, pull the portion of the stirrup that supports the calf backward. This then suspends the patient's leg by the heel. The legs are then well padded and protected from any metal parts.

The patient's left arm is kept close to the body and is wrapped and doubly protected using a pillowcase and gauze sponges. Usually in these situations, the patient's right arm is extended for access by the anesthesiologist. If absolutely necessary, it also can be placed at the patient's side.

Both the abdomen and the perineum are prepared and draped using a sterile technique. The instrument table can be positioned either between the legs (a European convention) or above the patient's head (as is done in the United States). Alternatively, instrument tables may be placed at both locations. Importantly, if the table is positioned above the patient's head, it must be placed well back; if it is only at chest level, when the table is placed in steep Trendelenburg, there will not be enough room to work in the abdomen. Another advantage of this position is that it allows a third operator to work between the patient's legs during the abdominal portion of the operation. Furthermore, it allows a second team to perform the perineal portion of the operation (i.e., excision of the rectum, endorectal mucosal resection or stapling) simultaneously. Another indication for the use of this position is if intraoperative colonoscopy is contemplated.

Supine Position

The supine position is used for all abdominal procedures that do not involve pelvic dissection. The arm position depends on the type of operation to be performed. For right-sided lesions, the left arm is out, and for left-sided operations, the right arm is out. It is also important to anchor the patient's ankles with an ankle strap in case steep Trendelenburg tilt is required.

Jackknife Prone Position

If general anesthesia is ordered, the patient is anesthetized on the cart. The patient, with arms at the sides, is then log-rolled onto the operating table. A pillow is placed beneath the head, chest rolls along the chest, and a pillow for the hips and legs. It is important that the hips be placed at the break in the table. It is also important to lift the legs up slightly, as illustrated in Figure 1-3. The buttocks may be taped apart. The arms are positioned as shown by carefully abducting the arms 90 degrees and flexing

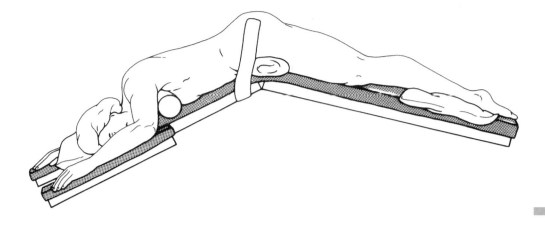

Figure 1-3.

the elbows to 90 degrees. The palms are placed down. We perform nearly all anal procedures using this position.

Lithotomy Position

The lithotomy position with stirrups (Fig. 1-4) is used for all examinations under anesthesia and for endoscopy when general anesthesia is required. Moreover, this position facilitates inhalational anesthesia. Because of the awkwardness of this position, Allen stirrups are substituted in procedures expected to take longer than a few minutes. Again, the buttocks are placed so that the perineum hangs off the end of the table. We perform no anal surgical procedures using this position because the anal tissues and perineum tend to become engorged with blood in this position, which would complicate such procedures as hemorrhoidectomy or fissurectomy.

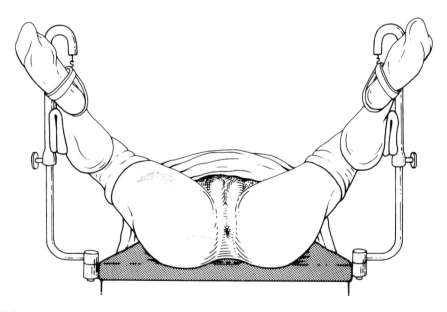

Figure 1-4.

Left Lateral Decubitus Positon

In the left lateral decubitus position (Fig. 1-5) it is important that the buttocks overhang the table by about 4 to 6 inches. The arms are positioned as shown. This position is used for abdominosacral approaches to low rectal cancers as popularized by Localio and others. A sigmoid incision is made in the abdomen in this position (Fig. 1-6A), thus facilitating mobilization of the abdominal contents. At the same time, a

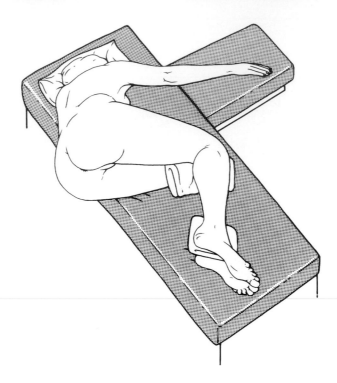

Figure 1-5. ▬▬▬▬▬▬

transcoccygeal incision (Fig. 1-6B) is made to gain access to the presacral space. This approach is included for completeness and interest only, as I know of very few surgeons who approach rectal tumors in this manner. A more contemporary use for the transsacral approach is as part of a laparoscopic low anterior resection.

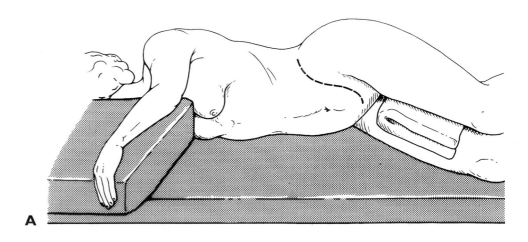

A

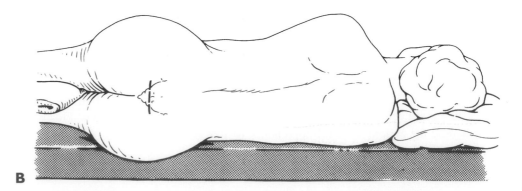

Figure 1-6. ▬▬▬▬▬▬ **B**

Incisions

Midline Incision

The midline incision is my incision of choice for all abdominal procedures, whether performed routinely or emergently. Whenever a laparotomy is performed as an emergency, such an incision seems mandatory. This incision provides unrestricted access regardless of the patient's size or shape.

An upper midline incision (Fig. 1-7A) is useful for operations on the stomach, esophagus, spleen, left lobe of the liver, and other exotic general surgical procedures. A mid-midline incision (Fig. 1-7B), straddling the umbilicus above and below, is the incision of choice for small bowel and right colon resection. A lower midline incision (Fig. 1-7C) extended above the umbilicus is the incision of choice for abdominal colectomy, proctocolectomy, left hemicolectomy, and sigmoid and rectal resection. One rule that I find most helpful in deciding whether to extend a lower midline incision above the umbilicus is this: If the stomach is not visible in the uppermost portion of the incision, then the splenic flexure will be too high to approach safely. Extension of the incision until the stomach can be visualized is warranted.

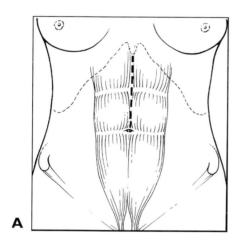

A

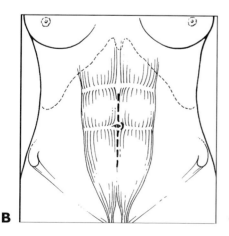

B

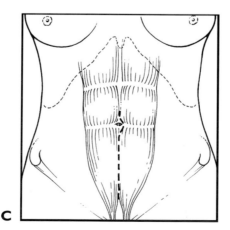

C

Figure 1-7.

Although it is the current fashion to nick the skin with a scalpel and then proceed with cautery, this seems a totally unnecessary exercise in wasting time (and blood). The rapid, simple, and nearly bloodless way to proceed is to use the scalpel all the way. As soon as the fat is exposed, the wound is spread with the fingers. By pulling on the wound and applying digital pressure, bleeding is minimized. The natural midline plane separates down to the fascia upon pulling (Fig. 1-8A). This is quite useful because often the midline is not obvious below the umbilicus. By the time the fascia has been incised, any bleeding from the skin and subcutaneous fat has stopped—without one joule of electrical energy being used (Fig. 1-8B).

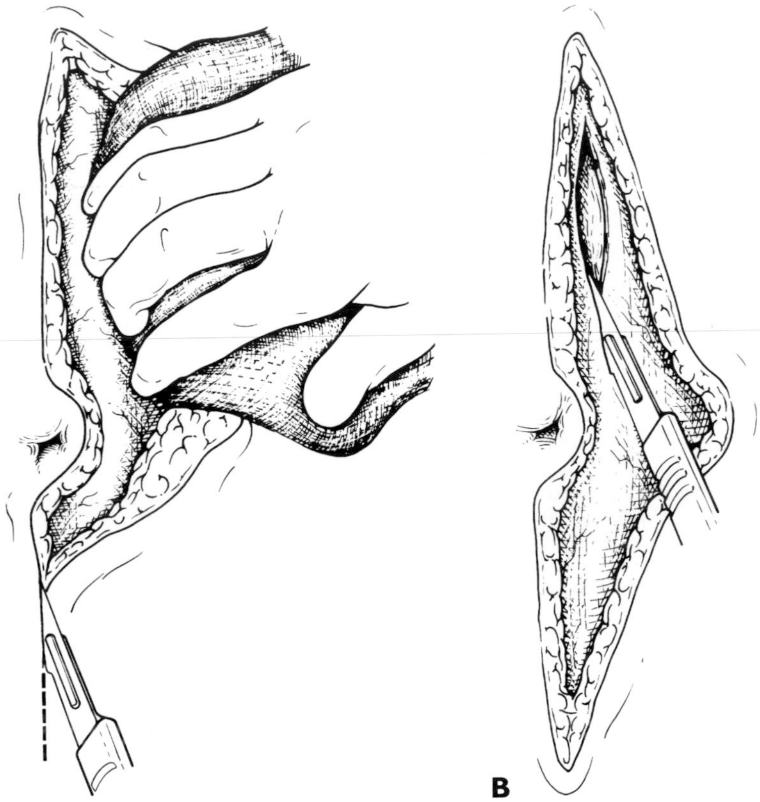

Figure 1-8. A B

Transverse Incision

The anterior superior iliac spine to anterior superior iliac spine, or smile, incision (Fig. 1-9) is an alternative to the midline incision. I have assisted in a procedure in which this incision was used on an obese patient.

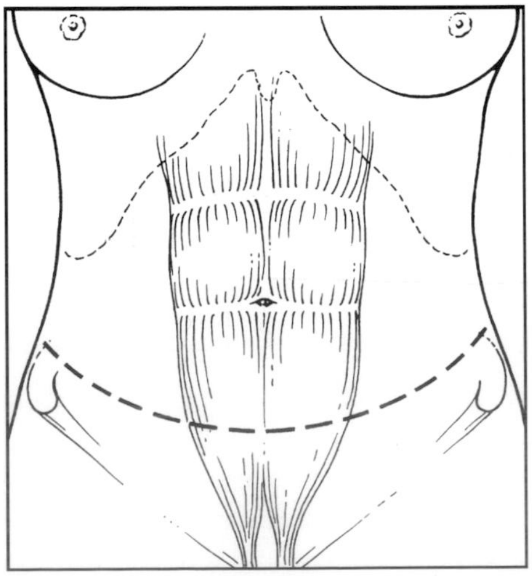

Figure 1-9.

Stoma Incisions

If at all possible, the stoma site should be chosen before the operation (see Ch. 4). A circular incision is made about the premarked site, excising the fat as a core down to the anterior fascia. A cruciate incision is made in the fascia, the muscle separated, and, if encountered, the epigastric vessels are ligated.

Approaches

Abdominoperineal Resection

Abdominal Approach. The patient is placed in the combined position (see Fig. 1-1) and prepared and draped. A lower midline incision is made skirting the umbilicus to the patient's right. The stoma site, marked preoperatively by a stoma therapist, is in the left lower quadrant. The incision is deepened into the perineal cavity and the abdominal portion of the operation performed as described in Chapter 10. At any time, a second surgeon may begin the perineal phase of the operation; this is usually best accomplished after most of the rectum has been mobilized intra-abdominally.

Figure 1-10 shows the incision to be made in the perineum; it is elliptical and made about the anus 3 to 4 cm from the anal verge. This need not be a huge incision. As seen in Figure 1-11, the levators can be incised radically or conservatively, irrespective of the width of the skin incision.

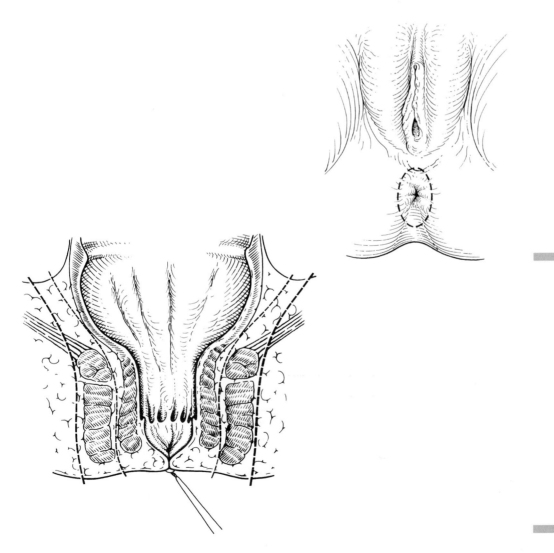

Figure 1-10.

Figure 1-11.

Perineal Approach. The anus is first closed with a heavy suture to prevent soilage. Figure 1-11 shows the intended resection via a coronal view. Note that the levators can be taken in any width. The dotted line shows an intrasphincteric approach used for resection of the rectum and anus in benign disease, whereas the dashed line illustrates the more standard approach used for rectal cancer.

After incising the skin, large Kraske rakes are used to provide exposure laterally. A smaller rake is used anteriorly. Using the cautery, the fat is incised circumferentially about the anus until the level of the anal coccygeal ligament is reached posteriorly. Rarely do vessels need to be ligated. At this point, I use a scissors positioned on my finger toward the coccyx posteriorly, pushing down and then cutting above my finger aggressively (Fig. 1-12). I cut directly into a laparotomy pad that has been packed firmly into the pelvis after the abdominal procedure, during which a circumferential dissection about the rectum down to the level of the levators has been performed.

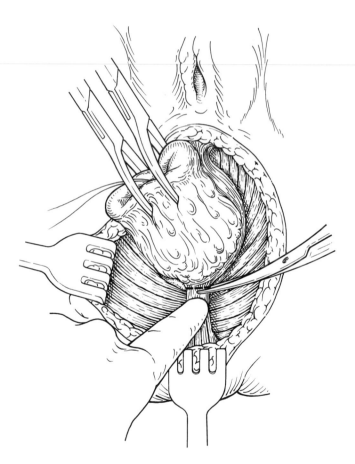

Figure 1-12.

Cautery is used to incise the levators. The fingers of the surgeon are inside the pelvic cavity above the level of the levators. They are used to guide the incision from the 6 o'clock position (directly posteriorly) to the 3 and 9 o'clock positions laterally. Figure 1-13 shows the dissection extended to the 9 o'clock position. At this point, the specimen has been passed down by the abdominal operator and is ready to be removed posteriorly.

Figure 1-14 shows the rectal specimen in the surgeon's left hand. The surgeon is seen dissecting the anterior attachments, principally those to the prostate or vagina. Either a clamp or cautery can be used to divide the puborectalis muscle at this level.

Hint: If a specimen is removed posteriorly, thus exposing the anterior structures by posterior tension, it is easy to make a mistake and extend the dissection deeply ante-

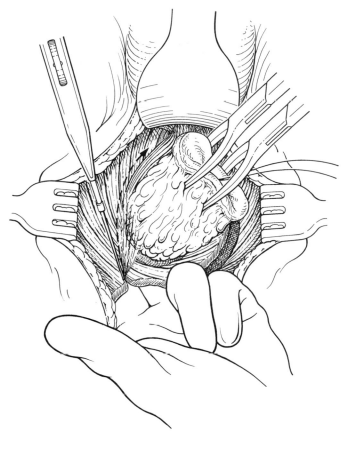

Figure 1-13.

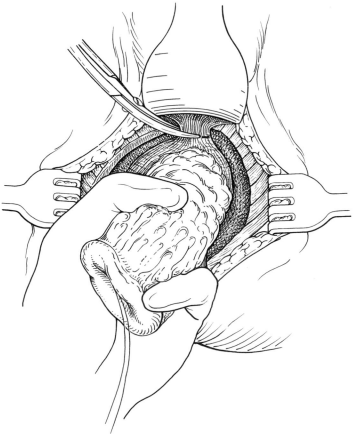

Figure 1-14.

riorly, thus placing the urethra in jeopardy. To prevent this, after maneuvering the specimen out posteriorly, <u>palpate the catheter lying in the urethra.</u> This will prevent any unintentional exposure of the catheter via the perineal incision.

The central principle then is to free up the rectum completely posteriorly and laterally to the 9 and 3 o'clock positions by incising the levators. This allows the specimen to be pulled out posteriorly and facilitates freeing the anterior attachments under direct vision. Once the specimen has been removed, two round suction drains are placed on either side of the perineal incision (Fig. 1-15A). The levators are then reapproximated using interrupted sutures of heavy Vicryl (Fig. 1-15B). The subcutaneous tissues are closed using lighter Vicryl while the skin is closed with a running subcuticular Vicryl suture.

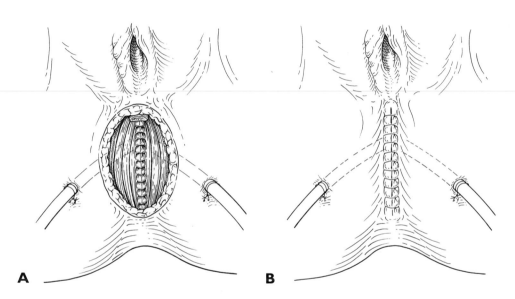

Figure 1-15.   **A**   **B**

Intersphincteric Approach. The principal difference between the standard perineal approach and an intersphincteric resection is that a large amount of muscle (external anal sphincter, puborectalis, and levators) is preserved. In order to accomplish this, the incision is made quite close to the anus and a plane is developed between the internal and external anal sphincters (Fig. 1-16A), which is followed to the top of the puborectalis muscle (Fig. 1-16B). This is usually very easy to perform but is sometimes more bloody than the standard dissection.

The remainder of the operation is the same as for the more aggressive standard approach. Obviously an intersphincteric approach is not recommended if a rectal cancer is located in the lower third of the rectum abutting the levators. The reason for performing a proctectomy is to achieve wide clearance. If wide clearance is not possible using an intersphincteric approach, then a standard wide resection of the levators is indicated. The principal usefulness of the intersphincteric proctectomy is in patients who have inflammatory bowel disease or familial adenomatous polyposis, and who are not candidates for restorative procedures.

Intra-Anal and Intrarectal Procedures

At our institution, patients are placed in the prone jackknife position (see Fig. 1-3) for intra-anal or intrarectal procedures. The biggest advantage of this position for these circumstances is that the rectum and anal canal are not continually engorged with blood, as they would be if the lithotomy position were used. However, posteriorly located polyps in a large man might better be approached using the lithotomy position.

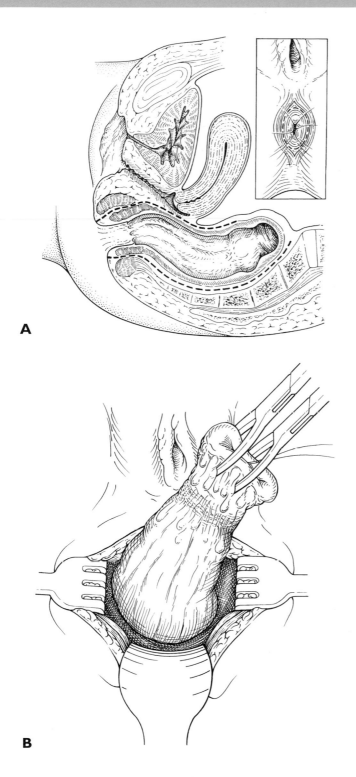

A

B

Figure 1-16.

Biopsies, removal of hypertrophied anal papilla, hemorrhoidectomy, anal fissure repair, drainage of abscess, and fistulotomy are all covered in detail elsewhere. Removal of a polyp in the low rectum (up to 6 to 8 cm above the dentate line) can usually be accomplished easily by a transanal approach (Fig. 1-17). Moreover, polyps can often be pulled down further, even from 7, 8, or 9 cm above the dentate line, especially in a woman (Fig. 1-18). The polyp is outlined as illustrated in Fig. 1-19A using the electrocautery to include a circumferential margin of about 0.5 cm. The polyp, if not hard or suspicious of cancer, is excised using the electrocautery, dissecting in the submucosal plane (Fig. 1-19B). If for any reason there is tethering, then a full-thickness excision is performed (Fig. 1-19C). It is best to begin suturing the resulting wound before the tumor is completely removed, because the polyp can act as a handle. The biggest problem is losing the apex of each side of the incision. As soon as the apex is achieved it should be sutured and tagged (Fig. 1-20). The suture material we use is either 2-0 chromic or 2-0 Vicryl on a special UR needle, which facilitates working in a tunnel. If the dissection is full thickness, then a two-layer closure should be used; if not then a one-layer interrupted closure may be used. It is important that the polyp be completely removed and then blocked out and oriented on a piece of filter paper for examination by the pathologist.

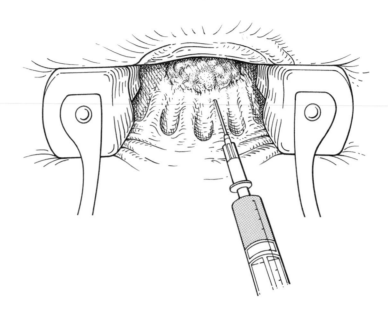

Figure 1-17.

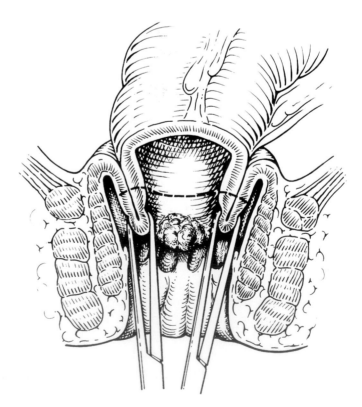

Figure 1-18.

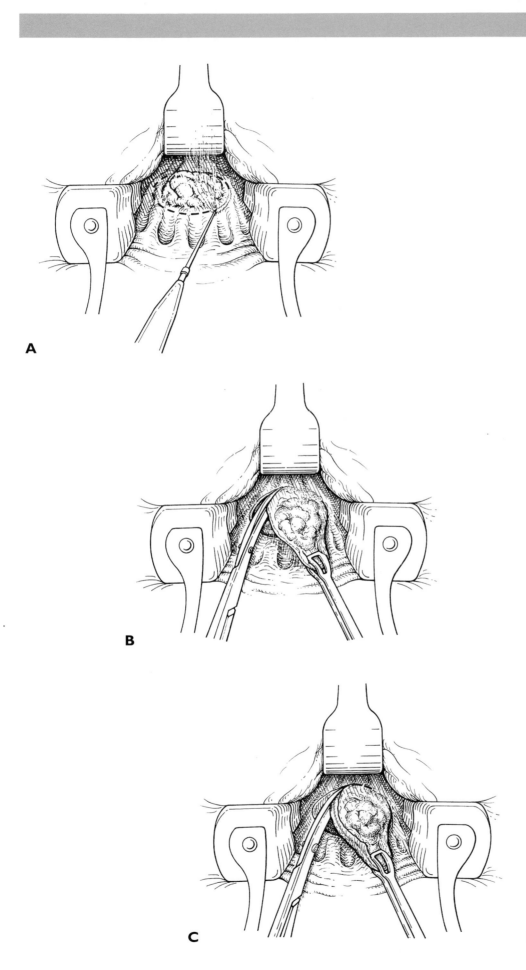

A

B

C

Figure 1-19.

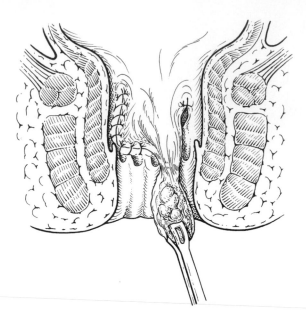

Figure 1-20.

We do not use the new operating proctoscope introduced in Germany (transanal endosocpic microsurgery [TEB]) because it seems to be unnecessarily complicated. It is used to remove polyps and tumors from the mid- and high rectum. This can be achieved in a more straightforward way using a posterior or transanal approach, or, if necessary, the standard abdominal approach. It may be a technique searching for an application.

Transsphincteric Exposure

A transsphincteric/parasacral approach is excellent for certain tumors polyps and fistulas of the midrectum(Fig. 1-21). Whereas the transsphincteric approach (Fig. 1-21A) may be unnecessarily invasive, the parasacral approach (Fig. 1-21B) is usually much easier to perform. Transsphincteric exposure is probably not indicated for low tumors,

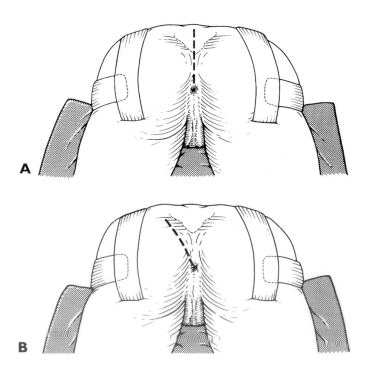

Figure 1-21.   **B**

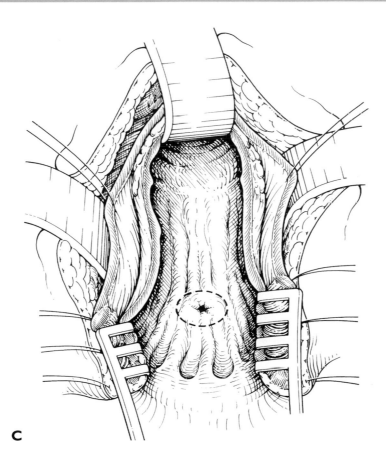

C

Figure 1-21.

because transanal approaches are adequate, and for higher tumors parasacral approaches are fine.

Parasacral Exposure

The patient is placed in the prone jackknife position, prepared, and draped. For the parasacral incision, the sacrum is outlined with a marker, as is the gluteal muscle. The major goals are to separate the gluteal muscle from the attachments to the sacrum during the dissection and to spare the external anal sphincter muscles. The incision is commenced with a knife, but electrocautery is used to enter deeper tissues. It is always a good idea to have the assistant push with a finger in the rectum posteriorly, which will give the operating surgeon information about the depth of the incision.

The first muscle encountered is the gluteus; this should be separated from its lower third attachments to the sacrum, exposing the levators. Upon transection of the levator (Fig. 1-22A) the rectal wall is easily visualized. It is not necessary to remove the coccyx unless there is a tumor in the presacral space and the coccyx needs to be removed together with the tumor. The rectum is then entered at about the S3-S4 level. Polyps and tumors can be removed easily from any location (Fig. 1-22B). The rectal wall is closed in two layers (Fig. 1-22C). The parasacral approach is also superb for repair of ureterorectal fistula. The secret here is that radiation damaged tissues may heal if stool and urine are diverted from the repair.

In brief, a parasacral incision is deepened to the rectal wall posteriorly. The rectal wall is incised to gain access to the anterior rectal wall. The fistula site is excised (Fig. 1-23A) and the wall mobilized in all directions (Fig. 1-23B). The urethral closure is separate from the rectal wall closure (Fig. 1-23C). The rectal wall closure is an overlapping one (Fig. 1-23C, inset).

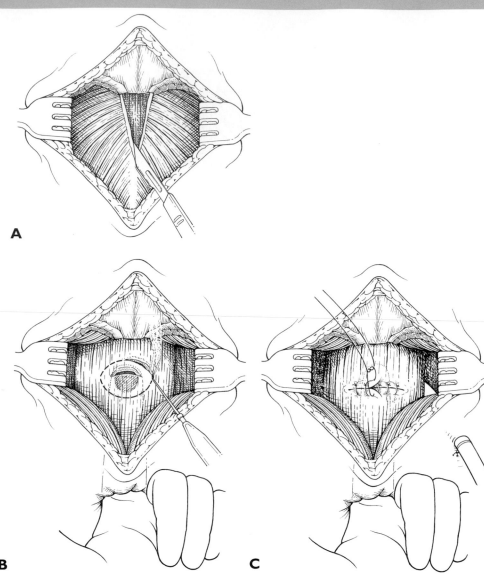

Figure 1-22. ▬▬▬▬ **B**   **C**

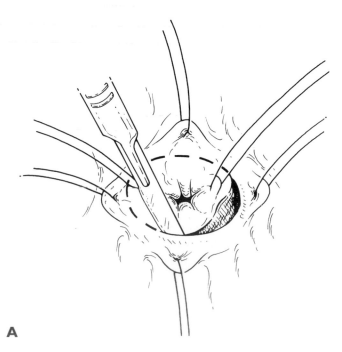

Figure 1-23. ▬▬▬▬   **A**

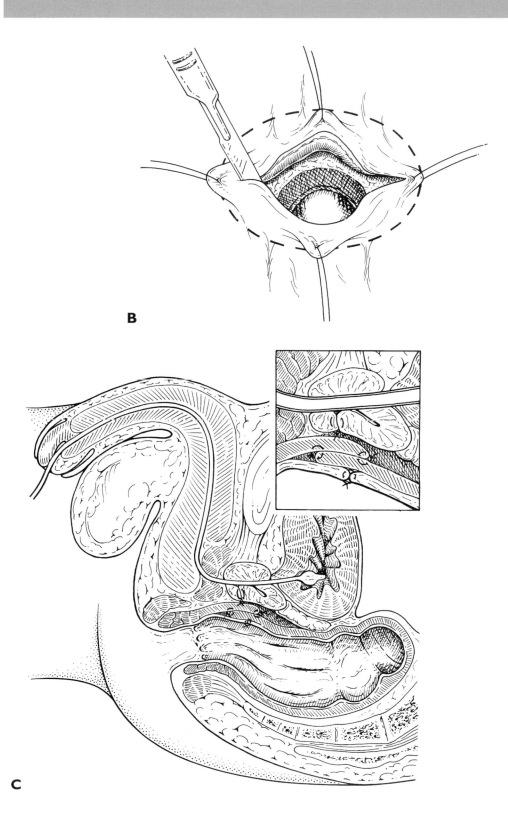

B

C

Figure 1-23.

Transsacral (Kraske) Approach

The idea of an abdominal/posterior approach for low-lying cancers is probably best known as a Kraske approach. A straightforward definition of a Kraske approach is difficult to determine. I do not perform this procedure for primary cancer of the rectum. Sacretomy, which is *not* a Kraske approach, is useful for recurrent rectal cancer.

Editorial Commentaries

In Birmingham there are few colorectal procedures that we do not now perform using the Lloyd-Davies combined abdominoperineal approach. The introduction of Allen stirrups has made the position easier to use, although somewhat longer to set up than the usual supine laparotomy approach. We entirely agree with Dr. Pemberton that, provided the buttocks are well over the bottom of the table, shoulder restraints are not necessary. We virtually always place a perineal tray below the buttocks so that if a combined procedure is necessary, instruments can be placed both on the Mayo table and between the legs. The use of a headlamp was not mentioned by Dr. Pemberton; in my own experience, it has totally revolutionized intra-anal procedures, perineal operations, and dissections in the pelvis. Furthermore, recent headlight developments allow excellent video transmission of the operating surgeon's field of view, which maintains active participation by the assistants and scrub nurses, as well as being a useful teaching model for trainees.

We increasingly use the jackknife position in preference to the lithotomy position for perineal procedures. Access to the rectovaginal septum and the anterior aspect of the anorectum is far better than in the lithotomy position. Because the tissues do not become engorged with blood in this position, it is now our preferred approach for hemorrhoidectomy, complex anal fistulas, and intrarectal excisions. We prefer to use a beanbag rather than a pillow to support the hips.

We never use the lateral decubitus position. We almost never use a transsphincter exposure and find that intra-anal excision and rectal excision from above are the preferred routes for midrectal lesions. We have no experience with the parasacral exposure. Like Dr. Pemberton, we find the operating (German) proctoscope a highly complicated instrument for surgical procedures that can nearly always be performed with a good anal speculum and a headlamp or should be treated by anterior resection.

We entirely concur that a midline laparotomy is the optimum incision in colorectal surgery. It provides quick access, is easy to close, can be repeatedly used, and, most important, does not compromise potential stoma sites. Although a transverse incision may appear to be more cosmetically acceptable, in our experience it is associated with more postoperative pain, usually compromises two potential stoma sites, and provides inadequate access to the splenic flexure or to the base of the pelvic floor. We are not impressed with the "smiling" incision!

Michael R. B. Keighley

My practice is to use the midline abdominal incision for most abdominal operations, the exception being cases where a paramedian incision has been made initially, in which case that incision rather than a new incision will be used. For abdominoperineal dissections, such as rectal resection or coloanal anastomosis, the modified Trendelenburg position is used and the patient's legs are placed in Lloyd-Davies or Allen stirrups. The prone jackknife posi-

(Continues)

tion is used for most anorectal procedures, the exception being simple incision and drainage of abscesses or insertion of setons; in the latter case, the conventional lithotomy position is used.

The stoma is positioned and marked preoperatively; positioning is performed with the patient supine and sitting. The principle of stoma site fashioning is to examine the surface of the right lower quadrant and to position the stoma over the rectus abdominus muscle in an area bounded superiorly by a transverse imaginary line passing to the right of the umbilicus, a vertical midline extending from the umbilicus downward, the lateral border of the rectus abdominus muscle, and the fold of the infraumbilical fat mound. The stoma site should be visible to the patient. In the event that the site selected is not visible to the patient because of obesity, the site should be relocated in a supraumbilical or paraumbilical area. The general principles here are that a disc of skin 3.5 cm in diameter can be excised and that there be a margin of undisturbed skin at least 2.5 to 3 cm beyond the excision to allow for the placement of an adherent skin barrier. In addition, the site chosen should be away from bony prominences, skin creases, previous scars, rib cage, and skin distorted by radiation or grafting.

In certain cases, because of multiple previous scars or the particular body habitus of the patient, a site extraneous to this optimal location must be chosen. In such circumstances, the first priority is that the stoma be located on the dominant part of the protruding abdomen in an area where there is a 1- to 2-inch radius of smooth skin beyond the stoma site. In certain cases this will be extraneous to the rectus abdominus muscle. Although such a patient is more susceptible to hernia, prolapse, and recession, this risk is relatively small compared to the certain risk of leakage from the stoma and skin barrier edges should the above criteria be ignored. The goal of stoma fashioning is to create an ostomy that will allow for maximum period of time between pouch and skin barrier changes (4 to 7 days in the case of an ileostomy). The enterostomal therapist will be a major resource in augmenting that interval with such devices as a convex faceplate and inserts, as well as stomahesive paste.

Because of the uncertainties of selecting a stoma site intraoperatively, it is our practice to use an indelible mark over the preoperatively selected stoma site so that abdominal skin preparation or body fluids on the abdominal wall surface during the operation will not eradicate the mark.

For abdominoperineal resection for malignancy, the perineal incision used is similar to that used by Dr. Pemberton; for benign disease, we prefer an intersphincteric operation, in which the circumferential incision is made just below the dentate line and carried between the internal and external sphincters up to the supralevator space. The perineum is then closed by sequential sutures of interrupted 0 Vicryl between the levators and then, in turn, the upper, middle, and lower portions of the external sphincter. The skin is usually closed with interrupted Dexon. An exception to this rule is the patient with both Crohn's disease and multiple perianal fistulas; in such cases, the fistulas are laid open or excised. This may preclude closure of the

(Continues)

skin. However, the levators are still closed as is the component of the external sphincter that allows for approximation. In the presence of sepsis, the perineal skin is either left open or only partly closed. In certain circumstances split-thickness skin graft will be required at a later date.

With the transsphincteric operation, the approach is similar to that described by Dr. Pemberton, and for similar indications the transsacral approach is essentially an obsolete operation except to get at or facilitate the dissection of presacral and sacral masses.

Victor W. Fazio

In Paris nearly all colorectal surgical procedures (except right colectomy) are now performed using the Lloyd-Davies combined abdominoperineal approach. This position offers many advantages, such as easy on-table colonic lavage and rectal washout, and colonoscopy if needed, but also the benefit of permitting an assistant to work between the legs of the patient. We always position the instrument table above the patient's head. To avoid the risk of ischemia of the anterior compartments of the leg muscles in a patient maintained in the steep Trendelenburg position for a long time, we bring the operating table back to horizontal for a few minutes every 2 hours.

The jackknife position is not frequently used in France. For anal procedures and transanal resection of villous tumors or polyps located posteriorly, we find the lithotomy position with peridural anesthesia very useful. To avoid blood stasis, it is possible to put the patient in the Trendelenburg position. We agree with Dr. Pemberton that it is often possible to pull down a polyp and that this may be done easily with the patient in the lithotomy position.

We also prefer the jackknife position for lesions located anteriorly, although for the highest ones we do not hesitate to use a parasacral exposure, which we find very useful for removing a large villous tumor located anteriorly in the midrectum.

We concur that a midline laparotomy is the optimum incision in colorectal surgery. In obese patients with a well-localized lesion near the hepatic or splenic flexure, we find a supraumbilical transverse right or left laparotomy satisfactory.

Regarding the perineal approach during abdominoperineal resection of the rectum, I believe that in the overwhelming majority of cases resection of the levator muscles is too great a procedure to permit a reapproximation at the time of closure. We prefer to mobilize the great omentum pediculized on the left gastroepiploic artery and to pull it down to the perineum before closing the skin in order to include it in the subcutaneous closure. This technique considerably diminishes postoperative perineal infection and delay in scar healing, especially after radiation therapy. Finally, for the comfort of the patient we prefer to have the drain come out of the perineum through the lateral abdominal wall.

Rolland Parc

2

Intestinal Anastomosis

Michael R. B. Keighley

Principles

The principles of intestinal anastomoses are that they should be leakproof, both bowel ends should have an adequate blood supply, they should be under no tension, and there should be minimal discrepancy in luminal size.

The strength of the intestinal anastomosis is dependent on the material used to approximate the circular muscle fibers of the intestinal tract. Because the mucosa itself has no inherent strength, the longitudinal fibers tend to split, and the peritoneal surface is too weak to be relied on as more than a buttress in an intestinal anastomosis (Fig. 2-1).

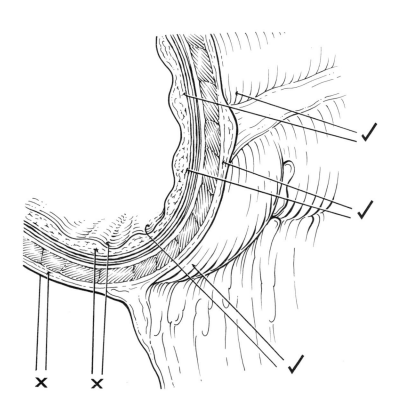

Figure 2-1.

21

The blood supply to the bowel ends must be adequate. A patent vascular arcade must have been demonstrated and the divided arcade at the site of anastomosis should bleed freely (Fig. 2-2). Tension at the anastomosis should not be a problem in mobile segments of bowel but may present a problem in low rectal and anal anastomoses.

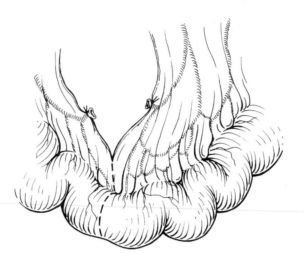

Figure 2-2.

Discrepancy in luminal size may be overcome in a number of ways. Bites of varying thickness can be taken from two bowel segments having different diameters, but this does not always achieve a satisfactory anastomosis and there may be an inadequate luminal diameter (Fig. 2-3). Other matching techniques include creating a Cheatle slit, a longitudinal incision along the antimesenteric border of the narrower segment (Fig. 2-4). Alternatively, an end-to-side anastomosis may be constructed, preferably by placing the wider bowel lumen onto the side of the smaller-diameter bowel segment or, in the case of a mobile segment and a fixed rectum, to join the side of the mobile bowel to the end of the rectum (Fig. 2-5). It may be wiser to perform a side-to-side anastomosis, having closed both bowel ends (Fig. 2-6). This forms the basis of the stapled functional end-to-end anastomosis.

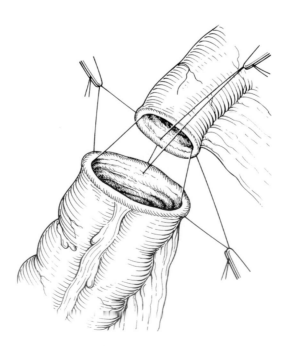

Figure 2-3.

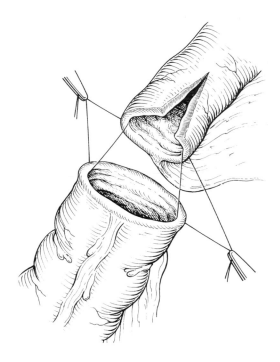

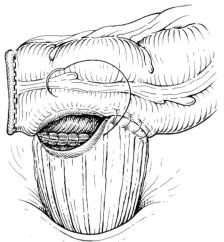

Figure 2-4.

Figure 2-5.

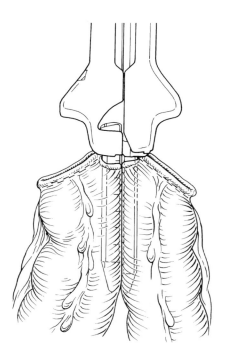

Figure 2-6.

If the luminal diameter of both bowel segments is narrow, a double Cheatle slit technique may be performed. A longitudinal incision is made along the antimesenteric border of the bowel ends; one bowel end is rotated through 180 degrees so that the blunt end of one segment is anastomosed to the apex of the Cheatle slit on the other (Fig. 2-7).

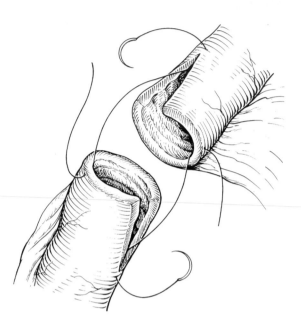

Figure 2-7.

Anastomosis of Two Mobile Segments: Ileoileal, Ileocolonic, and Colocolonic Anastomosis

Continuous Single-Layer Extramucosal Anastomosis

I generally prefer a single-layer extramucosal continuous anastomosis for mobile segments of bowel.

Meticulous hemostasis is achieved at both bowel ends. Two stay sutures are placed on the mesenteric and antimesenteric segments of bowel (Fig. 2-8A). The anastomosis commences in the middle of the posterior component of the two bowel ends. We prefer to use 3-0 PDS sutures with a needle at either end. If a double-needle suture is not available, two separate PSD sutures, each with a single needle, can be used. The full thickness of the bowel wall (i.e., submucosa, circular muscle fibers, longitudinal muscle, and serosa) of both segments is picked up by the needle and a knot is tied. If two separate sutures are used, identical sutures are placed adjacent to each other and the two free edges are tied together. If a double-needle suture is available, a single loop is tied simply to approximate the bowel ends. A continuous suture technique is then used toward the antimesenteric border of the bowel, taking large bites of the bowel wall but omitting the mucosa, until the antimesenteric border is reached (Fig. 2-8B). Similarly, extramucosal sutures are placed from the center point posteriorly to the back row of the anastomosis. The suturing then continues to approximate the anterior components of the bowel, with particular care taken to invert the bowel edges (Fig. 2-8C). The anastomosis is completed when the antimesenteric needle and the mesenteric needle meet in the midanterior portion of the anastomosis. The two sutures are then tied, after it has been ascertained that the lumen is adequate, and the mesenteric defect is closed as appropriate.

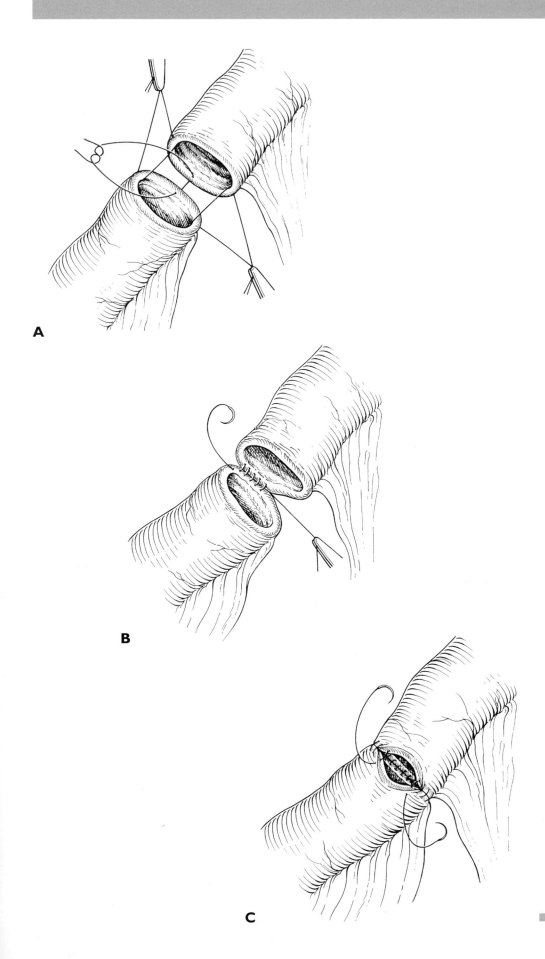

A

B

C

Figure 2-8.

Interrupted Single-Layer Extramucosal Anastomosis

The principles of the interrupted extramucosal anastomosis are exactly the same as those described above, except that instead of using a continuous suture technique, a series of interrupted sutures are placed between the bowel ends, leaving the sutures long so that each can be tied when they have all been appropriately placed. The anastomosis starts in the midline posteriorly (Fig. 2-9A). Once the posterior sutures are placed, tied, and cut, a series of interrupted extramucosal sutures are placed between the bowel ends and subsequently tied (Fig. 2-9B).

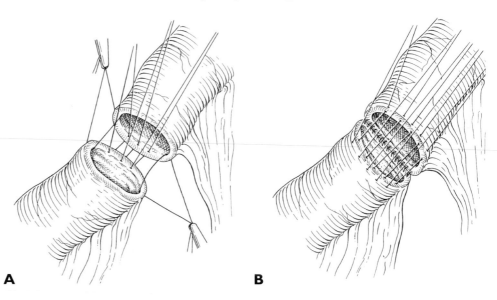

Figure 2-9.   **A**   **B**

Two-Layer Anastomosis

The principle of the two-layer technique is to <u>ensure complete inversion</u> by performing a continuous or interrupted full-thickness anastomosis between the two bowel ends and then applying a few interrupted serosal sutures (Fig. 2-10). <u>The strength of the anastomosis, however, lies in the full-thickness sutures.</u>

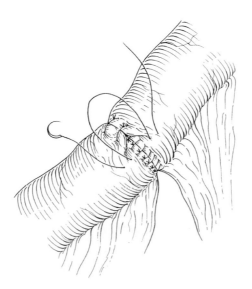

Figure 2-10.

The anastomosis commences in the midline posteriorly. A double-ended 3-0 PDS suture is preferred. Full-thickness bites of both bowel ends are taken, working from the midline posteriorly to the antimesenteric and mesenteric borders. It is usually advisable to continue the sutures around the mesenteric and antimesenteric borders in order to ensure full inversion after completion of the corners. The two sutures meet in the midline anteriorly and are tied. If a continuous suture technique is used, once the inner layer is completed, the needle is brought to the outside of the bowel in preparation for the start of the outer layer. A second layer of interrupted Vicryl or PDS sutures completes the fully inverted anastomosis.

End-to-Side Anastomosis

If there is a discrepancy in the luminal diameters of the two bowel ends it may be preferable to perform an end-to-side anastomosis. The end of the narrow-diameter bowel is closed with sutures or staples. Stapled closure may be performed with a TA or RL instrument, which provides a double row of staples (Fig. 2-11A). Alternatively, the bowel end may be closed with a continuous PDS suture or a double row of sutures.

An antimesenteric enterotomy is made, the length of which is determined by the diameter of the bowel end (Fig. 2-11B). Hemostasis is achieved and an end-to-side anastomosis is constructed using the continuous extramucosal suture technique or the two-layer suture technique, as depicted in Figure 2-5.

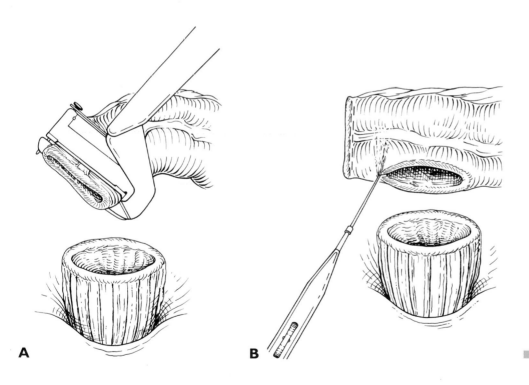

A   **B**   *Figure 2-11.*

Side-to-Side Anastomosis

If both bowel lumina are narrow, it may be wiser to consider a side-to-side anastomosis rather than the double-Cheatle slit rotated end-to-end anastomosis. Both bowel ends are closed, either with staples or with sutures, as described for the end-to-side anastomosis. Two antimesenteric enterotomies measuring approximately 3 cm in diameter are made between stay sutures. Meticulous hemostasis is achieved in both enterotomies and a side-to-side anastomosis is performed using an extramucosal single-layer technique (Fig. 2-12), an extramucosal interrupted suture technique, or a two-layer technique.

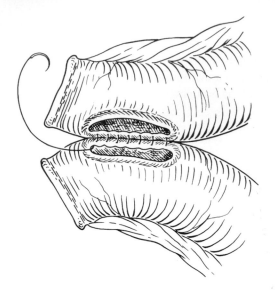

Figure 2-12.

Stapled Anastomoses for Mobile Bowel Segments: Ileoileal, Ileocolonic, and Colocolonic Anastomoses

A functional anastomosis may be fashioned either during or after resection.

Functional Stapled Side-to-Side Anastomosis During Bowel Resection. The limit of the resection is first determined and the mesentery with its intestinal blood supply is divided up to the limits of resection so that all mesenteric attachments to both limbs of bowel have been cleared. Two small enterotomies are made within the segment to be resected about 1 cm beyond the site of vascular division (Fig. 2-13A). A series of stay sutures are placed to approximate the antimesenteric borders of both bowel segments. A side-to-side anastomosis is then fashioned using a linear staple cutter (PLC or GIA), preferably one with a length exceeding 5 cm. The limbs of the staple cutter are passed through the enterotomies and the knife blade advanced, creating a row of staples and a side-to-side anastomosis (Fig. 2-13B). After the staple cutter is withdrawn, two stay sutures are placed on each enterotomy and the two bowel ends are transected just beyond the site of the anastomosis, either with a TA or RL instrument, which produces a double line of staples, or with a linear staple cutter (GIA or PLC) (Fig. 2-13C). The length of the staple instrument will depend on the luminal diameter of the two bowel ends. If a double staple line is used, a bowel clamp will need to be applied across the specimen prior to bowel resection.

Functional Side-to-Side Anastomosis After Bowel Resection. After intestinal resection the two open ends of bowel should be protected by noncrushing clamps. A linear staple cutter (PLC or GIA), preferably one equipped with a cartridge exceeding 5 cm in length, is inserted through the open bowel ends and fired (Fig. 2-14A). Once the staple cutter has been removed, stay sutures are placed over the two bowel ends and a staple cutter (TA or RL) of sufficient length is used to complete closure of the two bowel ends (Fig. 2-14B). Hemostasis is then assessed; if bleeding continues, the staple line may be oversewn.

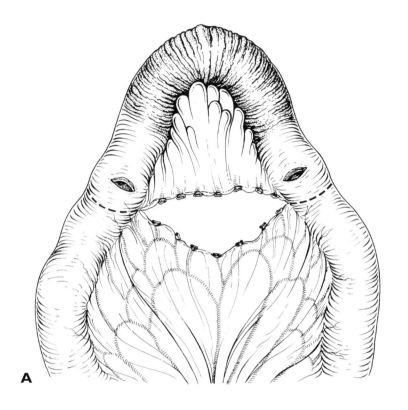

A

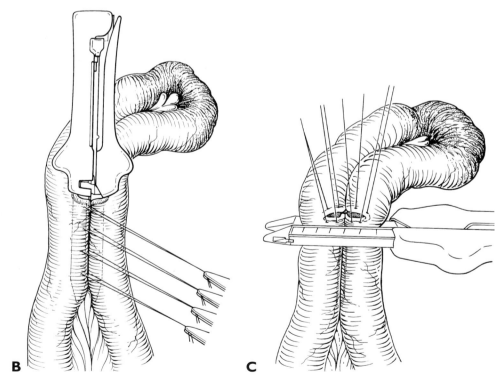

B   **C**

Figure 2-13.

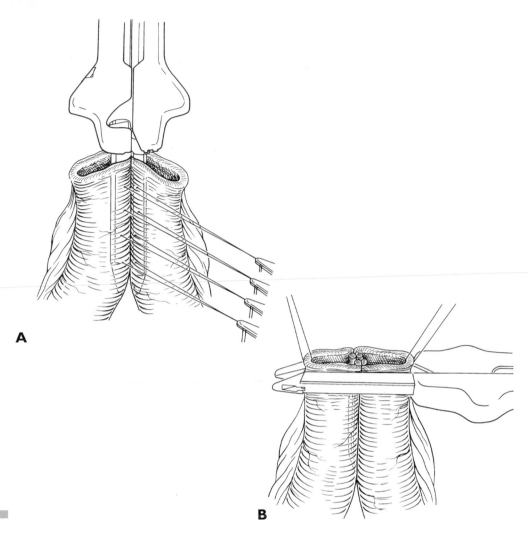

Figure 2-14.

Anastomosis of Mobile to Nonmobile Segments: Ileorectal and Colorectal Anastomosis

Continuous Single-Layer Extramucosal Anastomosis

Continuous extramucosal anastomosis is a feasible option if there is no gross disparity between the luminal diameters of the rectum and the end of the ileum or colon and if the anastomosis is at the pelvic brim. The technique is generally used for colorectal anastomosis but is less applicable to ileorectal anastomosis because the ileal lumen is generally much smaller than the lumen of the rectum. Using a double-ended suture, preferably of 3-0 PDS, and taking bites of the proximal bowel and rectum, each suture is worked from the midline posteriorly to the lateral edges of the anastomosis (Fig. 2-15A). The sutures exclude the mucosa but take in all other layers of bowel wall. The suturing is continued, ensuring that the mucosa is inverted and that hemostasis is achieved. Both sutures meet in the midline anteriorly, the needles are excised, and the two free ends are tied (Fig. 2-15B).

Interrupted Single-Layer Extramucosal Anastomosis

When a rectal anastomosis is being fashioned, the interrupted single-layer extramucosal anastomosis is often much more difficult than the full-thickness single-layer anastomosis described below. Interrupted extramucosal bites are taken starting in the

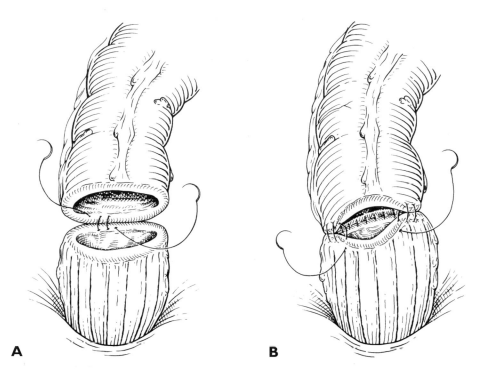

A   **B**   *Figure 2-15.*

midline posteriorly. Each suture is clipped and left long and untied until all of the posterior sutures have been correctly aligned. A Cheatle slit may be needed, particularly if an ileorectal anastomosis is being fashioned. It is usually wise to place the lateral sutures first to help display the posterior suture line. A series of posterior sutures are then placed but not tied until all of the sutures have been correctly positioned (Fig. 2-16A). Once the sutures have been ligated and tied, the interrupted extramucosal technique is used anteriorly to complete the anastomosis (Fig. 2-16B).

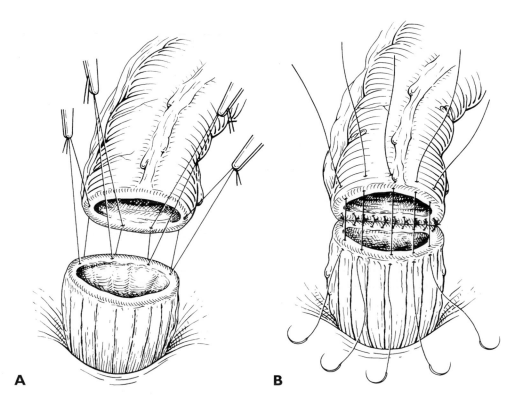

A   **B**   *Figure 2-16.*

Interrupted Single-Layer Full-Thickness Anastomosis

The interrupted single-layer full thickness anastomosis is particularly useful if the anastomosis must be placed in the middle or lower third of the rectum. Under these circumstances, the bowel ends may need to be widely separated in order to ensure that the sutures are correctly placed before the bowel ends are railroaded together and the sutures are tied. As in other techniques, the first suture is made from the proximal bowel to the rectum in the midline posteriorly (Fig. 2-17A). A full-thickness bite of proximal bowel is taken from within out; the needle is then replaced in the needle holder and a full-thickness bite of rectum is taken from without in so that at the completion of the anastomosis the knots lie on the mucosa. All sutures are clipped and held after excising the needle. The two most lateral sutures are then placed from the proximal colon from within out, then through the full thickness of the rectum from without in. The sutures are again clipped and left untied to serve as retractors. The next sutures should divide the space between the midline posteriorly and the lateral extent of the anastomosis on both sides. A similar technique of placing subsequent sutures such that each space is evenly divided ensures that any discrepancy in luminal diameter is overcome and that a sound anastomosis is achieved (Fig. 2-17B). It is a good idea to place the clips holding each suture onto some sort of mount. We usually use a long straight artery forceps that is attached to the towels with a towel clip. We prefer to use 3-0 PDS sutures for this technique. If Vicryl sutures are used, it is wise to lubricate them with liquid paraffin to facilitate sliding the two segments together. Once all of the posterior sutures are correctly placed, they are held up by an assistant and the proximal bowel slowly advanced onto the posterior aspect of the rectum by the surgeon. Once this is accomplished so that there is no tension on the bowel and an adequate blood supply to both segments is assured, the sutures can be tied and all except the lateral sutures ligated above the knots (Fig. 2-17C).

An alternative technique is to use vertical mattress sutures for the posterior aspect of the anastomosis (Fig. 2-17D). It is entirely possible to use this technique even for coloanal anastomosis, but in very low anastomoses it is often advisable to have an assistant press on the perineum in order to display the upper end of the anus or low rectum to facilitate placement of the sutures (Fig. 2-17E). It is also much easier to perform the anastomosis before the rectum is completely divided. The anterior portion that is left attached acts as an upward retractor, and is left undivided until the posterior suture line has been completed (Fig. 2-17F). The anterior anastomosis is constructed using the Lembert technique, the principle of which is to place the suture in the proximal bowel from outside in, through the full thickness of the bowel wall; the needle is then rotated and held by the needle holder so that a more medially placed bite can be taken from without in at a site closer to the bowel end. The needle is again rotated and replaced in the needle holder so that a full-thickness bite of adjacent rectum can be taken from the outside in at a site reasonably close to the bowel end. The needle is then rotated and replaced in the needle holder, and a more lateral bite of rectum slightly farther away from the bowel is taken from within out, leaving two loops of suture on the mucosa. In this way the mucosa is inverted (Fig. 2-17G).

When using the Lembert technique, it is essential that each suture be clipped and the needle excised so that the sutures are tied only when they have all been correctly aligned. If there is any discrepancy in the lumina of the segments it is a good idea to place an anterior Lembert suture in the midline and then to use the technique of dividing between the space to complete the anterior suture line. If there is no discrepancy it may be acceptable to place sutures serially from one end of the bowel to the other. Once all of the anterior Lembert sutures have been correctly placed they are tied and ligated (Fig. 2-17H).

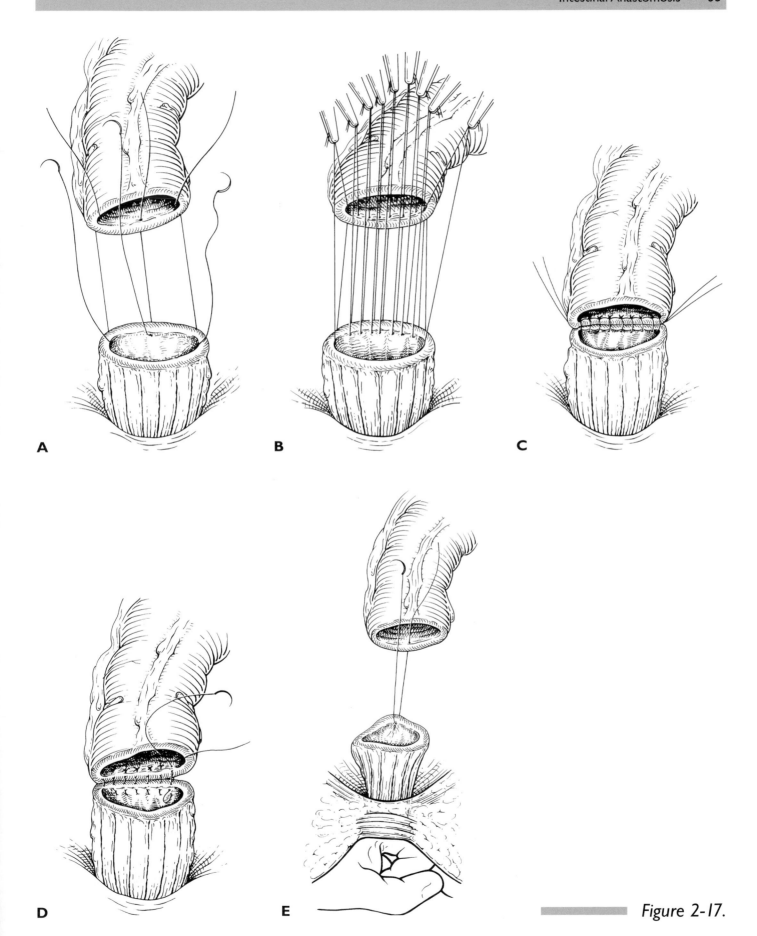

A

B

C

D

E

Figure 2-17.

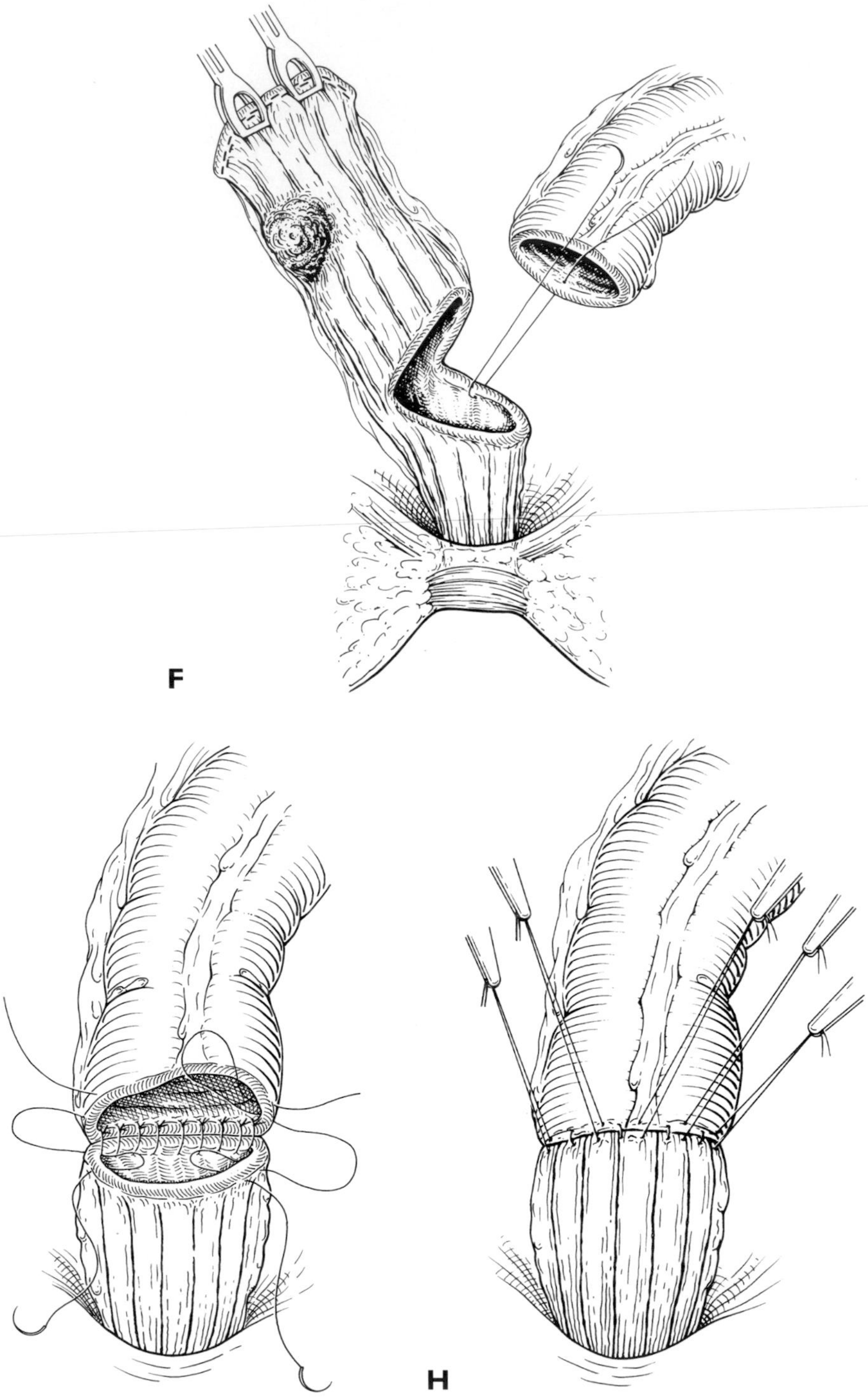

F

Figure 2-17.   G   H

Two-Layer Full-Thickness Anastomosis

A two-layer anastomosis is only feasible if the rectum has been divided at the sacral promontory. It is a technique that we do not advise, as there is no evidence that the strength of an anastomosis to the rectum is increased by using a two-layer technique and it is also technically more difficult to place sutures accurately using a two-layer as opposed to a single-layer technique. It is also more likely to compromise the lumen of the bowel.

Usually a continuous full-thickness anastomotic technique reinforced with interrupted seromuscular sutures is used. Alternatively, an interrupted full-thickness anastomosis may be constructed as already described and then reinforced by further seromuscular sutures (Fig. 2-18).

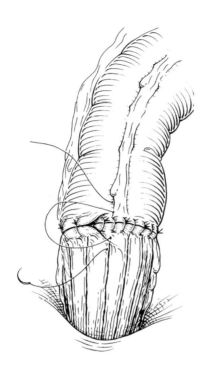

Figure 2-18.

Stapled End-to-End Anastomosis Using Circular Stapling Devices

Principles

Stapled end-to-end anastomosis using a circular stapling device is widely performed after resections for malignant disease; it can also be applied to resections for inflammatory disease. It is not particularly applicable if there is gross discrepancy in the luminal diameters of the bowel ends and thus is not frequently applied to ileorectal anastomosis, although it is commonly used in colorectal anastomosis. As in all other intestinal anastomoses, it is absolutely essential to ensure that there is an adequate blood supply to the two bowel ends. If a colorectal anastomosis is to be used, it is wise to take down the splenic flexure so that the wider-diameter descending colon can be approximated to the rectum. For low rectal anastomosis using the descending colon it will be necessary to totally mobilize the splenic flexure so that the blood supply of the descending colon is based on the middle colic artery and its marginal vessels (Fig. 2-19A). There is usually no technical difficulty in placing a pursestring suture around the proximal colon because the colon is mobile and easily accessible. However, the placement of a pursestring in the rectal stump may pose greater problems, particularly if the anastomosis is placed in the lower third of the rectum or in the anus. Therefore, in low rectal anastomoses it is wise to place the pursestring suture in the rectum before totally dividing the distal resection margin (Fig. 2-19B). The technique of cut and sew is particularly applicable under these circumstances; thus the lateral aspect of the rectum is divided, a pursestring suture is started posteriorly, and the remainder of the posterior rectal division is undertaken during placement of the posterior aspect of the pursestring suture. Similarly, anteriorly the suture needle follows the scissors or diathermy as the pursestring suture is completed and the lower resection margin divided (Fig. 2-19C). Using this technique it may be necessary to secure hemostasis in the submucosal vessels during division of the rectum and before applying the pursestring suture at that particular site.

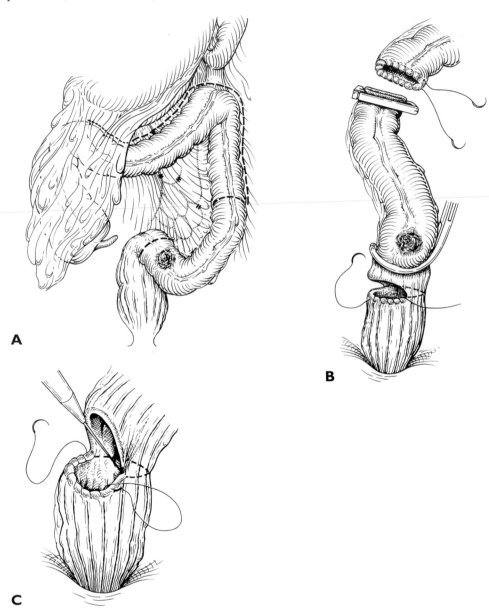

Figure 2-19.   A

B

C

Double-Pursestring Circular End-to-End Anastomosis

The proximal pursestring suture is first completed using 0 Prolene on a 30- or 40-mm needle. Satisfactory hemostasis should be secured before starting the pursestring suture. A bite is taken through the full thickness of the proximal bowel from outside in and an over-and-over technique is used so that the next bite of the needle is also from outside in. The space between each suture should not exceed 2 mm. When the whole of the bowel end is encircled, the pursestring is completed by passing the last suture from inside out, adjacent to the end of the suture that is clipped (Fig. 2-19B). At this point, it is wise to ensure that the pursestring suture will run freely through the bowel. The distal pursestring is then placed through the divided or partially divided rectum in the same manner (Fig. 2-20A). However, it is easier to place a low rectal pursestring by using the technique of divide and suture before the anterior bowel end is divided. Again, pressure on the perineum may assist in the placement of the lower pursestring. Once the pursestring has been checked to ensure that it will run freely through the rectum, it is clipped. The alternative technique using a Furness clamp is only appropriate for high anastomoses and is rarely used by us (Fig. 2-20B).

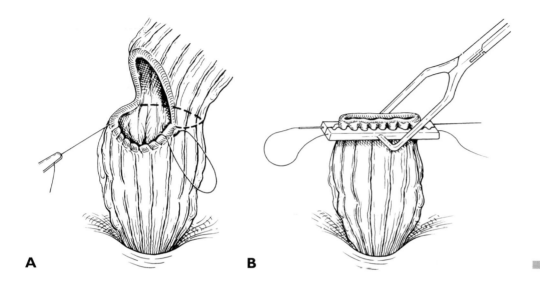

A   **B**   *Figure 2-20.*

The stapling technique depends on the type of stapler used. First, the size of the stapler should be carefully chosen. The widest diameter staple should be used. When the descending colon is used for anastomosis, the luminal diameter of the descending colon is almost always the limiting factor in determining the appropriate size staple. If there is any doubt about the most appropriate staple gun to use, the pursestring on the proximal bowel should be loosened, and a single finger and then a second finger gently inserted inside the bowel to dilate the bowel end and smooth out the puckering caused by the pursestring so that the bowel diameter can be measured. If the diameter is more than 31 mm, a large staple gun can almost always be used without risk of damage to the bowel wall (Fig. 2-21).

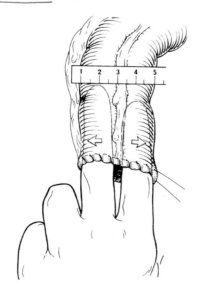

Figure 2-21.

Modern staple guns have detachable anvils that can be spring-loaded through the central spine onto the cartridge-holding section. Nondetachable circular staplers have become virtually extinct; therefore, the technique described herein will involve the detachable-anvil circular stapler. The anvil is gently advanced through the pursestring of the proximal colon and the suture ends tied onto the central spindle adjacent to a notched segment specifically designed to engage the pursestring suture and its knot (Fig. 2-22A). Several knots must be applied to the Prolene suture, which is left long and clipped. The lubricated smooth, rounded end of the staple gun is passed via the dilated anus into the low rectum with its central spindle retracted (Fig. 2-22B). This step should be done with great care. When the cartridge section reaches the lower pursestring, any fecal material is sucked away. The central spindle is then advanced through the rectal pursestring by the perineal operator by opening the wing nut on the cartridge holder to its maximum extent. The central spindle of the anvil in the proximal bowel is engaged into the central spindle of the cartridge holder. Engagement is assured by an audible "snap." The lower pursestring is then tied as securely as possible against the central spindle of the cartridge holder (Fig. 2-22C). The perineal surgeon then closes the circular staple gun by rotating the wing nut clockwise until the staple head adjustment color zone becomes visible in the hub of the instrument. When the two bowel ends are satisfactorily approximated, and with the knots of the pursestring outside of the staple line that will be created, the perineal surgeon closes the gun and fires the cartridge. The two pursestring sutures are both transected by the cutting blade within the instrument as it is fired. The anvil is then disengaged from the cartridge holder by three counterclockwise rotations of the wing nut. The circular stapling device is then rotated 360 degrees and gently withdrawn, either by the perineal surgeon with the abdominal surgeon holding the proximal colon to ensure that it does not become distracted or by the abdominal surgeon who leans over the patient's left groin in order to check that the gun is withdrawn without any trauma to the proximal colon (Fig. 2-22D). The presence of two complete circles of tissue within the opened gun will indicate a successful anastomosis (Fig. 2-22E).

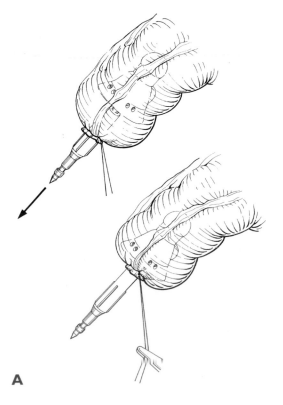

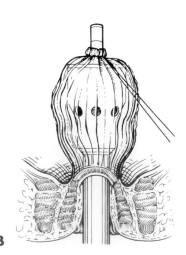

Figure 2-22.   ▬▬▬▬   **A**   **B**

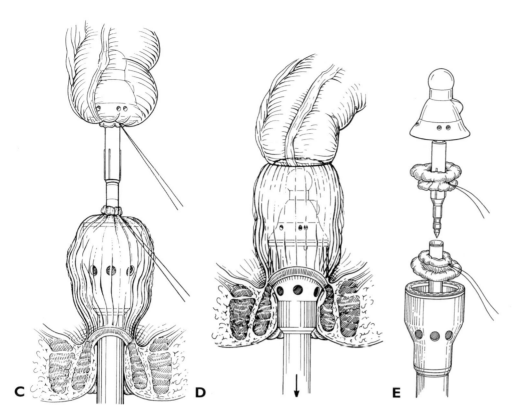

C   D   E   *Figure 2-22.*

There are two circular stapler types, the Ethicon ILS and the Autosuture Premium
CEEA (Fig. 2-23A). Each instrument design has its own modifications but the principles of their use are as described above. In high rectal anastomoses it may be wiser
to use the nondetachable anvil (Fig. 2-23B), because the plastic anvil on the cartridge section has less potential to cause trauma during its passage through the long
rectal stump, and the pursestring may be easier to secure and the instrument easier to
withdraw (Fig. 2-23B, inset). If the conventional nondetachable anvil is used, or if
the detachable anvil has not already been inserted into the proximal bowel, the
proximal colon can be levered over the anvil using three Allis forceps (Fig. 2-24).

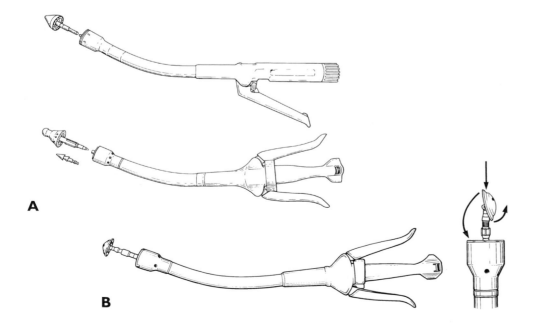

A

B   *Figure 2-23.*

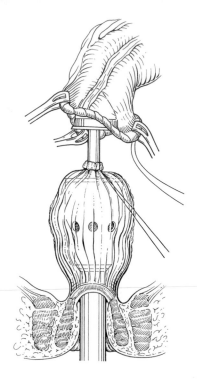

Figure 2-24. ▬▬▬▬

Double Stapled End-to-End Rectal Anastomosis

It is sometimes preferable to use double stapling, a technique that minimizes the degree of contamination from the rectal stump as the staple gun is advanced through the rectum and also avoids having to place a potentially difficult pursestring in the low rectum or anus. The principle is that a double row of staggered staples is placed across the rectum or anal canal. The rectum must have been completely mobilized and the mesorectum divided adjacent to the bowel wall before the staple gun is used to transect it. The Ethicon RL series may be used, but the 3M stapling device or the Autosuture TA series may be preferred. The Ethicon and 3M instruments have a pin that engages the rectum, thus facilitating correct application of the stapling device adjacent to the bowel end (Fig. 2-25). Unfortunately, this design is not available on the Autosuture instrument. The size of the stapler will depend on the diameter of the rectum. Usually a TA 55 or RL 50 stapler is adequate, but even wider instruments may have to be used if the rectum is very large.

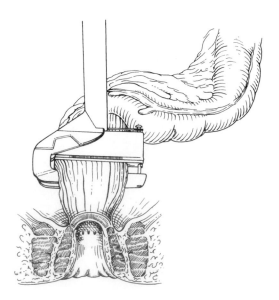

Figure 2-25. ▬▬▬▬

Double-Stapled Circular End-to-End Anastomosis

Using a linear stapler, a double row of staples is applied to the lower rectum, which is then divided above the staple lines. A 0-0 Prolene pursestring suture is placed in the proximal bowel end as already described. A circular stapling device with a detachable anvil is selected for use. The anvil is inserted as previously described into the proximal colon beyond the pursestring, which is tied around the central plastic spindle of the anvil (Fig. 2-26A). The plastic spindle is then engaged into the central spindle of the Premium CEEA instrument. In the ILS device the central spindle is an integral feature of the staple gun. The shoulders of the cartridge-holding section are lubricated by the perineal operator and gently advanced through the anal canal into the low rectum. The abdominal operator must then ensure that the free circular edge of the cartridge-holding section is at the transected staple line. This is often best achieved by the abdominal surgeon grasping the shaft of the staple gun with the left hand. The cartridge-holding container must be lined up so that the rectal staple line divides its center, which will ensure that when the central spindle is advanced by the perineal surgeon, it will transect the center of the staple line. The perineal surgeon then proceeds to fully advance the central spindle while the abdominal surgeon pushes the staple line against the central spindle. If the Premium CEEA device is used, the plastic pin is withdrawn and the central spindle of the anvil is advanced onto the central spindle of the cartridge-holding section. If the ILS instrument is used, the central pin does not have to be withdrawn, as the central spindle of the anvil can be slid over it to engage the two components of the circular stapler instrument. The circular staple gun is then closed by the perineal surgeon, who rotates the wing nut clockwise to a distance that seems most appropriate for the thickness of tissue, and the circular knife blade and staples engage. This maneuver usually cuts the pursestring suture on the proximal bowel (Fig. 2-26B). The perineal surgeon disengages the anvil by three counterclockwise rotations of the wing nuts. The staple gun is rotated 360 degrees to ensure that it is not adherent at any position. The abdominal and perineal surgeons gently ease the circular stapler through the anastomosis and out of the anorectum. The presence of two complete tissue rings is checked. Once the gun has been withdrawn and fully opened the lower ring may be quite difficult to display, hence we generally advise further testing of the anastomosis, as described in the next section.

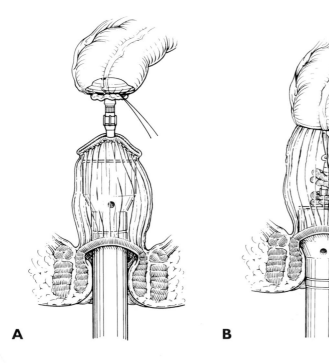

A   B   *Figure 2-26.*

Testing the Anastomosis

We generally recommend testing all rectal and anal anastomoses. It is not always necessary to test the anastomosis of two mobile ends of bowel unless there has been technical difficulty with the anastomosis or the entire small bowel has had to be mobilized because of extensive adhesions where there may have been iatrogenic damage above or below the anastomosis.

Testing of Mobile Anastomoses for Damage to the Small Bowel

The simplest method of testing a small bowel anastomosis is to milk a segment of air across the anastomosis while holding the line of anastomosis submerged in the fluid-filled peritoneum. The appearance of air bubbles will indicate the presence of a leak (Fig. 2-27). Sometimes, however, this technique is not possible because there is insufficient air within the small intestine. Hence if there is real concern about the possibility of iatrogenic damage, it is wise to have the anesthesiologist pass a nasogastric tube, which is then fed through the upper jejunum, and inflate the bowel with carbon dioxide, having first applied a crushing clamp to the ileocecal valve. The test then proceeds in the saline-filled peritoneal cavity.

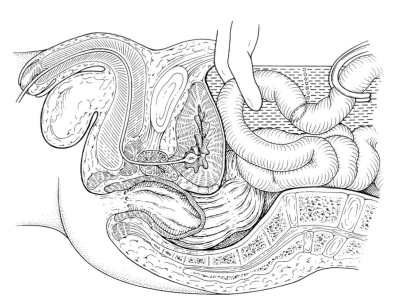

Figure 2-27.

Testing of Anastomoses in Mobile Colon

The simplest way of testing an anastomosis of the colon is again by milking air across the anastomosis while holding the anastomosed segment under water. If there is insufficient air within the bowel, air may be introduced from below using a Foley catheter in the rectum (Fig. 2-28A). Alternatively, if carbon dioxide insufflation has been used to check for leaks in the small bowel, the noncrushing clamp can be removed and the gas milked through the ileocecal valve into the colon (Fig. 2-28B). As described above, the anastomotic site is submerged in the saline-filled peritoneal cavity and the surgeon looks for evidence of air leakage.

Testing of Lower Rectal Anastomoses

All rectal anastomoses are usually checked within a fluid-filled pelvis by passing a 30-Fr catheter through the anal sphincter into the low rectum. A 50-ml syringe is then used to insufflate the rectum while the area above the rectal anastomosis is held by a noncrushing clamp. If an anal anastomosis is being checked, the anastomotic line is simply inflated by placing the nozzle of a 50-ml syringe through the anus (Fig. 2-29).

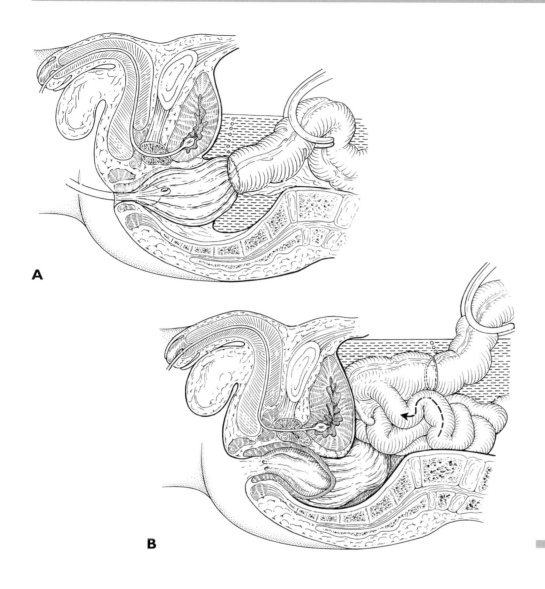

A

B

Figure 2-28.

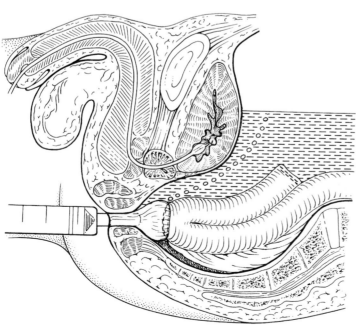

Figure 2-29.

Management of Leaks

If a localized leak is detected and the anastomosis otherwise appears to be sound, a pursestring suture or one or two interrupted buttressing sutures should be placed at the site of the leak and the anastomosis rechecked after the sutures have been tied. If there is any doubt about the integrity of the anastomosis, a proximal stoma should always be raised. If on repeat testing no further air leakage is detected despite the injection under pressure air across the anastomosis, then in our view a proximal stoma might not be necessary.

Editorial Commentaries

Dr. Keighley's descriptions of intraperitoneal and extraperitoneal (pelvic) anastomoses, both hand sewn and stapled, are simple and therefore utterly useful. The principles enunciated by Dr. Keighley so exhaustingly in this chapter are basic ones and should be understood by all surgeons.

There are as many anastomotic techniques and suture materials as there are surgeons; thus comments on the specifics of intraperitoneal and extraperitoneal hand-sewn techniques are valueless. Basically, the principles described need to be followed by every surgeon. I particularly enjoyed the sections on stapling and completely agree with the details.

The only comment I would make about ileorectal anastomosis is that usually the luminal discrepancies are so large that I perform a side-to-end ileorectal anastomosis using a hand-sewn technique. By the way, nearly all of my anastomoses, when hand sewn, are done using a two-layered technique. I understand that this is hopelessly archaic in the eyes of my European colleagues, but nonetheless, this is my technique.

Finally, I, too, check the anastomosis after stapled low anterior resection using insufflation, but I do it using a proctoscope.

John H. Pemberton

I make few comments relating to the fashioning of anastomoses because I have outlined the techniques of anastomosis for bowel resection for certain specific conditions in other chapters. In general, our group has favored stapled anastomoses where feasible because of the greater rapidity of fashioning of the anastomosis and, therefore, shorter operating room time. For low anastomoses to the rectum or upper anal canal as well, stapled operations have a singular advantage because of greater safety as well as speed. In the case of coloanal anastomosis, where it is feasible, stapled operations are used because of the enhanced sphincter function occurring to the patient thereafter (compared to hand sewn).

The principles of hand-sewn anastomosis intraperitoneally have been well outlined. Our preference has been to use a Cheatle slit to equilibrate the caliber of the bowel ends. Quarantining of the bowel content is carried out by placing an umbilical tape on the proximal side of the anastomosis to minimize intraoperative contamination. To minimize the placement of forceps on the bowel end as well as to allow for accurate apposition of the bowel edges, stay sutures of 4-0 chromic or Vicryl are placed at the 2, 4, 8, and 10 o'clock positions on each side of the bowel and tagged with a hemostat. A one-layer anastomosis is carried out posteriorly. This is done with 3-0 Vicryl using a mattress suture. When the sutures have reached the 4 and 8 o'clock positions; the mattress suture is stopped and seromuscular sutures are used. The mattress suture consists of full-thickness stitch starting from inside the lumen of the bowel, in the midline posteriorly, passing full thickness through the bowel, through the fat, and into the corresponding sections on the adjacent bowel end. The suture is then brought back between the mucosa and submucosa and passed through the same mucosa and submucosal junction on the proximal bowel end and then tied.

The seromuscular sutures are placed in turn toward the midline of the antimesenteric margin. The last three or four stitches are placed and not tied to allow for more accurate placement of such sutures, always attempting to keep the mucosa turned in.

In the case of an intraperitoneal stapled anastomosis (e.g., with an ileoileal anastomosis), the bowel ends are stapled and divided using a linear cutter stapler, such as the GIA-60. Similar quarantining tapes are placed proximal and distal to the sites to be anastomosed. The two ends are lined up side by side, or in certain circumstances simply offset (see Ch. 12). Enterotomies are made using a cutting cautery and the enterotomy is completed using a hemostat ensuring quarantining the anastomosis with packs. The cartridge and anvil of the stapler are serially inserted. The assistant's role is to maintain the approximation of the antimesenteric margins on each side while using forward traction to bring the ends of the bowel up onto the hub of the instrument. When such alignment has been deemed satisfactory, the instrument is fired, which allows for stapling and cutting at the same time.

All such anastomoses have a tendency to bleed, albeit usually in a minor fashion. This can be checked by placing a small right-angled retractor into the opened enterotomy and examining the posterior layer of the anastomosis. In certain circumstances, light touching with the electric cautery suffices to control bleeding; however, this must be used with caution because the metal staples will transmit the electrical impulse onto adjacent tissues. Should there be any arterial-type bleeding or a small pumper, then this posterior layer can be simply reinforced using a running 30 Vicryl. Upon completion of this, the enterotomy is then closed. A linear stapler (e.g., the TA-55) is sometimes used to close the enterotomy. Although the double-stapling technique is used in certain circumstances, as a general rule, it should be avoided. In this case, it is simple to avoid by using a continuous 30 Vicryl as a seromuscular suture to occlude the enterotomy opening. In this particular circumstance, I tend to reinforce this closure using interrupted 30 Vicryl outside of the continuous layer. The mesenteric defect is closed with 0-chromic catgut; the quarantining tapes are then removed.

With respect to the stapled end-to-end anastomosis between the colon and rectum, there are two excellent staplers available: the EEA and the Ethicon ILS. Techniques of mobilization and ensuring the blood supply and quarantining the bowel ends have been discussed previously. As a general

(Continues)

rule, the largest size stapler head that will allow for an anastomosis to be made without tearing or injuring the bowel end because of inequalities in size should be used.

With respect to placement of the pursestring sutures, it is important to start the suturing on the antimesenteric aspect of the bowel and to use very small bites of the bowel edge. Specifically, this means passing the needle (0 Prolene) into the serosa of the bowel approximately 2 mm from its cut edge and then attempting to pick up a wisp (1 mm) of mucosa before passing onto the next placement of the suture. It is also important to space the sutures adequately, that is, at 1.0-cm intervals. Intervals closer than this, especially for a wide anastomosis, may mean that pulling up on the pursestring fails to allow the suture to run and causes a bunching of the bowel edge on the shaft of the instrument. Taking more tissue than that described above will cause an excessive amount of tissue to be encompassed within the stapler, between the anvil and the cartridge. After placing the suture, the anvil and cartridge are inserted. The ties are tied down over the respective shafts, and the instrument is closed and fired.

A few points on the distal pursestring. In the case of a high colorectal anastomosis (i.e., to the intraperitoneal rectum), this poses no special challenges. It is wise to have the rectum packed away with quarantining packs and to have aspirated out rectal mucous and stool preoperatively or just before the passage of the staple gun. The rectum may be further quarantined by placement of a vascular clamp below the planned area or placement of the sutures. This is optional because such a clamp can be inconvenient at times.

For the anastomosis being made in the midrectum, especially for a patient who is somewhat obese, the placement of the rectal pursestring can be a challenge. In such circumstances, a useful technique is to have the assistant, who is standing on the right side of the patient looking down at the pelvis, make an incision with the cutting cautery across the anterior third of the rectum. A Babcock clamp may be placed on one edge that has been thus exposed. The abdominal operator stands on the left side of the patient with 0 Prolene placed on a needle holder, in a backhand fashion, and commences to start the placement of the pursestring. As this is proceeding, cephalad traction of the specimen will allow for displacement of the anterior edge from the main specimen, facilitating the placement of the pursestring suture. Because the incision is then taken around to the right anterior aspect of the proctotomy, these sutures can be placed forehand. In this fashion continuous traction is maintained and serial incisions are made in the rectal wall allowing for the operator to continue to place the pursestring sutures with exactitude, until the bowel has been completely transected and the specimen delivered. Babcock clamps can be placed on the four quadrants or stay sutures to either check for hemostasis or the accuracy of placement of these sutures.

During the course of passage of the stapler transanally, it is sometimes difficult for the perineal operator to judge the correct angle of passing the instrument. In such cases it is always best for the abdominal operator to place a gloved index finger into the open end of the rectum from the abdominal aspect, placed into the lumen and use this to act as a guide for the further cephalad passage of the instrument. During this time copious mucous can come out, so it is worthwhile having this area quarantined and suction ready.

With the very low anastomosis, placement of the pursestring suture can be achieved commonly by the technique described above. In such circumstances having available lighted retracting instruments, such as the Goligher or lighted Dever, is invaluable in helping to facilitate fashioning this anastomosis. In certain special cases (e.g., ileo-pouch-anal anastomosis) it is worthwhile using the double-stapled technique. This consists of passing a linear stapler around the rectal stump prior to its transection. The preferred instrument in this instance is that of the PI30 (30 mm). After placement around the rectum, the pin that allows encompassing of the specimen into the instrument is pressed home. The instrument can then be slid down the denuded rectum to the level of the upper border of the levators while maintaining proximal traction of the rectal specimen. The instrument can then be fired and the rectum divided with a long-bladed knife. Upon release of the stapler, the specimen will commonly retreat within the muscle groups of the levators. At this point the EEA stapler is passed to the perineal operator.

Effacement of the anal verge is carried out with the placement of three or four Allis clamps. The anvil is replaced by the white trocar, which is placed into the central shaft of the cartridge and withdrawn within the housing of the cartridge. At this point manipulation of the cartridge is used to allow for passage of the instrument into the lower portion of the anal canal. Slight cephalad traction as well as elevation of the handle will cause effacement of the divided and stapled anorectal end. During this time, exposure is facilitated with straight lighted retractors in the pelvis. In all cases, it is preferable to have the trochar pass through the staple line posterior to the staple line, especially in women. In this way the ultimate anastomosis is far less likely to cause injury to the posterior vaginal wall. On passing the trochar through the anorectal stump, this is then detached and the proximal end of the bowel with its now attached anvil is delivered down to the pelvis and mated with the open shaft of the cartridge component of the stapler. The remaining details of the use of the instrument are as discussed by Dr. Keighley.

Testing the anastomosis is always done either with passage of air by an asepto syringe into the opened anal canal while saline fills the pelvis, or with the use of betadine injection into the low rectum while observing the presacral space for any possible leaks. The tissue rings are examined carefully to ensure their integrity.

Victor W. Fazio

Dr. Keighley's descriptions of intraperitoneal and pelvic anastomoses are readily understandable and I agree with nearly all of his statements. I would like to add a few comments.

My almost unique technique of hand-sewn anastomosis is a continuous single-layer full-thickness technique using polyglactin sutures on a 26-mm needle. This technique is easy to perform and to teach, as well as very safe.

(Continues)

Prior to carrying out the anastomosis, one must ensure two essential conditions in order to prevent leakage: (1) the absence of any tension on either the anastomosis itself or on the mesentery; and (2) a sufficient blood supply to both bowel ends. For this reason we mobilize the splenic flexure nearly always for a high colorectal anastomosis and always for low colorectal and coloanal anastomoses. The only exceptions are in aged or arteriosclerotic patients, in whom mesenteric arterial flow is essential. In the vast majority of patients, once the tumor is deemed resectable, the procedure begins with mobilization of the splenic flexure in order to ensure that the question of tension will not be neglected by the surgeon. In patients submitted to tumor resection with curative intent, this maneuver has to be followed immediately by ligation and division of the inferior mesenteric vessels (i.e., the vein behind the body of the pancreas and the artery at its origin on the aorta). After completion of this step, the total mobilization of the left colon guarantees against tension on the anastomosis. The mesentery has to be as floppy as the colon. The section of its vascular parts from the line of knotting results in even more length and even less tension. We consider mobilization of the colon to be sufficient when, after completion of the anastomosis, the colon can be easily raised 20 to 30 cm above the level of the abdominal wall. The colon can thus fall down freely, filling the pelvic cavity. We are thus confident that there will be no tension on the anastomosis during the early postoperative period despite edema and intestinal distension.

The colon should be divided at a point where blood supply is sufficient. We usually determine this by cutting the pedicle of fat appendix just distal to the point chosen for the intestinal section. This simple and inexpensive method appears safe.

The spillage of feces is avoided by closing off the bowel 10 cm above the section line with a tape. The bowel is then divided and washed out up to the tape. After a crushing clamp is applied to the rectum just below the tumor, or to the rectosigmoid junction in diverticular disease, placing the patient in the Lloyd-Davies position allows the rectum to be washed out up to the level of the clamp through the anus.

When choosing a hand-sewn colorectal anastomosis, a Satinsky clamp should be applied as distally as possible to both the rectum and its mesentery to assist in bringing up the rectal stump and to avoid retraction on the muscular layer, particularly on the posterior wall. There is usually no need for hemostasis of the intestinal ends because we use continuous and full-thickness sutures.

We usually take large (5 to 6 mm) bites from both ends. The technique of suturing by itself is quite easy to do and to teach. The first stitch, taking the full thickness of bowel, is placed opposite to the surgeon (i.e., on the right corner). It is tightened on the mucosa, inside the bowel lumen. A stitch is then placed on the left corner of the colon segment to keep it open. The following bites from the posterior layer are executed toward the left in the same way, taking the colon first from within out. The needle is then replaced in the needle holder and, after checking that the muscular layer has not slipped away, a full-thickness bite is taken from the rectum from without in. The bites are spaced out 3 to 4 mm apart symmetrically on both ends. With the assistant holding the suture tail and applying gentle tension, a running suture is performed. Once the needle is totally through the rectal wall, the stitch is taken with the needle holder to a point about 2 mm above the point where it comes out from the rectal wall. This allows the thread to be regularly spaced while keeping constant tension on the suture. A satisfactory appearance is given to the posterior layer by overlapping the colonic layer with the rectal layer. Once the posterior part of the anastomosis is done, the needle is passed through the colon wall and the suture is gently stretched. A single stitch is passed and tied outside the lumen, the knot being placed on the rectum. The posterior running suture is then tied with this stitch. Using this stitch, two backhand passages, taking the rectum first and then the colon, are made from the left to the right. This thread is then secured with a clip to maintain tension. Most of the anterior layer is made from the right corner toward the left. The starting stitch is tied outside the lumen and the Satinsky clamp is usually opened at this moment. The anterior part of the anastomosis is made in the same manner as the posterior part. The suture is tied with the suture coming from the left. During completion of the anterior part, one must avoid invaginating the rectal mucosa. We overcome this problem using Gawke points: At each passage the needle goes through the rectal mucosa and the rectal wall separately and in the opposite direction.

For very low colorectal anastomosis, we prefer the double-stapled procedure. Moreover, this is the only anastomosis we test in the way described by Dr. Keighley.

Rolland Parc

3

Laparoscopic-Assisted Operations

Heidi Nelson
John H. Pemberton

The field of minimally invasive surgery is at once exciting and frustrating. The very thought of tiny incisions, anatomically correct colorectal resections, and discharge from the hospital within 3 to 4 days would energize even the most recalcitrant surgeon, yet the tools and methods to accomplish the task are somewhat primitive. Proponents of laparoscopic colon surgery have an uphill fight on their hands to prove that such a technique is clinically and cost effective.

It is common to discuss the "learning curve" every time a new surgical procedure is introduced. We saw this with ileoanal anastomosis and coloanal anastomosis, and are now seeing it with laparoscopic colectomy. Whereas the other curves were indeed akin to a curve, laparoscopic colectomy's learning curve is closer to a cliff—it is tough. Whether it is worth it will be judged over time, but as of now, yes, it is worth it. Each continent has its promoters. It will be an interesting 2 or 3 years.

Positioning

The position of the patient depends on the portion of the colon requiring resection. The patient is placed supine for right and left resections, whereas the combined position is used for sigmoid colon and proximal rectal resections. The "golden rule" when setting up for these procedures is to avoid creating a "reverse image environment."

Resection of the Right Side of the Colon

With the patient supine, equipment and personnel are positioned as detailed in Figure 3-1. The one monitor is placed on the patient's right at the head of the table; the scrub nurse is also on the patient's right side, but at the foot of the table, while the operating surgeon and the camera operator stand to the patient's left, with the surgeon above.

The patient is then placed in 20 to 30 degrees of Trendelenburg and an infraumbilical incision is made. A Veress needle technique is almost always used to establish a pneumoperitoneum (Fig. 3-2). By elevating the abdominal wall and directing the

51

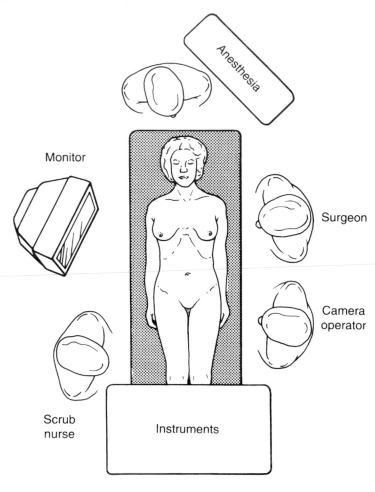

Figure 3-1.

needle toward the pelvis, injuries to the bowel and major vascular structures are avoided. Hasson's open approach is quite useful for patients who have had previous operations. The abdomen is next insufflated with carbon dioxide to 12 to 15 mmHg. A 10-mm trochar/cannula is used to gain camera access to the abdomen through the umbilical incision. Additional 10- to 12-mm cannulas are placed under direct vision at the sites shown in Figure 3-3. The precise position of the cannulas among individ-

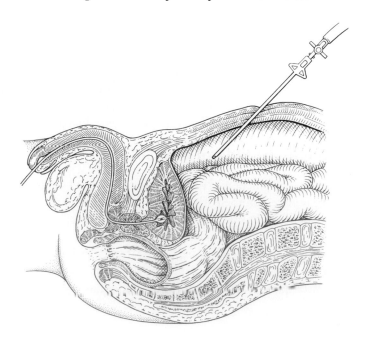

Figure 3-2.

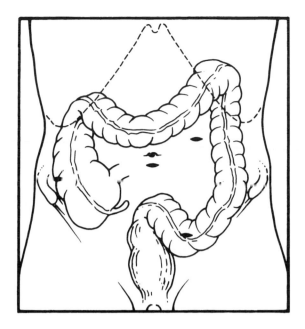

Figure 3-3.

ual patients depends on the patient's stature. In short, stout patients, the access sites need to be spaced further apart to prevent "sword fights"; in tall patients the sites must be spaced more closely together to ensure that the instruments reach.

Next, the laparoscope is replaced in the left upper paramedian site. With the assistant controlling the laparoscope and the table positioned head down, left side down, the cecum is retracted cephalad and to the left. The assistant retracts the peritoneal reflection in the opposite direction. Dissection proceeds along the peritoneum of the ileum, where the proper plane can readily be identified. Traction is key to all types of surgery; in laparoscopic surgery, it is utterly central. This dissection progresses to the hepatic flexure (Fig. 3-4A). The right ureter should now be identified. It is not uncommon for adhesions from an appendectomy to hinder progress; particularly bad adhesions should prompt conversion to an open procedure.

Once the hepatic flexure is reached, the scope is moved to the left lower paramedian site. The operating table is repositioned head up, left side down. The ascending colon and hepatic flexure are retracted by the surgeon with one hand while dissection with hook cautery or scissors is performed with the other. The ascending colon and transverse colon can be retracted in such a way (inferiorly and medially) that the omentum is separated from the colon relatively easily (Fig. 3-4B). The surgeon should be able to see the duodenum and right ureter during this dissection.

The right colon and a portion of the transverse colon are now mobilized. The mesentery is placed on tension, which facilitates identification of the superior mesenteric, ileocolic, right colic, and middle colic vessels. The primary vascular bundle that needs to be ligated laparoscopically is the ileocolic arcade (Fig. 3-4C). Vessels are double-clipped and endolooped. Once the ileocolic vascular pedicle is ligated, the bowel is fully mobile and is exteriorized easily.

Usually the mobile right colon reaches to the abdominal wall at the site of the right abdominal cannula; thus, the 4- to 6-cm transverse incision should be made there. After bringing the bowel through the incision, the right branch of the middle colic artery may be ligated readily. The operation from this point on does not differ from a standard resection and anastomosis (Fig. 3-4D). The bowel is returned to the peritoneal cavity and the abdominal wound is closed in two layers. The pneumoperitoneum is then reestablished and the laparoscope is reinserted to inspect for bleeding. The abdomen is irrigated thoroughly. The cannulas are removed under direct vision. The cannula sites are closed using a single figure-of-eight suture in the fascicular layer and a subcuticular suture in the skin.

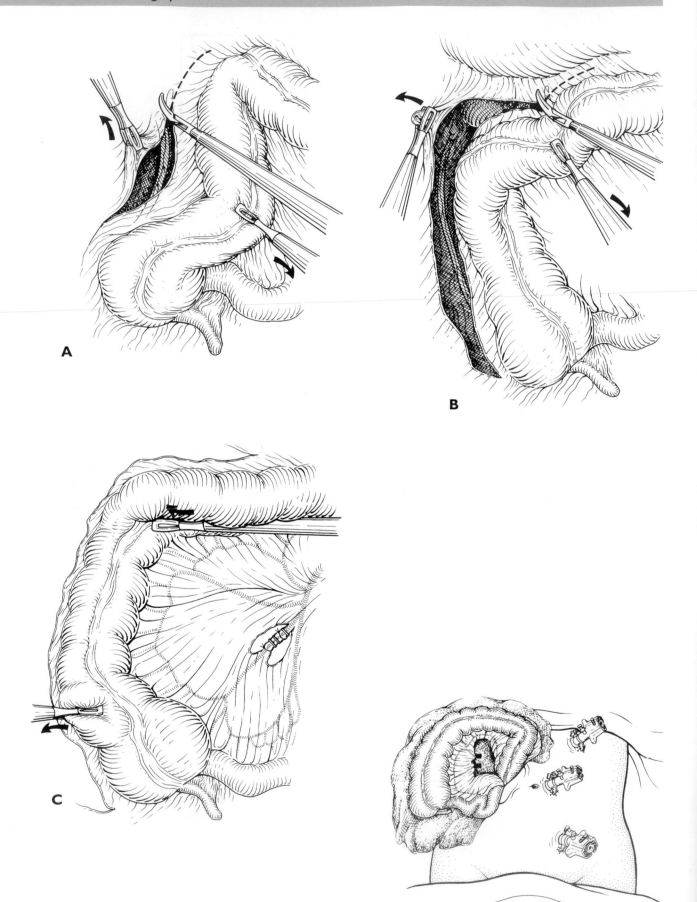

Figure 3-4.

Resection of the Left Colon

The patient is supine. The equipment and personnel are positioned as follows. One monitor is placed on the patient's right and one at the left at the head of the table; the scrub nurse is on the patient's left side, at the foot of the table, and the surgeon and the camera operator stand on the patient's right side, with the surgeon closer to the patient's head. After the pneumoperitoneum is established, the scope is placed infraumbilically, and 10- to 12-mm cannulas are positioned in the left lower abdomen and in the right upper and right lower paramedian positions.

The laparoscope is then removed from the infraumbilical port and replaced into the cannula at the right upper paramedian site. The table is placed head down, right side down. The descending colon is retracted in the opposite direction. Cautery then frees the left lateral peritoneal reflections of the sigmoid and descending colon. The ureter is then identified.

Next, the scope is placed into the right paramedian cannula and the surgeon and the assistant exchange positions. The operating table is then repositioned head up, right side down. The descending colon and transverse colon are retracted in an inferomedial direction, facilitating anorectal mobilization.

The pedicle containing the sigmoidal, superior hemorrhoidal, and left colic vessels is dissected and divided using clips and endolooped. The exteriorizing incision (4 to 6 cm in length) is made over the left abdominal cannula site. An extracorporeal anastomosis is then performed. Closure is the same as for the right colon procedure.

Resection of the Sigmoid Colon

The patient is placed in the combined position (see Ch. 1). Equipment and personnel are positioned as shown in Figure 3-5. The Hasson technique is used to place the first cannula in the left upper abdomen. Once pneumoperitoneum is achieved, additional 10- to 12-mm cannulas are positioned as shown in Figure 3-6.

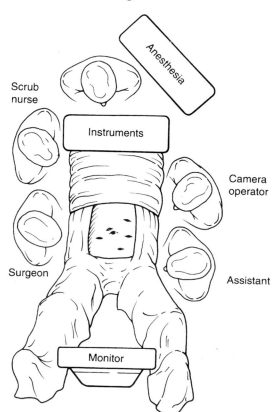

Figure 3-5.

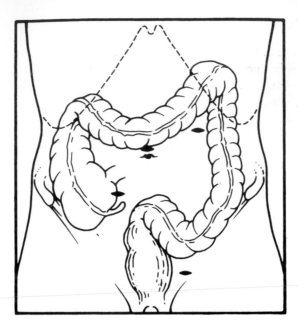

Figure 3-6.

The table is positioned head down, right side down. The scope is positioned through the left upper quadrant cannula. The assistant grasps the descending colon with one hand and retracts the peritoneal attachments of the sigmoid colon with the other. The surgeon elevates the sigmoid colon in a cephalad direction and to the right using one hand, while the peritoneal attachments are divided with cautery using the other (Fig. 3-7A). The ureter is now identified. If the colon pathology needs to be localized precisely, the colonoscope is inserted through the anus and advanced proximally. The sigmoid colon is easily transilluminated and the site of pathology marked.

The sigmoid dissection may be continued as far caudally as needed. The distal dissection requires rectal mobilization. By retracting the sigmoid colon cephalad and to the right, the presacral window, under the superior hemorrhoidal vessels, can be opened. The superior hemorrhoidal vessels are then identified, dissected, and removed. To mobilize the descending colon and splenic flexure to obtain needed length, the camera is positioned in the left lower quadrant and the dissection commenced as described for the hepatic flexure.

Once the bowel is mobilized and the sigmoid/superior hemorrhoidal vascular pedicle ligated, the proximal rectum is divided using one (or more) applications of the 60-mm linear stapler (Fig. 3-7B). A 20-mm cannula is required for this stapler and is placed through the right lower abdominal cannula site. The proximal bowel is then exteriorized, usually through a transverse incision no more than 6 cm long at the left midabdominal cannula site. After the bowel is resected, the anvil of a circular stapler is secured in the proximal bowel (Fig. 3-7C). The bowel and anvil are then returned to the abdominal cavity. The circular stapler is then introduced per anus and a double-stapled anterior resection performed in a manner no different from the conventional open technique described in Chapter 2 (Fig. 3-7D). The Autosuture CEEA circular stapler may be used (Fig. 3-7C–F); alternatively, the Ethicon ILS device may be used. A Kraske-type approach has also been used to perform the anastomosis near the levators after laparoscopic mobilization and transection of the rectum.

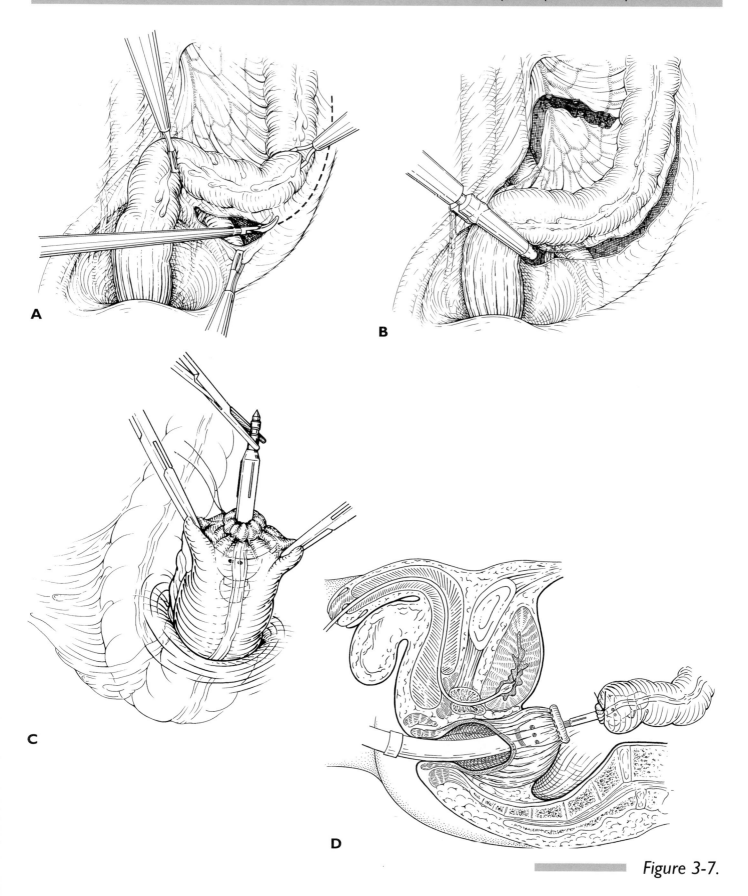

A

B

C

D

Figure 3-7.

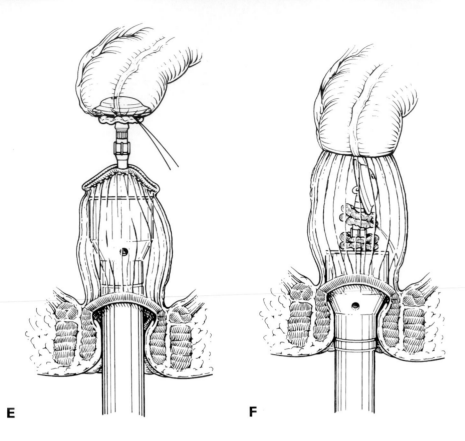

Figure 3-7. ▬▬▬▬   E   F

Abdominoperineal Resection

In order to perform an abdominoperineal resection laparoscopically, the steps described above are performed identically, except that the rectal dissection is carried downward to the levators laterally, to the anococcygeal ligament posteriorly, and to the midvagina or midprostate anteriorly. This is accomplished relatively easily in thin patients. Progress of the dissection is observed by placing the finger (or proctoscope) into the vagina and rectum (in women) or rectum (in men) while visualizing their movements through the laparoscope. This is not an easy mobilization. There is also a tendency to stay close to the wall of the rectum, which may have implications with regard to adequate margins. When the rectum is completely mobilized, the 60-mm linear stapler is used to transect the bowel. A 3-cm circular incision is made over the trochar site in the left lower quadrant and the stapled bowel end is pulled through for colostomy. The colostomy stoma is matured as the last step of the operation. Attention is then turned to the perineum, where the rectum and anus are removed as described in Chapters 1 and 10.

It is interesting to visit patients the morning after an abdominoperineal resection; they behave as if little or nothing was done at all!

Laparoscopic Appendectomy

The appendix lends itself to laparoscopic removal readily. There is little question, however, that an inflamed, enlarged appendix or an appendiceal mass makes for a difficult laparoscopic appendectomy; thus, the threshold for converting from a laparoscopic to an open procedure should be very low. Moreover, if the appendiceal cecal junction cannot be visualized easily and with absolute certainty, a standard open appendectomy should be performed. All of the standard preoperative measures (fluids, antibiotics, general anesthesia, bladder catheterization) apply.

A Veress needle approach is used to establish the pneumoperitoneum. Access sites are shown in Figure 3-8. The surgeon and camera operator stay on the same side of the table on the patient's left. Through the suprapubic port the mesoappendix is grasped with a Babcock grasper. The appendiceal artery must be clearly definable. It can be dissected with the hook electrode. It is doubly clipped and/or stapled across with a vascular stapler (Fig. 3-9A). Once the appendix has been dissected to the appendiceal-cecal junction, the base is doubly ligated with 0-chromic endoloops. A total of three such endoloops are used on the appendix, as illustrated in Figure 3-9B. The appendix is then divided, the mucosa cauterized, and the appendix placed in a retrieval bag and removed from the abdominal cavity. The area is irrigated and the endoloops are visualized to ensure hemostasis.

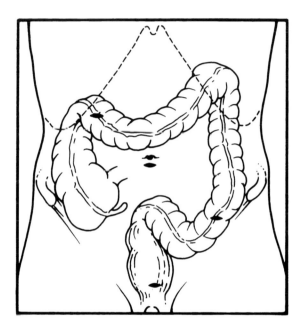

Figure 3-8.

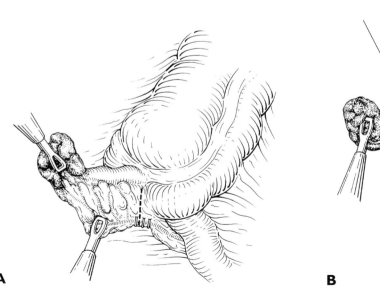
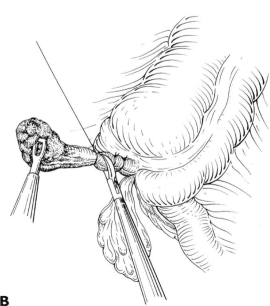

A

B

Figure 3-9.

It is good practice to remove the pneumoperitoneum for about 3 to 4 minutes and then to reestablish the pneumoperitoneum to see if there is any pooling of blood in the right lower quadrant. Pneumoperitoneum of 14 to 15 mmHg is sufficient to tamponade venous bleeding.

Whether laparoscopic appendectomy is a rational operative technique to pursue in large numbers is unknown. Standard open appendectomy is associated with a very short (2 day) hospital stay, and whether laparoscopic techniques can appreciably alter this, while at the same time not requiring excessive expenditure on instrumentation, remains to be seen. It is currently being studied at our institution in a randomized prospective manner.

Editorial Commentaries

We challenge the concept of laparoscopic colorectal surgery for the following reasons:

1. It still requires much more operating room time and is therefore much more costly, operating time being at a high premium in terms of availability and cost.
2. There is no evidence to date that laparoscopically assisted colorectal resections result in shorter hospital stays than open operations.
3. More rapid return to work in our experience is entirely related to patient motivation and not to the method of surgical excision.
4. There is an increased incidence of iatrogenic damage to vital structures (ureters, blood vessels, etc.) using laparoscopic techniques compared to open operations.
5. The reported incidence of the wrong segment of bowel being resected laparoscopically is alarming.
6. The concept of mincing up tumors in order to deliver them through mini-incisions contravenes standard oncologic surgical principles of no-touch technique.

Despite these rather dogmatic views, we believe that laparoscopic rectopexy and laparoscopic-assisted subtotal colectomy and ileorectal anastomosis for slow-transit constipation, and even laparoscopic restorative proctocolectomy for familial adenomatous polyposis, could have considerable psychological advantage (if they can be justified on cost-benefit terms) in the future because operations can be completed through small transverse suprapubic incisions. In our experience, laparoscopic-assisted resections for Crohn's disease are generally ill-advised both because of the presence of adhesions and, more important, because the thickened mesentery with enlarged lymph glands together with the fistulous communications between the affected segment of bowel and other structures make laparoscopic resections difficult and potentially dangerous.

Michael R. B. Keighley

4

Stomas

Michael R. B. Keighley

Principles

The optimum stoma site is identified and marked by the stoma therapist preoperatively. The stoma therapist should evaluate the potential stoma sites with the patient supine, upright, and sitting. The optimum site is influenced by the patient's normal clothing habit (e.g., whether loose- or tight-fitting clothing is worn at the waist).

The abdominal trephine is begun by excising a disc of skin over the stoma site. A Littlewood forceps is used to grasp and raise the skin in preparation for excision (Fig. 4-1A). A disc of subcutaneous fat is then excised, exposing the anterior rectus sheath. A cruciate incision is then made over the anterior rectus sheath to expose the muscle belly (Fig. 4-1B).

The muscle belly is delivered to the abdominal wall by placing a curved Kocher forceps beneath it. Partial division of the muscle belly, which allows any vessels within the muscle to be identified, is then performed with coagulation diathermy

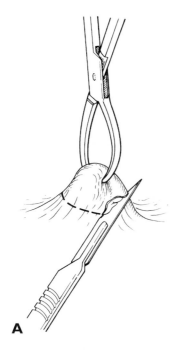

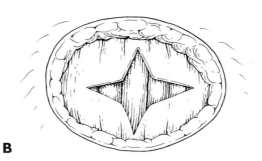

A   B

Figure 4-1.

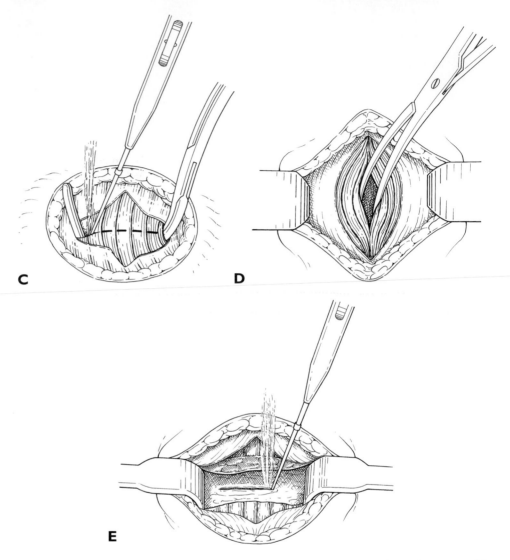

Figure 4-1. ▬▬▬▬

(Fig. 4-1C); some surgeons prefer to split the muscle longitudinally with scissors (Fig. 4-1D). Langenbeck retractors are used to expose the posterior rectus sheath and the peritoneum, which are then opened by diathermy (Fig. 4-1E). Complete hemostasis must be achieved after every step of the procedure. Upon completion of the trephine, we generally place gauze within the trephine to secure hemostasis.

Ileostomy

End Ileostomy

The stoma is usually sited over the right rectus muscle, as far as possible from the anterior superior iliac spine and the umbilicus in the lower abdomen, and avoiding any scars or depressions (Fig. 4-2). It is essential that all ileostomies be placed through the rectus muscle and not lateral to it. If the patient usually wears loose-fitting clothes, a higher site may be identified; those who wear tighter-fitting clothing around the waist may need a lower ileostomy site.

The distal end of the ileum is divided using a linear staple cutter or by dividing the bowel between two Potts clamps. Use of the staple cutter ensures that there will be no contamination of the abdominal wall as the bowel end is delivered through it. An adequate blood supply to the ileum may be ensured by examining the vascular

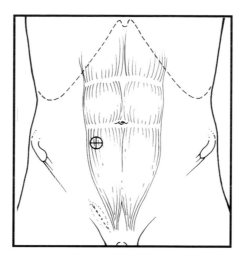

Figure 4-2.

arcades (Fig. 4-3). If the mesentery is very thick, reduction of its bulk, if possible without impairing the blood supply to the ileum, might be advisable.

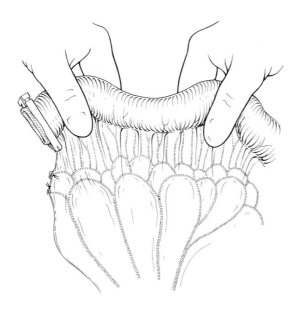

Figure 4-3.

The ileum is delivered through the trephine and onto the skin surface. Delivery of a 5-cm length of terminal ileum will ensure that, upon eversion, a 2.5-cm long ileostomy will result. Some surgeons place sutures from the peritoneum to the serosa of the ileum, and then to the anterior rectus sheath after the bowel has been delivered (Fig. 4-4). We do not generally advise this practice, except in the patient who has had a previously unstable ileostomy. If stabilizing sutures do seem necessary, it is far better to place them before delivering the bowel so that the serosal component of the sutures can be applied after the bowel has been everted.

Once the abdominal wound has been securely closed and covered, the bowel is opened (by removing the Potts clamp or excising the staple line) and the stoma everted. We always advise closing the laparotomy wound prior to opening the bowel to avoid contaminating the abdominal wound. Closure of the lateral gutter is rarely performed but is more fully discussed in Chapter 12. Meticulous hemostasis of the

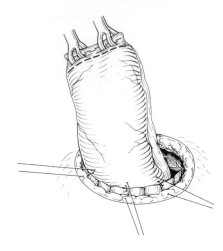

Figure 4-4.

ileal end is essential. A pair of Allis forceps is introduced into the stoma lumen and applied to the midpoint of the antimesenteric portion of the ileum (Fig. 4-5A). Two or three additional Allis forceps are applied to the free edge of the ileum to facilitate full eversion of the stoma. Once the stomas has been everted, mucocutaneous sutures are placed using 4-0 Prolene on a cutting needle. We try to avoid suturing too close to the edge of the trephine, because if the sutures lie too close to the mucocutaneous junction, they may be difficult to remove (Fig. 4-5B). Many surgeons prefer to use an absorbable suture material, such as 3-0 plain catgut, making suture removal unnecessary. It is our policy to include the ileal serosa in the mucocutaneous suture; hence, the needle is first passed through the skin into subcutaneous tissues and through the adjacent serosa of the ileum, and then a second tuck of ileal wall is taken before tying the suture to the skin edge (Fig. 4-5C). This procedure is repeated around the circumference of the ileum until six to eight sutures have been placed. The sutures are then clipped but left untied until correct positioning is verified. Once positioning is correct, the sutures should be loosely tied to prevent damage to the bowel during the usual period of postoperative edema.

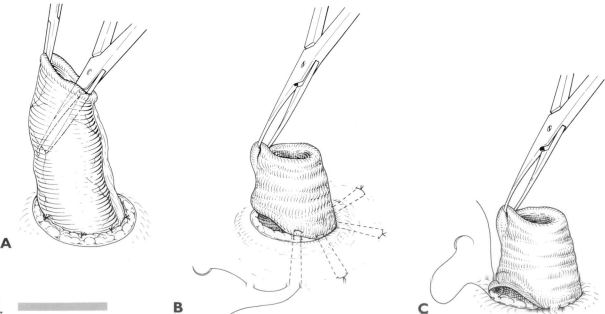

A   B   C

Figure 4-5.

Loop Ileostomy

A loop ileostomy is usually constructed at the time of laparotomy to divert the fecal stream. Occasionally a loop ileostomy may be constructed without a full laparotomy, the end of the ileum visualized directly through the abdominal wall trephine or laparoscopically in order to deliver it to the skin surface (see Ch. 3). If a laparotomy is not used, identification of the bloodless fold of Treves will define the distal loop so that the proximal end only is everted. Construction of a loop ileostomy without a laparotomy is only feasible in thin patients in whom the orientation of the terminal ileum can be clearly displayed and in whom laparotomy itself is contraindicated.

A trephine is made exactly as previously described. The rectus muscle is partially divided or split and the peritoneal cavity widely opened using Langenbeck retractors. The terminal ileum is defined (by the bloodless fold of Treves) and the distal limb marked with a suture. A nylon tape is placed around the bowel through a mesenteric window made adjacent to the wall of the terminal ileum and the loop is delivered through the abdominal wall. An enterotomy is made in the distal limb and the proximal lip is everted (Fig. 4-6A). Direct mucocutaneous sutures using interrupted 4-0 Prolene or plain catgut are then placed to secure the stoma (Fig. 4-6B).

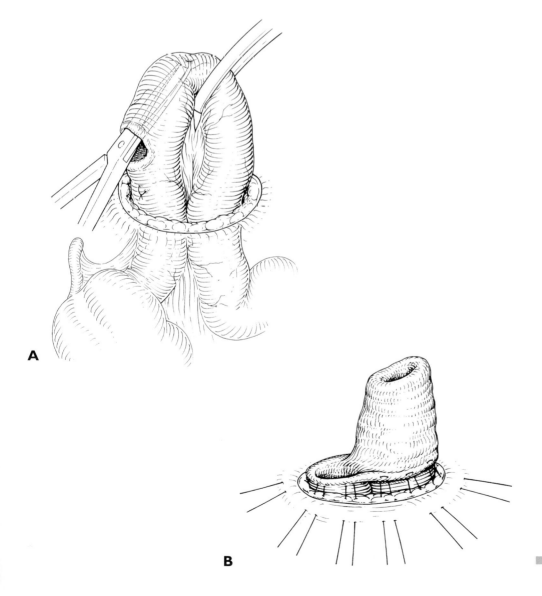

A

B

Figure 4-6.

Construction of a loop ileostomy at laparotomy involves identification of a loop of ileum suitable for delivery without tension to the abdominal wall. A tape is placed around the ileum and the distal end is marked. The trephine, made as previously described, must admit two fingers to ensure that there will be no obstruction to the blood supply of the bowel. If there is difficulty in delivering the ileum through the abdominal wall, it may be advisable to place a small rod, such as 1-mm polyethylene intravenous tubing, underneath the bowel through the mesenteric window made for the nylon tape. The rod is trimmed so that its ends just appear beyond the edge of the bowel and is then secured to the skin with sutures (Fig. 4-7). A small enterotomy is made over the distal limb of the bowel at the junction of the ileum and the skin. It is important that the enterotomy is not too large, as it will act as a collar to ensure that the stoma remains everted. Once the enterotomy is made, the antimesenteric border of the ileum is grasped at its apex and the proximal limb is everted. Three or four mucocutaneous sutures are made to secure the distal limb to the skin, and the everted stoma is sutured as described for end ileostomy.

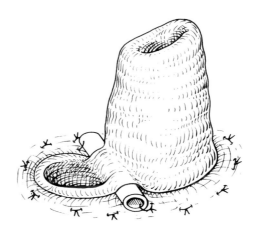

Figure 4-7.

Closure

Digital assessment of the anal sphincters together with endoscopic or radiologic examination of the distal anastomosis is necessary to establish that the anal sphincters are functioning satisfactorily and that there is no distal obstruction before closure of the loop ileostomy. A simple test to exclude distal obstruction is to verify the free passage of air from a sigmoidoscope into the loop ileostomy bag.

Preoperative mechanical bowel preparation (a distal ileostomy washout and a rectal washout) may be necessary, particularly to clear out any inspissated fecal material distal to the loop ileostomy. Antimicrobial cover is ensured preoperatively. With the patient under general anesthesia, a circumstomal incision is made around the mucocutaneous junction with a small blade. The edge of the ileum is grasped with tissue forceps. With a combination of sharp and scissor dissection, the two limbs of ileum are dissected from the skin, subcutaneous fat, and the rectus sheath. It is sometimes advisable to place a stay suture on either side of the rectus sheath (Fig. 4-8A). The entire circumference of the ileostomy should be freed from the abdominal wall so as to allow the loop of ileum to be delivered completely from the peritoneal cavity onto the abdominal wall. The everted proximal loop is rolled back by dissecting between the two serosal surfaces of the gut (Fig. 4-8B). The edge of ileum is excised to remove any adherent skin and hemostasis is achieved. Various techniques may be used for

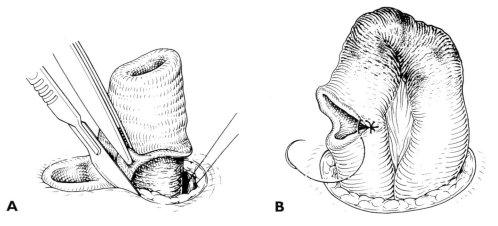

A   **B**

Figure 4-8.

closure, including single-layer continuous extramucosal suture, two-layer suture, and stapled closure with construction of a functional end-to-end anastomosis.

Single-Layer Extramucosal Closure. Having established that there is no evidence of damage to either loop of bowel and having freshened the edge of the mucocutaneous junction, the enterotomy is closed transversely using a continuous extramucosal 3-0 PDS suture, which fully inverts the mucosa and establishes hemostasis (Fig. 4-9). This technique is identical to that of strictureplasty (see Ch. 12).

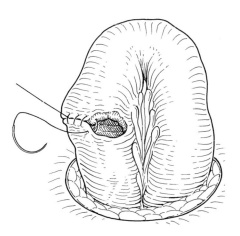

Figure 4-9.

Two-Layer Closure. An extramucosal continuous suture is reinforced by returning to the point of origin and inverting the closure line by picking up seromuscular bites from the ileum, the second layer being tied to the starting suture. Alternatively, reinforcement may be achieved with interrupted seromuscular sutures.

Stapled Closure. If a stapled closure technique is to be used, it is absolutely essential that at least 15 cm of small bowel can be delivered from the peritoneal cavity to the skin surface. A series of antimesenteric stay sutures are placed on the serosa of the small bowel ends to bring them into close apposition. Using a PLC 75 linear staple cutter, a side-to-side ileoileal anastomosis is constructed (Fig. 4-10A). Then, while grasping the open end of the ileum by stay sutures or tissue-holding forceps, the linear staple cutter (PLC 75 or GIA 70) is applied a second time (Fig. 4-10B). The result is a functional end-to-end anastomosis that is quite bulky, hence care must be taken in replacing the bowel into the peritoneal cavity.

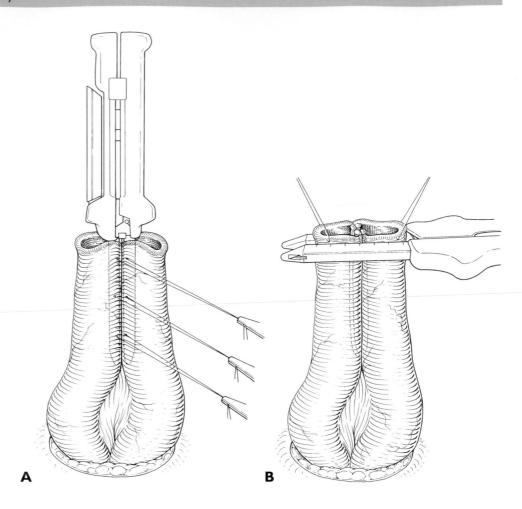

Figure 4-10.   **A**   **B**

Resection and End-to-End Anastomosis. It is sometimes preferable, particularly if there is considerable fibrosis around the ileostomy stoma, to resect the loop and perform an end-to-end anastomosis (Fig. 4-11). This does not necessarily require complete resection of the mesenteric surface of the gut. In other situations it may be preferable to perform a full resection and an end-to-end anastomosis using the single-layer continuous extramucosal, single-layer interrupted full-thickness, or two-layer closure technique, all of which are described in Chapter 2. Alternatively, a stapled procedure may be adopted to provide a functional end-to-end anastomosis, as already described.

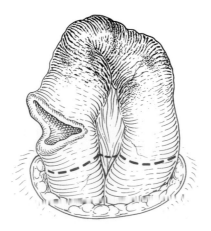

Figure 4-11.

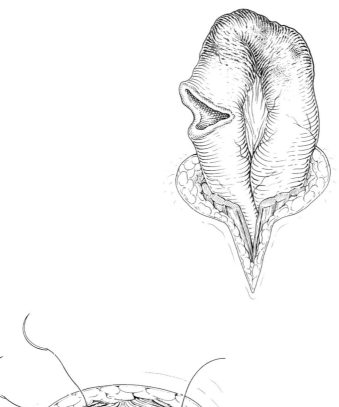

Figure 4-12.

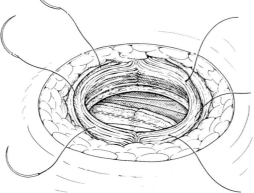

Figure 4-13.

Access and Abdominal Wall Closure. Occasionally, it is necessary to make a lateral incision through the skin and rectus muscle in order to gain full access to the ileum for safe closure (Fig. 4-12). When the stoma has been closed and the bowel replaced, the abdominal wall defect is closed using 0-0 Prolene sutures through the rectus and its sheath (Fig. 4-13) prior to skin closure.

Colostomy

End Colostomy

End colostomies are usually constructed during laparotomy. The precise location in the large intestine will depend on the operation being performed. Generally, an end colostomy site lies on the left side and must be made through the rectus muscle. There should be no tension on the bowel and the blood supply to the bowel must be good. The lumen of the colon should pursue a straight course from the stoma site along the bowel in order to facilitate colostomy irrigation (Fig. 4-14).

Once the site has been chosen and the integrity of the vascular supply via the marginal vessels ensured, the colon is divided using a linear staple cutter (PLC or GIA), which minimizes the potential for contamination, or divided between two Potts clamps. The abdominal trephine is sited (Fig. 4-14, inset) and made in the manner described previously (see Fig. 4-1), and the colon is delivered through the abdominal wall (Fig. 4-15A). The laparotomy wound is closed before the colostomy is sutured. It is rarely, if ever, necessary to apply sutures from the rectus sheath to the serosa of the colon. A series of interrupted mucocutaneous sutures are used to mature the stoma (Fig. 4-15B); some surgeons prefer nonabsorbable 3-0 or 4-0 Prolene sutures, whereas others prefer to use plain 3-0 catgut on a cutting needle so that future removal of sutures is unnecessary.

Loop Colostomy

Loop colostomies are performed much less frequently today than they were 10 to 15 years ago. It is generally agreed that defunction of a colonic end anastomosis is better achieved using a loop ileostomy than a loop colostomy. Loop ileostomy does not

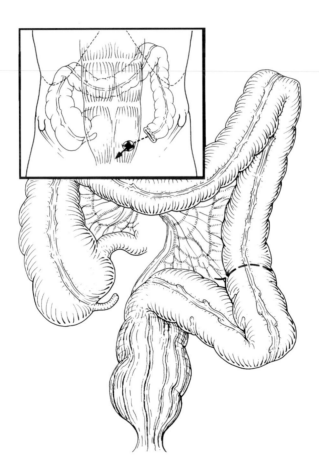

Figure 4-14. ▬▬▬▬

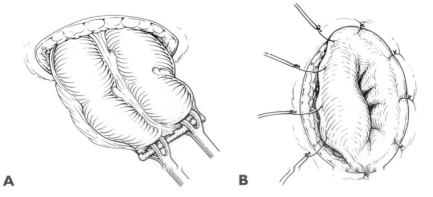

Figure 4-15. ▬▬▬▬ **A**   **B**

have the potential to impair the blood supply of the distal colon; it is easier to manage, odorless, and generally easier to close. Its disadvantage compared to loop colostomy is that there may be a long segment of colon containing considerable fecal residue between the stoma and the anastomosis; however, if a satisfactory preoperative bowel preparation has been achieved, this argument is no longer relevant.

A loop colostomy may be sited in the transverse colon on the left or the right side of the abdomen, or it may be placed in the sigmoid colon (Fig. 4-16). Loop colostomy is still an important method of managing acute large bowel obstruction (see Ch. 13). The loop of bowel may be delivered through the trephine used for stoma construction and a laparotomy avoided provided there are no other reasons for performing a laparotomy at the time. A trephine in the right rectus muscle is usually used for a right transverse colostomy, the left rectus muscle above the umbilicus for a left transverse colostomy, and the lower part of the left rectus muscle for a sigmoid loop colostomy.

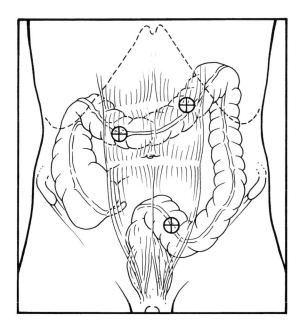

Figure 4-16.

The principles of constructing a loop colostomy are independent of its site in the colon. The construction of the loop colostomy is the same as that of loop ileostomy; however, the diameter of the trephine must be substantially greater than that for an ileostomy—it must be large enough to accommodate three fingers in patients with large bowel obstruction. Once the peritoneal cavity is opened, the loop of bowel to be used for decompression is selected. A window is constructed in the mesentery just underneath the bowel serosa and a nylon tape is threaded through the window to serve as a retractor. In the case of the transverse colostomy, the omentum will have to be dissected off the bowel and the transverse mesocolon to secure a mesenteric window (Fig. 4-17A). The colon is then incised longitudinally over the taenia and hemostasis is achieved (Fig. 4-17B). If there is any tension on the bowel, it is wise to replace the nylon tape with a piece of polyethylene tubing that is sutured to the skin as described earlier. Nonabsorbable 3-0 or 4-0 Prolene, or plain catgut, is then used to secure the mucocutaneous junction of the bowel and skin (Fig. 4-18).

Double-Barreled Colostomy

In certain circumstances, particularly in sigmoid volvulus, obstruction in the sigmoid, or occasionally in perforated diverticular disease, a double-barreled colostomy

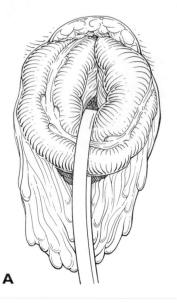
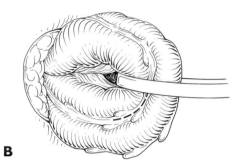

Figure 4-17. ▬▬▬▬▬   **A**   **B**

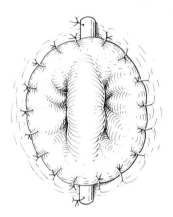

Figure 4-18. ▬▬▬▬▬

may be a useful procedure (see Chs. 11 and 13). In most cases, however, the sigmoid colon is not sufficiently mobile for this to be a feasible option.

The diseased segment of colon is resected through a laparotomy incision. The proximal and distal limbs, which are transected with a linear staple cutter or between two Potts clamps, must be completely mobilized (Fig. 4-19). The trephine is made in the rectus muscle as described earlier and must be of sufficient diameter to accommodate the two limbs of colon. The limbs of colon are delivered through the trephine to the skin surface. It is advisable to suture the adjacent limbs together, as this will secure hemostasis (Fig. 4-20A). The free portions of both limbs are left for mucocutaneous suture with absorbable plain catgut or nonabsorbable Prolene (Fig. 4-20B).

Closure

It is essential to verify that there is no obstruction distal to the loop colostomy and that any distal anastomosis is patent prior to closure. The distal bowel may be assessed by sigmoidoscopy, colonoscopy, and contrast radiography, and the anal sphincters tested digitally if there is any question of incontinence. A full mechanical bowel preparation is administered to clear the proximal colon and a rectal washout is performed to remove any residual fecal material beyond the stoma. Perioperative antibiotic cover is necessary and the operation is performed with the patient under general anesthesia.

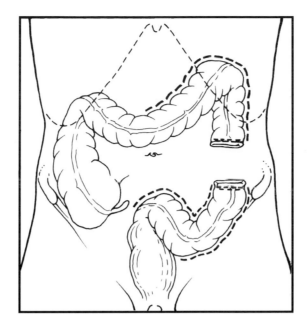

Figure 4-19.

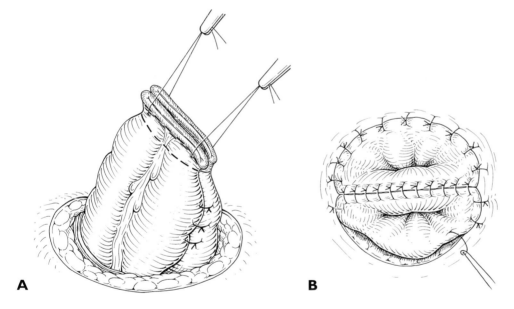

A   B

Figure 4-20.

A circumstomal incision is used to mobilize the loop of colon from the skin, sub-cutaneous tissue, and rectus muscle. It is essential to clear the colon from the rectus muscle and to enter the peritoneal cavity around the full circumference of the bowel before attempting closure (Fig. 4-21). Closure may be achieved with a single-layer extramucosal suture, single-layer full-thickness interrupted sutures (Fig. 4-22A), con-tinuous closure reinforced by interrupted seromuscular sutures, or stapling to con-struct a functional end-to-end anastomosis (Fig. 4-22B).

The techniques of closure are identical to those described for loop ileostomy. It may be necessary to resect the colostomy if there is extensive fibrosis around the stoma or if there has been any damage to the colon during mobilization (Fig. 4-23). Under these circumstances, the colostomy is resected in its entirety and an end-to-end colocolonic anastomosis is performed; alternatively, the antimesenteric surface of the colon is excised and closed as a long strictureplasty using a a single-layer or a two-layer technique. The principles are identical to those described for resection in ileostomy closure.

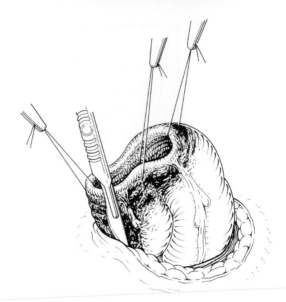

Figure 4-21.

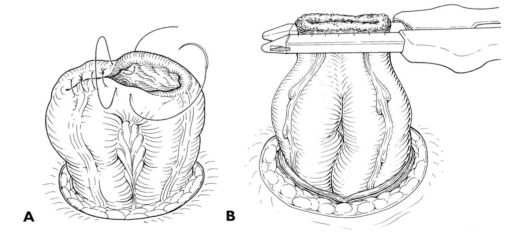

Figure 4-22.   **A**   **B**

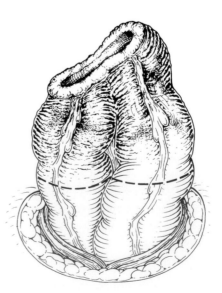

Figure 4-23.

Cecostomy and Appendicostomy

I do not recommend the use of cecostomy or appendicostomy as a means of decompression when other methods, such as loop ileostomy, are available. They will therefore not be described here.

Common Stoma Complications

Parastomal Hernia

Most parastomal hernias are due to a badly sited stoma, usually outside the rectus abdominus. The best means of managing such hernias is by resiting the stoma. Resiting operations almost always require a laparotomy. Although resiting has been described without laparotomy using extensive intraperitoneal mobilization, in our experience this practice is rarely feasible and usually does not provide a satisfactory result, as the bowel is distorted and is of insufficient length. Occasionally, despite optimal siting, a hernia may develop because of poor abdominal musculature, too wide an initial trephine, parastomal sepsis, ascites, or tumor recurrence. In such cases, if other previously optimal stoma sites have been rendered unsuitable by scarring, a local repair procedure may be attempted. Generally, however, local repair procedures give inferior results to that of laparotomy and resiting.

Resiting. The new stoma site must be marked preoperatively. Adequate mechanical bowel preparation is essential and perioperative antibiotic cover should be given. A peristomal incision is used to mobilize the stoma from the skin, subcutaneous tissues, abdominal wall musculature, and peritoneal cavity. A laparotomy incision is then made and the bowel is thoroughly mobilized (Fig. 4-24). If there is any doubt about the viability of the end of the bowel (i.e., potential ischemia or stenosis), inflammatory or distorted bowel should be resected. The bowel is divided by stapling or between Potts clamps. A trephine is made at the newly selected optimal stoma site, and must be through the rectus muscle. The technique is described earlier in this chapter; however, the rectus is usually not divided but merely split in the line of its fibers. Once the peritoneal cavity is opened, the transected bowel is then delivered through the trephine and sutured as previously described, preferably after laparotomy closure and repair of the defect in the abdominal wall left by the parastomal hernia, using 0-0 nylon (Fig. 4-25A & B). If there has been any gross contamination at the parastomal hernia repair site, the skin should not be closed; rather, it should be left open to granulate. In the absence of contamination, the previous stoma site may be closed with staples or sutures.

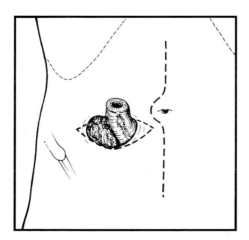

Figure 4-24.

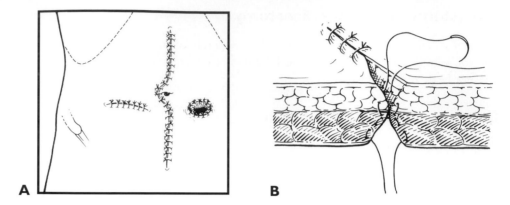

Figure 4-25.   **A**   **B**

Local Repair. If stoma resiting is not the optimum option and the stoma is placed through the rectus muscle, local repair may be feasible. Under these circumstances, a peristomal incision is made, and the bowel is thoroughly mobilized from the subcutaneous tissues, the abdominal wall musculature, and the peritoneal cavity. There may be adherent omentum in the peritoneal sac, which must be mobilized also (Fig. 4-26A). It is advisable where possible to remove any redundant peritoneal sac adjacent to the stoma, leaving healthy rectus sheath and muscle with a wide defect adjacent to the bowel. In our experience, it is then preferable to repair the muscular defect using interrupted nylon sutures, incorporating the rectus muscle (Fig. 4-26B). These sutures must not be tied until the optimum diameter of the abdominal wall orifice that will accommodate the bowel has been determined. Preferably, sutures are taken from either side of the bowel to repair the defect. There is a tendency to close the abdominal wall defect too efficiently; the enthusiasm for achieving a satisfactory hernia repair should be balanced against the risk of stenosis to the emerging bowel. A

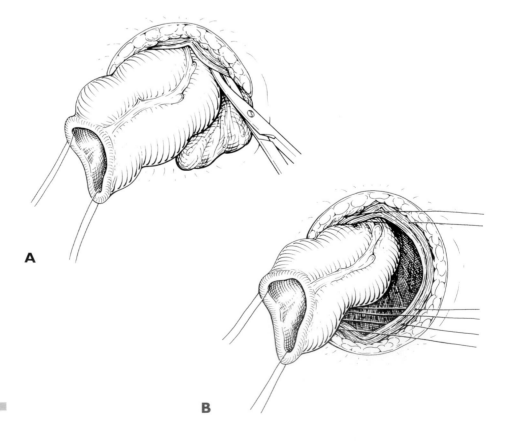

A

B

Figure 4-26.

finger placed in the bowel after the sutures have been tied will determine whether there is any stenosis; if the bowel is found to have been narrowed, one or two of the repair sutures adjacent to the bowel must be removed. It is preferable to place the knot in the nylon repair deep to the rectus sheath.

Occasionally, foreign material may be used to repair a defect in the abdominal wall. It is our practice to resist the use of foreign material because of the risk of infection, particularly when nonabsorbable mesh is placed adjacent to the colon. Absorbable meshes provide an occasional compromise; however, in our experience, with appropriate mobilization, mesh implants are rarely required.

If the defect in the abdominal wall is very extensive, it may be necessary to enlarge the parastomal incision medially or laterally to gain better access to the abdominal wall. We recognize that this technique is sometimes necessary, but avoid using it, particularly in repairing a paraileostomy hernia, because a lateral scar adjacent to the mucocutaneous junction may make stoma management difficult.

Stomal Prolapse

A stomal prolapse is much more common in a loop colostomy than an end colostomy. It is also much more common in a loop colostomy compared with a loop ileostomy, and it is rare in an end ileostomy. A prolapsed stoma is usually due to a wide defect in the abdominal wall. It is also associated with poor fixation of the bowel to abdominal wall structures and to excessive peristalsis. Stomal prolapse is unsightly, may bleed, and may pose difficulty with applying stoma bags. If it occurs in a temporary loop stoma (Fig. 4-27), it is best managed by closing the loop colostomy or ileostomy as already described. If closure of the loop stoma is not feasible, it might be worth considering dividing the bowel, oversewing the distal portion of the bowel,

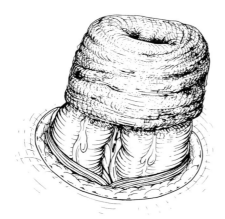

Figure 4-27.

and constructing an end stoma. Under these circumstances, it is probably wiser to construct an entirely new trephine for an end colostomy or ileostomy, with a second new trephine for a mucous fistula; if so, the mesentery will have to be widely divided. Alternatively, the distal end of the bowel may be closed with staples or sutures (Fig. 4-28A & B). Prolapse occurring in an end stoma almost always signifies too large a defect in the abdominal wall; hence, the optimum management is to resite the stoma and construct a much smaller abdominal wall defect in a new site (Fig. 4-29A & B). The original abdominal wall defect can then be closed as described for repair of parastomal hernia.

Particular attention may need to be paid to the fixation sutures between the serosa of the bowel and the rectus sheath when constructing the new stoma. During resiting of a prolapsed stoma, it may be necessary to resect redundant bowel, particularly

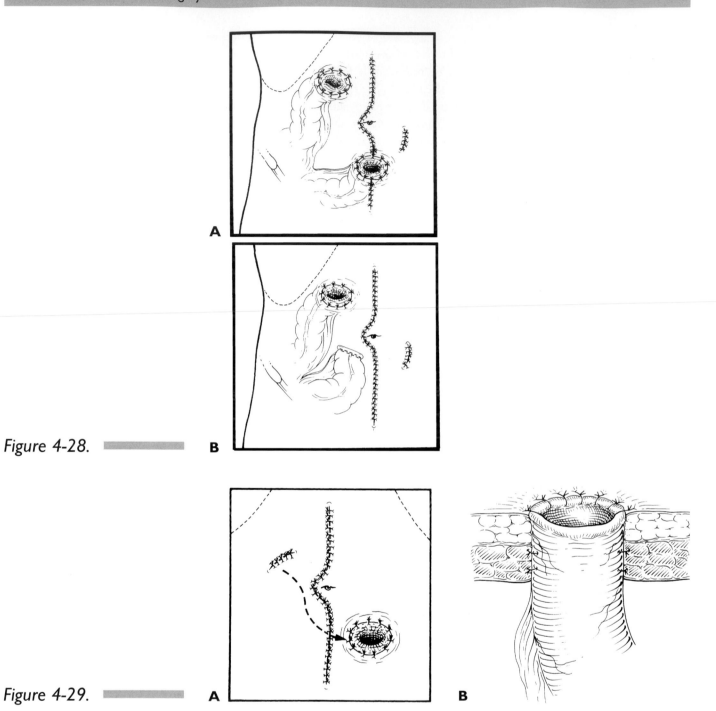

Figure 4-28.

Figure 4-29.

colon, to provide a relatively narrow-caliber segment of bowel that will be admitted through the narrow new abdominal wall trephine (Fig. 4-30).

Recurrent Disease in the Stoma

Rarely, malignancy may recur in a colostomy. In such cases, surgical treatment is generally only palliative.

Crohn's disease may recur just proximal to the abdominal wall in patients treated with ileostomy, but recurrence rates are generally low. Patients often present with bleeding, distortion of the stoma, ulceration on its surface, or obstructive symptoms. Treatment is by resection of the terminal ileum and construction of a new ileostomy,

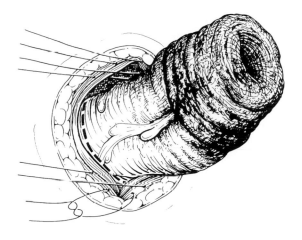

Figure 4-30.

which usually can be brought out through the old defect in the abdominal wall (Fig. 4-31). If colostomy has been used to treat Crohn's disease or ulcerative colitis, recurrent disease may present with bleeding, liquid effluent, anorexia, weight loss, and protein-calorie malnutrition. Under these circumstances, the remaining colon is usually badly diseased and resection with an end ileostomy is required.

Stoma Retraction

Stoma retraction is only a problem with end or loop ileostomies, because colostomies are generally flush and do not need to be everted. A retracted, flush ileostomy is usually associated with leakage, excoriation, and difficulty in applying the base plates;

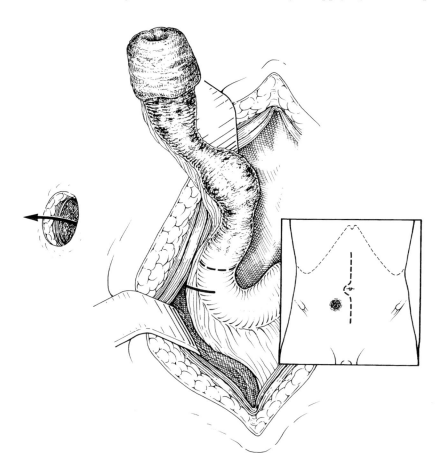

Figure 4-31.

hence, some sort of revision is usually necessary. Retraction is usually due to instability owing to excessive laxity between the abdominal wall and the ileum. This may be the result of a badly sited stoma (i.e., outside the rectus abdominis), a wide defect in the abdominal wall, excessive intestinal peristalsis, or inadequate fixation of the bowel to parietal structures. Simple stapling or suturing may be adequate treatment if the trephine is through the rectus muscle and is not too wide. If, on the other hand, the stoma is badly placed, it is preferable to resite the stoma through the rectus muscle and to fix the ileum to the parietal structures. Occasionally, reconstruction may be a problem with loop ileostomy, causing spillover of intestinal contents into the distal limb of the ileum and thus incomplete fecal diversion. Inadequate diversion may be dangerous if the loop stoma was constructed to protect a distal anastomosis or an anastomosis that had already leaked, or to manage distal intestinal fistula. Retraction of a loop ileostomy may be managed by closing the loop ileostomy if it is safe to do so; if it is not, it may be necessary to convert the loop ileostomy to an end ileostomy, oversewing the distal limb, and constructing a mucous fistula. The long-term results of local revision procedures for retraction are generally poor.

Staple Fixation. Staple fixation is a simple method of controlling a flush stoma. It is generally suitable only for an end ileostomy. Staple fixation of a loop ileostomy necessitates resection when the loop ileostomy is to be closed, hence it is generally used only if the loop is serving long-term function.

The operation does not require general anesthesia and may be undertaken using intravenous analgesia and sedation. The ileostomy must first be everted again. This can be accomplished by grasping three quadrants of the bowel with Allis forceps to deliver the stoma so that its apex is approximately 2 cm in length from the skin surface. Failure to achieve this degree of eversion foretells that the technique will be unsuccessful and that some other method will have to be used to stabilize the stoma. Once a good length of ileostomy bud has been everted, the two limbs of bowel are stapled together using a linear stapler without a cutter (PLC or GIA). It is important to avoid stapling the blood supply to the ileum, hence the mesentery should be avoided. Three rows of staples can generally be applied (Fig. 4-32). Although the

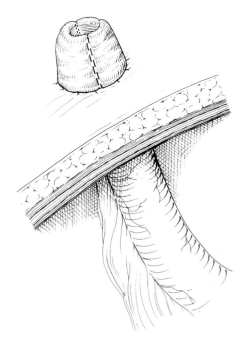

Figure 4-32.

functional outcome is quite satisfactory, the end result often is rather unesthetic; however, the staples darken with time and eventually are hardly visible at all.

Sutured Revision. A circumstomal incision is made, the ileostomy is thoroughly mobilized from the subcutaneous tissue, rectus muscle, and rectus sheath, and the peritoneal cavity is entered. A sufficient length of ileum is delivered for eversion (Fig. 4-33). A series of interrupted sutures are placed between the rectus sheath and the serosa of the bowel. The ileostomy is then everted and sutured to the skin in the usual manner. Any redundant ileum will need to be resected.

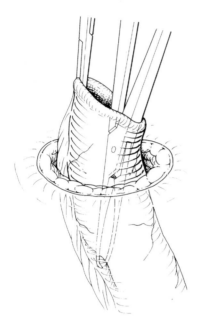

Figure 4-33.

Peristomal Varices

Portosystemic communications may develop between systemic veins of the abdominal wall and portal veins of the gut. Peristomal varices frequently occur in portal hypertension and either underlying liver disease or portal vein thrombosis; they may be associated with ascites and impaired liver function. Owing to the higher incidence of liver disease associated with inflammatory bowel disorders, peristomal varices are more common complicating an ileostomy for colitis than after construction of a colostomy. Bleeding may be catastrophic or intermittent and repeated. Control of hemorrhage may be achieved by suture ligation of the bleeding varix; alternatively, the entire stoma may be mobilized from the skin using a circumstomal incision and the free edge of the ileum oversewn and a series of new interrupted mucocutaneous sutures applied (Fig. 4-34).

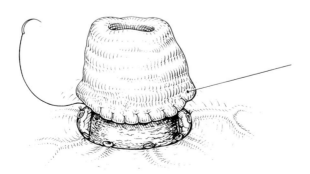

Figure 4-34.

Peristomal Abscess

An abscess may develop early after stoma construction. Making a small incision at the mucocutaneous junction to allow drainage into the stoma appliance is usually sufficient treatment. This technique avoids distortion of the peristomal skin, which could lead to difficulty with affixing future appliances. Occasionally, a catheter may be inserted to facilitate drainage (Fig. 4-35).

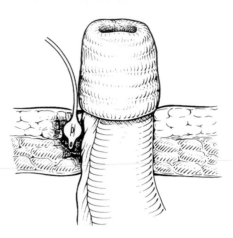

Figure 4-35.

Late peristomal sepsis is due to either an infection around a foreign body, such as a nonabsorbable suture knot or a mesh implant, in which case the foreign material should be removed and the sepsis drained (Fig. 4-36), or recurrent bowel disease, particularly Crohn's disease, in which case resection and reconstruction of a new stoma will be necessary (see Fig. 4-31).

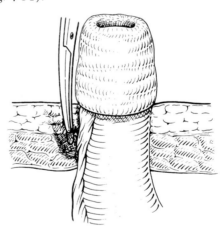

Figure 4-36.

Stomal Ischemia

Acute ischemia is more common following end colostomy than end ileostomy. It may resolve spontaneously, may progress to infarction, or may result in late stenosis. Infarction requires urgent laparotomy and resection of the infarcted bowel, with formation of a new stoma (Fig. 4-37A & B). Ischemia of a loop stoma suggests that the abdominal wall trephine is too tight; hence, treatment should be directed at relieving the obstruction in the abdominal wall. Early abdominal wall decompression usually results in total resolution. Late stenosis may be due to a previous ischemic episode that only partially resolved, and may be managed by gentle dilatation (Fig. 4-38), but if it persists, the end of the bowel should be resected and a new stoma constructed, usually in the same site (see Fig. 4-31).

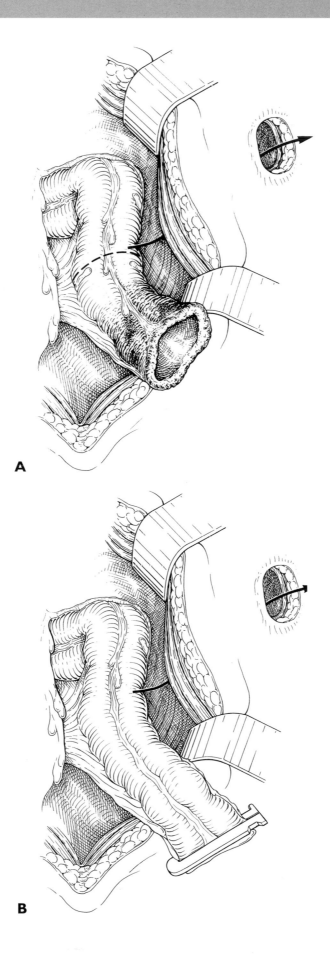

A

B

Figure 4-37.

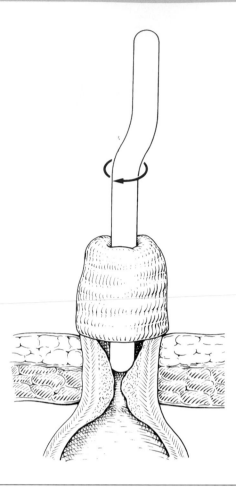

Figure 4-38.

Editorial Commentaries

End Ileostomy. I agree completely with Professor Keighley that stapling the ends of the ileum in preparation for end ileostomy is important, because it eliminates the possibility of contamination of the abdominal cavity and, more important, of the subcutaneous tissues at the time of ileostomy construction. I agree, too, that a disc of skin and fat should be removed (we do that in a block) down to the fascia. I think that Professor Keighley's method of determining the placement of the stoma is correct, as are his descriptions of the cruciate incision and splitting of the muscle fibers.

The end ileostomy should extend 5 to 6 cm above the level of the skin so as to allow for the creation of a stoma 2 to 3 cm in length when it is matured. The trephine at the stoma site should be the width of two fingers—three if the surgeon's fingers are small. I do not suture the stoma to the rectal sheath or to the peritoneum, and I only rarely close the lateral gutter. I agree that the midline incision should be closed before the stoma is matured. I use chromic or Vicryl sutures to mature the ostomy. If the patient is immunocompromised, however, I use permanent sutures to construct the stoma. I have had several quite difficult experiences with patients who were receiving cyclosporine, azathioprine, or more than 80 mg of prednisone per day.

Loop Ileostomy. A few comments regarding loop ileostomy. If the colon is in place and a loop ileostomy is constructed to divert the fecal stream from the colon, I choose to pull a loop of ileum about 15 to 20 cm proximal to the ileocecal valve to facilitate simple mobilization and closure of the loop when intestinal continuity is reestablished. The construction techniques described, especially the use of a tape to pull the loop through, are ones I use too. In the extremely obese patient, a loop ileostomy is often easier to construct and has a better blood supply than an end ileostomy.

At the Mayo Clinic closure of the loop ileostomy is done in either of two ways: The ileostomy is folded over and closed, or all extraperitoneal bowel is excised and an ileoileostomy is performed. I usually excise the bowel and perform an anastomosis. I do not use a stapler to close the ileostomy; the use of staples where the bowel is abnormally thick (as in bowel proximal to the loop stoma) or abnormally thin (as in bowel distal to the loop stoma) is less than reliable.

If a stoma site has to be constructed in an emergency and an enterostomal therapist is not available to determine the optimal site preoperatively, the stoma should be placed so as to allow for a good fit for the stoma device: close to the midline and approximately 3 to 4 cm below the umbilicus. Avoiding the anterosuperior iliac spine is extremely important. The surgeon can be assured of proper placement by drawing a line between the umbilicus and the anterosuperior iliac spine and placing the stoma close to the umbilicus along that line. All incisions in the abdominal wall are closed with interrupted sutures of Vicryl or running doubled No. 1 PDS. Finally, if the epigastric artery and vein are visible near the stoma site, they are ligated.

Colostomy. I agree with Professor Keighley's construction techniques completely. We construct the stoma to appear as a rosebud, that is, slightly elevated and everted (approximately 0.5 cm). With regard to loop colostomy, I also agree entirely that a loop ileostomy is better for diversion of the fecal stream than a loop colostomy. The loop construction technique described is the same as mine.

Cecostomy. I do not generally perform cecostomies; however, I do use a tube cecostomy in one situation, and that is for colonic decompression in the patient with Ogilvie syndrome whose colon will not stay decompressed despite multiple endoscopies. After a small midline incision is made, the cecum anterior cecal tinea is identified and a large, mushroom-tipped catheter is placed, with a portion of the omentum wrapped around it. The tube should be placed in the right lower quadrant about where an appendectomy incision might lie. I agree that appendicostomy is rarely indicated.

Double-Barreled Colostomy. I agree entirely with the technique and the indications described. Sometimes, however, I will separate the stomas, placing the mucous fistula on the left side well below the colostomy site, or alter-

(Continues)

natively, pulling the stapled end of the mucous fistula through with the proximal colostomy stoma and suturing the end of it to a portion of the skin defect. This is kind of a neat trick!

Stomal Herniation. Nearly all peristomal hernias, prolapses, and retractions require resiting. Local repairs can be performed if the original siting was correct, but usually the results are inferior. I, too, resist the use of mesh for stoma repair.

Peristomal Varices. My experiences with peristomal varices have been horrible. Thus, to avoid the possibility that stomal varices will form, I perform ileoanal anastomosis, if at all possible, in all patients with sclerosing cholangitis who require a colectomy.

Final Comments. A hint on how to manage an ischemic stoma: At the bedside, take a test tube, lubricate it, and slip it into the stoma. By shining a flashlight down the test tube, you can pinpoint the level of ischemia precisely.

John H. Pemberton

Commentary was made earlier with respect to the desiderata of constructing the stoma. This is true whether one is dealing with an ileostomy, jejunostomy, colostomy, or urinary conduit. With respect to the technical aspects of making or fashioning the stoma aperture, there is substantial agreement with the technique described by Dr. Keighley and as it was described originally by Rupert B. Turnbull, Jr. Because it is possible to have occult injury to the epigastric vessels, I place a large Kelly clamp through the trephine defect and raise it from the medial aspect while observing the internal ileostomy aperture for excessive bleeding. Relaxation on the instrument is allowed so any occult bleeders will be recognized and can be sutured from the internal abdominal aspect. It is important to release the chordee effect of the tethering of the terminal ileum and ileostomy by the final branches of the vasa recti. Otherwise, a curved spout to the ileostomy occurs. The ileum is delivered through the abdominal aperture for a distance of 3 cm in a fashion so that the mesentery lies in a cephalad direction. The internal mesenteric defect is obliterated using the Turnbull technique. This consists of placement of sutures from the cephalad end of the ileostomy aperture extending in a cephalad direction. Sutures of O chromic are placed between the peritoneum of the anterior abdominal wall approximately 1 inch to the right of the incision and sutured to the cut end of the small bowel mesentery. This is carried cephalad to the falciform ligament, which is then included in the closure to the apical component of the mesentery of the small bowel. In this way, the right side of the abdomen is separated from the left side of the abdomen by the small bowel mesentery and it makes it impossible for a volvulus of the small bowel to occur.

In certain circumstances, it is impossible to occlude this defect. In that case, it is always useful to place two or three sutures between the internal ileostomy aperture and the mesentery of the end of the ileum to help support this structure. Specifically, we do not use sutures between the serosa of the bowel and the internal ileostomy aperture, nor do we place them between the serosa of the bowel and the anterior sheath. Both practices can lead to development of early fistula from the ileostomy—a complication that is particularly difficult to treat. Primary maturation of the stoma is carried out in all cases, but not until the abdomen itself is closed and the wound and incision quarantined. Interrupted sutures of 30 chromic are placed between the cut end of the small intestine and the subcuticular layer of skin. In this way, the risk of implantation of islands of ileal mucosa, which could cause secretion and premature separation of the stoma plate from the skin, is avoided. The practice of placing a suture through the cut end of the small bowel, then to the serosa of the ileum at the level of the skin, and then to the skin itself, is mentioned only to condemn this practice as this again will run the risk of fistula.

Loop ileostomy or Turnbull ileostomy is described by Dr. Keighley on page 65. In essence, this is very similar to the end ileostomy in that the stoma aperture is identical. The loop is brought through the abdominal wall in such a way that the functioning end is clearly demarcated with a characterizing suture and the nonfunctioning end with a different color suture. We use a blue Vicryl suture for the proximal end, and approximately 1 cm from this on the apex of the loop a brown chromic catgut for the distal end as markers. In this way, it renders it impossible to make the enterotomy on the "wrong" side. For loop ileostomies placed in continuity above an anastomosis, we prefer the proximal functioning end to be cephalad in cases protecting ileorectal anastomosis or ileo-pouch anal anastomosis. In most other cases, the orientation is reversed through 180 degrees (e.g., for loop ileostomy proximal to an ileo-transverse colon anastomosis as this tends to be the way in which the bowel wants to lie). A plastic rod is used to support the loop. Primary maturation is carried out as for the end ileostomy. The exception to this, of course, is that an enterotomy is made on the nonfunctioning side of the stoma approximately one-half to 1 cm from the skin edge. If this is placed too flush, then mucous from the downstream end can escape at skin level, undermine the skin barrier, and cause premature separation of the faceplate. Thus, it is useful to have a small amount of eversion even on the distal nonfunctioning side.

In certain circumstances a loop end ileostomy is desirable. This is usually for patients who are obese, who require permanent stoma, but in whom an end ileostomy may become ischemic due to undercutting of the mesentery. In such cases a loop end ileostomy can be used to advantage. Our closure of the loop ileostomy has no substantial difference from that described by Dr. Keighley.

In most cases, when constructing an end colostomy, we will generally use an elliptical-shaped excision of skin located in the left lower quadrant. The stoma site is chosen with the same considerations as for an ileostomy. In the majority of cases, closure of the mesenteric defect is not used. Although volvulus is a theoretic possibility, this is rare.

(Continues)

Loop colostomies are generally placed in the left or right upper abdomen through a transrectus splitting rather than a cutting incision. The reputation of loop colostomy is poor. Not only is it more difficult for a patient to look after (odor, liquid discharge, leakage, prolapse) but also there is an extraordinarily high rate of subsequent hernia at the closure site.

Cecostomy is an extremely uncommon operation. We confine this operation to patients who have a simple stab wound of the cecum without contamination and for high-risk patients who have cecal volvulus without compromise of the vascularity of the cecum.

With respect to closure of the loop colostomy, the most significant difference to that described is the avoidance of any stapled instruments for this procedure.

The options available to the patient in the management of parastomal hernia include local repair or local repair with relocation of the stoma. Local repair is generally used by placing a circumferential incision around the mucocutaneous junction of the stoma. A tennis racquet-type extension is then carried out laterally for a distance of 3 or 4 inches. The dissection is carried down to expose the hernial sac, which is then excised in toto. It is useful to use cutting and coagulating cautery for this part of the procedure. Upon exposing the edges of the defect, one can then proceed to use one of several alternatives. In certain cases, it is possible to identify the fact that the stoma is actually coming through that portion of the abdominal wall peripheral to the rectus abdominus muscle. It is also quite feasible in these cases to fashion a new aperture through the belly of the rectus abdominus muscle and reroute the colon or ileum through this particular section. In this way, the primary defect in the hernia (i.e., fascia) is relatively easy to close using interrupted No. 1 Prolene sutures in a figure-of-eight fashion. In the event that this aperture is too large to close, then mesh repair is used (Gortex). The stoma is then brought out through the same ostomy aperture. Extensive hemostasis with copious irrigation is carried out. A subcutaneous drain is placed and brought out through a stab incision peripheral to the main suture line and placed to suction. Antibiotics are continued for 2 to 3 days. The stoma is matured primarily.

In the case of relocation of the stoma, this is usually done with laparotomy. In such cases, it is usual to require both a type of incision mentioned above for local repair of parastomal hernia as well as a midline abdominal incision. This helps facilitate dissection of adhesions to allow for the safe transposition of the bowel across to the newly marked location. This is a formidable operation and one that the patient understands is of greater magnitude. It is implied as well that this operation is reserved for patients who are generally considered fit for anesthesia. In our hands, reoperation rates for these two procedures are somewhat different (20 percent for relocation and 30 percent for local repair). However, the detectable rate of recurrence of the hernia is 40 percent for relocated ostomies and 50 percent for local repair.

In certain circumstances the patient is encountered who has had multiple repairs of parastomal hernias. In such cases, the tissue used in the fascial repair is of such poor quality that predictably a further hernia will form. In such cases, mesh repair is used and our preference is to use Gortex mesh making a trephine through the center of the mesh and bringing the stoma through this. To prevent sliding hernia, we will place a number of sutures between the mesentery of the bowel and the cut edge of the trephine in the mesh itself.

The ideal treatment to manage the prolapsed stoma is that of simple closure of the stoma. In the event this is not feasible (e.g., radiation rectovaginal fistula), then a range of procedures is available depending on the relative risks and magnitude of each of these procedures to the patient concerned. For the extraordinarily high-risk patient who can tolerate anesthesia poorly, perhaps the best alternative is that of "simple" resection of the prolapse and tightening of the enlarged fascial defect through which the colostomy is passing. As an alternative, it is possible to reduce the prolapse and transect the colon, stapling the distal end and dropping it back inside (this distal end is the one that usually prolapses). The proximal colon is then brought out through the aperture, attempting to eradicate any proximal redundancy of the colon.

The third alternative, and perhaps the best, is that of closing the colostomy and making a loop ileostomy through a previously marked ileostomy site in the right lower quadrant. The main colostomy fascial defect is then closed and a new ileostomy is created. This has been my preferred procedure for patients who can tolerate a laparotomy of the magnitude required to allow relocation.

I have no substantial comments to add to those of Dr. Keighley on the management of recurrent disease and intestinal stoma.

With respect to stapled fixation of retracted ileostomy, I find no role for the use of staples in this particular situation. For ileostomy recession, my preferred approach has been that of circumferential detachment of the ileostomy from the skin itself with mobilization into the peritoneal cavity. The ileostomy is then withdrawn out to a suitable length and fixation of the mesentery is carried out with several sutures between the cephalad component of the mesentery at the fascial level. Two or three sutures of 20-Vicryl are used in this fashion. A two-directional myotomy to expose the subserosa musculature or submucosa itself is then performed. This will produce adherence upon itself to essentially fix this ileum and prevent ileostomy recession from occurring again.

For the patient who develops a late recession of the stoma associated with ulcerative colitis surgery in the remote past, then there is a place for doing the Turnbull-Crile procedure of "mucosal grafted" ileostomy. There has never been a single case reported of recurrence of recession after this procedure. The disadvantages are that it is time consuming and risks enterotomy of the small bowel, hence the rarity with which it is used.

Our preferred technique for dealing with parastomal varices is to detach the mucocutaneous junction of the stoma and suture ligate any varices observed. The stoma is then rematured. Although rebleeding is the rule rather than the exception, this may not occur for a year or two.

(Continues)

While an assistant holds the proctoscope, the surgeon grasps the mucosa above the hemorrhoids and pulls the mucosa through the ring of the ligator. The ligator is advanced upward and two rubber bands are delivered from the cylinder of the ligator by squeezing the applicator handle, which advances the outer cylinder carrying the rubber bands over the inner cylinder (Fig. 5-6C). The patient should be forewarned that the applicator makes a noise and that there may be transient discomfort as the bands are applied. Severe pain, however, is caused by the rubber band being applied too low; should such an event occur, the rubber band should be removed as soon as possible with a Beever cataract knife. Two or three hemorrhoids may be treated during one procedure. Additional treatments, if necessary, may be performed after a 2- to 4-week interval. We have recently begun using the suction band applicator; the technique is very quick and it does not always require an assistant.

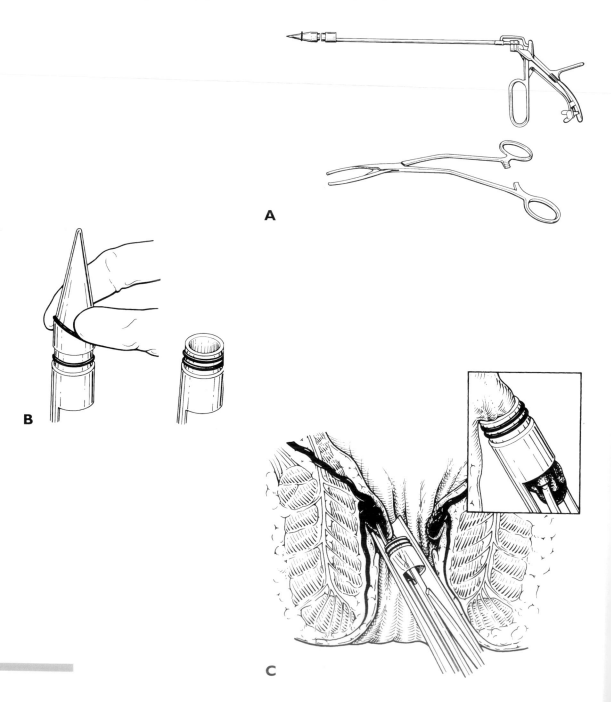

Figure 5-6.

Cryotherapy

Cryotherapy freezes tissue rapidly, resulting in thrombosis of submucosal veins. The applications of liquid nitrogen or nitrous oxide should be made well above the hemorrhoid if severe pain is to be avoided (Fig. 5-7). The drawbacks of cryotherapy are that excessive mucous discharge is common and the extent of tissue damage is quite considerable.

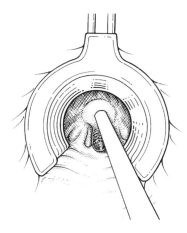

Figure 5-7.

Day-Case Management with Anal Dilatation

Anal dilatation may be performed on an awake patient using an inferior pudendal nerve block and perianal infiltration; however, most surgeons continue to use general anesthesia for the procedure. With the patient in the lateral recumbent position (Fig. 5-8), a manual and a sigmoidoscopic examination are performed. The anal canal is very gently stretched, first with one, then with two fingers using a sweeping movement around the anal canal (Fig. 5-9A). A third finger is then inserted and the sweeping motion is repeated. The three fingers are left in situ for at least 2 minutes (Fig. 5-9B). Finally, if anal pathology is severe and if there is no history of incontinence or severe obstetric trauma, a four-finger dilatation may be performed, thereby stretching the internal anal sphincter and hemorrhoid. Anal dilatation should be used cautiously in women, particularly if there is a history of obstetric damage.

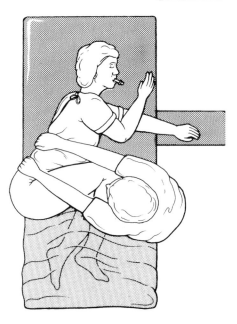

Figure 5-8.

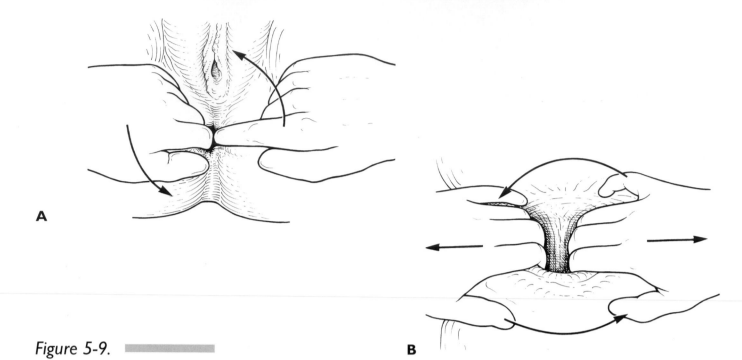

A

B

Figure 5-9.

Combined Anal Dilatation and Outpatient Techniques

In patients with mucosal laxity and internal sphincter overactivity, there is a real advantage to the combined use of a topical treatment, such as rubber band ligation, and gentle anal dilatation.

Open Hemorrhoidectomy

The traditional method of treating hemorrhoids in the United Kingdom is by the time-honored technique of Milligan-Morgan hemorrhoidectomy. The principles of the operation are to excise the skin tag and the internal hemorrhoid from the internal anal sphincter leaving the wounds open to freely drain, complete healing occurring by secondary intention. The operation is often performed with a gentle anal dilatation.

The sites of hemorrhoidal hypertrophy are carefully identified together with any associated skin tags. Generally, there is a large left lateral hemorrhoid at 3 o'clock, a large right posterior hemorrhoid at 7 o'clock, and a moderate-size right posterior hemorrhoid at 11 o'clock. However, secondary hemorrhoids may occur between the sites of primary hemorrhoids. In many patients only two hemorrhoids predominate.

Preoperative bowel preparation, generally using a disposable enema, is always advised. The patient is placed in the lithotomy position with the legs in stirrups. The operation is usually performed with general anesthesia, although regional anesthesia, particularly caudal anesthesia with inferior pudendal nerve block and local infiltration, is increasingly used (Fig. 5-10A). Perioperative antibiotic cover is generally not prescribed. Even if the operation is being performed under general anesthetic, it is almost always advisable to infiltrate the perianal skin around the skin tag in the submucosal region of the hemorrhoid and the intersphincteric plane with a combination of local anesthetic and a weak epinephrine solution. This practice reduces the amount of intraoperative bleeding as well as decreases the analgesic requirements in the first 4 to 6 hours.

The operation commences by grasping the skin tag superficial to the left lateral hemorrhoid (Fig. 5-10B). A second tissue forceps is applied to the hemorrhoidal tissue itself (Fig. 5-10C). A V-shaped segment of skin with the apex lying peripherally is cut with a pair of scissors around the margin of the skin tag (Fig. 5-10D). This incision usually exposes the distal margin of the internal anal sphincter once the skin has been divided (Fig. 5-10E). The hemorrhoidal tissue is then gently dissected from the internal anal sphincter in a cephalad direction. Whenever possible the dissection should lie close to the internal sphincter so that all the hemorrhoidal tissue is excised (Fig. 5-10F). The mucosa on either side of the hemorrhoid is also divided, leaving the proximal pedicle, which is generally secured by fixation (Fig. 5-10G). Two curved artery forceps are applied across the pedicle, which is divided and the hemorrhoid discarded (Fig. 5-10H). 2-0 chromic catgut or 2-0 Vicryl transfixation sutures are used to ligate the pedicle. The transfixation sutures are left long and clipped (Fig. 5-10I). Any bleeding from the perianal skin or from submucosal veins is secured by diathermy. Once complete hemostasis is achieved the right lateral and finally the right anterior hemorrhoid are excised in an identical manner. The traditional method of hemorrhoidectomy involves grasping the tissue forceps in the left hand with the left index finger extended for the left lateral hemorrhoid (Fig. 5-10D); dissection of the right lateral hemorrhoid is performed with the left hand holding the hemorrhoidal tissue with the right hand and the left index finger extended. Although this practice facilitates dissection of the hemorrhoid, it is not necessary. Many surgeons today prefer to use an intra-anal speculum, which gives better exposure of the anal canal and leaves both hands free to perform the operation.

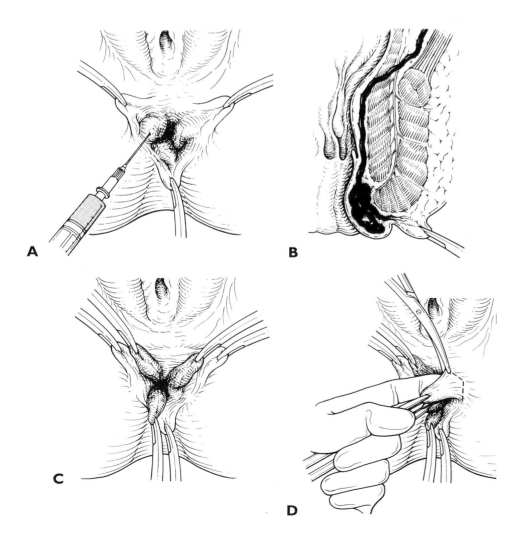

A

B

C

D

Figure 5-10.

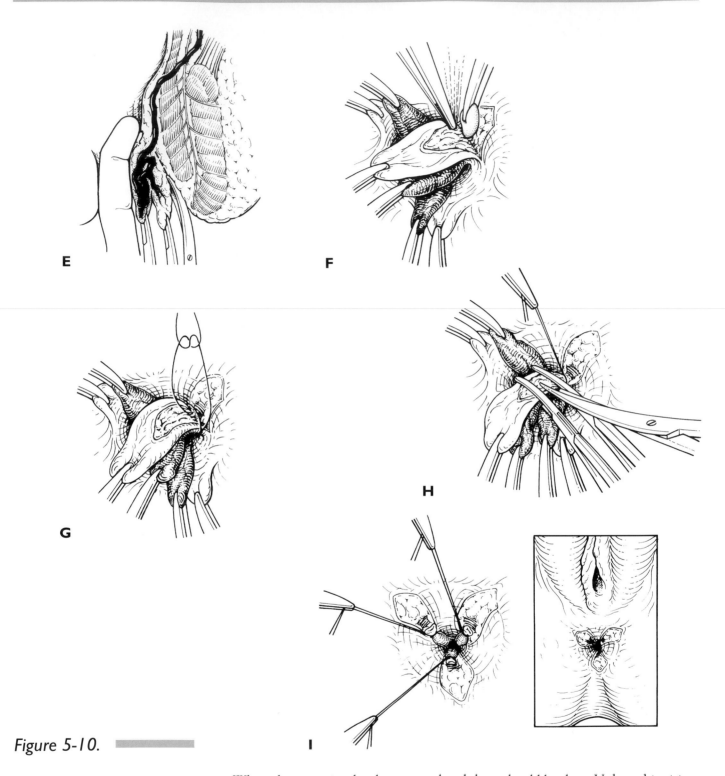

Figure 5-10.

When the operation has been completed there should be three V-shaped incisions at the site of the primary hemorrhoids, with three complete skin bridges between the incisions (Fig. 5-10I, inset). No attempt is made to close these defects; indeed, the rationale of the operation is to leave them open so that if there should be any reactionary hemorrhage blood can discharge freely through the open wounds, thereby avoiding a hematoma. The patient should be mobilized on the first postoperative day and started on a mild bulking agent and possibly an osmotic preparation to keep the stool soft. Most patients are discharged on the second or third postoperative day.

Closed Hemorrhoidectomy

The philosophy of closed hemorrhoidectomy is altogether different from that of the open technique. The aim of this operation is to excise all the hemorrhoidal tissue and the skin tag and to primarily close the defect in the anorectum.

A disposable enema is given on the day of the operation. No perioperative antibiotic cover is prescribed and the patient usually has a general anesthetic. The operation is usually performed with the patient in the prone jackknife position (Fig. 5-11). The position of the patient is crucial: 45 degrees of flexion of the hips with a steep head-down tilt will provide optimum exposure of the anorectum. The buttocks are strapped apart. The use of infiltration of epinephrine and a local anesthetic solution (approximately 15 ml at each site) is an integral part of the procedure, as the infiltration displays the hemorrhoidal tissue, lifts the mucosa from the internal anal sphincter, and displays the anatomy (Fig. 5-12). Although the operation may be feasible under local anesthetic, it is usually performed with general anesthesia owing to the degree of anal dilatation necessary.

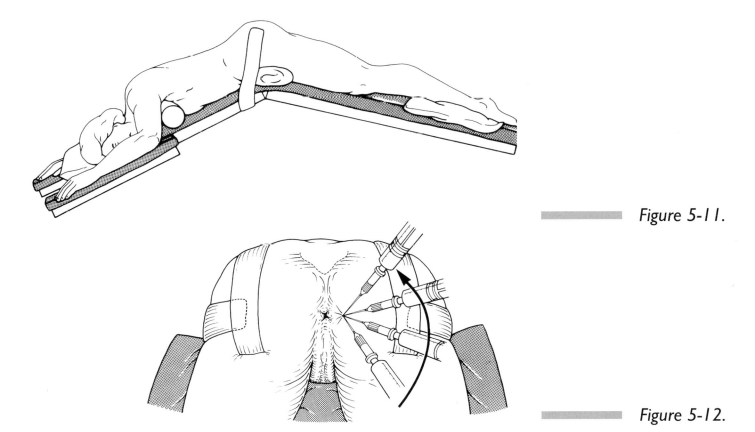

Figure 5-11.

Figure 5-12.

A large Pratt retractor is used to locate the hemorrhoids (Fig. 5-13A), while a Fauster anoscope (Fig. 5-13B) acts as an anal dilator and thoroughly exposes the anorectum. The skin tag is grasped with tissue forceps and is excised with a pair of curved Mayo scissors directed inward toward the anal canal (Fig. 5-14A), exposing the internal anal sphincter. Continued division with the scissors inside the anal canal allows excision of most of the hemorrhoidal tissue such that the apex of the hemorrhoid is completely divided. In this technique no attempt is made to transfix the pedicle of the hemorrhoid. The width of skin and mucosa within the anal canal that is divided should be fairly narrow to facilitate primary closure, but wide enough to allow adequate clearance of hemorrhoidal tissue (Fig. 5-14B). Because some residual hemorrhoidal tissue may remain the mucosa inside the anal canal is lifted upward with a pair of tissue forceps to expose any residual hemorrhoidal tissue, which can be secondarily excised after the primary excision has been completed (Fig. 5-14C). This maneuver is performed on either side of the mucosal defect, thus completing the hemorrhoidectomy. Following meticulous hemostasis, the defect is closed (Fig. 5-14D). We prefer to use 3-0 catgut on a 25-mm round-bodied needle. The apical stitch is crucial because it must encompass the divided mucosa, any residual hemorrhoidal tissue at the apex, and the circular muscular wall of the anorectum. A continuous locking suture is then used to close the mucosa of the anal canal. Finally, the retractor is then gently withdrawn and the skin defect is sutured. We return toward the anal canal and tie the suture at the point where it can be buried under the mucosa so that it does not cause discomfort when the patient sits down after the operation. The identical technique is repeated for all three hemorrhoidal sites. At the end of the operation the Pratt retractor is reinserted to check that there is complete hemostasis. The postoperative regimen is as previously described for the Milligan-Morgan open procedure. Most patients can be discharged on the first or second postoperative day.

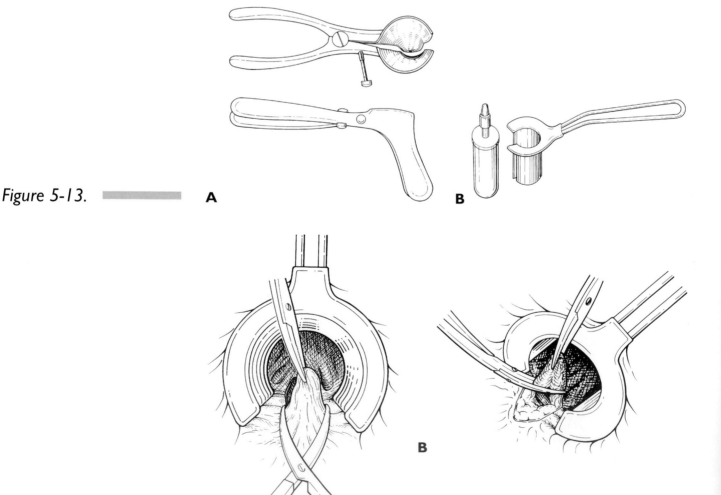

Figure 5-13. ▬▬▬ **A**   **B**

Figure 5-14. ▬▬▬ **A**

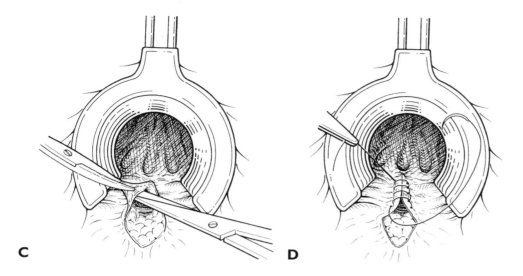

C   **D**   *Figure 5-14.*

Editorial Commentaries

Hemorrhoidal symptoms consist of bloody mucous discharge, frank bleeding fullness, and problems of anal hygiene. Hemorrhoids *do not* hurt; if the patient complains of anal pain, a fissure is likely present.

For patients complaining of these symptoms but with no prolapse (i.e., with first- or second-degree hemorrhoids), medical management with sitz baths and stool bulking agents will eliminate symptoms in fully 85 percent of cases. If symptoms are not alleviated in patients with first- or second-degree hemorrhoidal problems, then rubber band ligation (two per session as necessary) is performed. ✓

I do not perform injection sclerotherapy, cryotherapy, or anal dilatation, thus I cannot comment on these treatments. Laser hemorrhoidectomy is not performed, period. Rubber band ligation is performed in exactly the same manner as described by Professor Keighley.

At the Mayo Clinic, the time-honored technique of treating hemorrhoids requiring surgical excision is the closed technique. In reading Professor Keighley's description of the closed technique, I find little with which to argue; the principles and practice described are nearly identical to mine. Parenthetically, almost all anal surgery performed at Mayo is performed in the prone jackknife position; if you have not yet tried it, try it—you won't go back to the lithotomy position again.

John H. Pemberton

In the past two decades, there has been a progressive decrease in the frequency with which intervention—especially surgical intervention—is required in the treatment of hemorrhoids. Many patients respond to medical management, sitz baths, bulking agents, and dietary modification. Excisional surgery is reserved for patients who have third- or fourth-degree hemorrhoids, or certain second-degree hemorrhoids that have failed to respond to

(Continues)

conventional measures (e.g., infrared coagulation and rubber band ligation). Rubber band ligation is the most common procedure used for hemorrhoids at the Cleveland Clinic. We have abandoned cryotherapy because of the excessive tissue destruction engendered by that procedure. Infrared coagulation seems particularly suitable for patients who have symptomatic hemorrhoids, especially bleeding hemorrhoids clustered close to the anal outlet and in a form that does not allow for the creation of a pedicle (which would otherwise allow rubber band ligation to be used). The operative technique described by Dr. Keighley regarding hemorrhoidectomy is the one used by us. Specific points include the use of the prone jackknife position as opposed to the lithotomy position, dilute epinephrine, infusion of the submucosa, use of cutting cautery to excise the hemorrhoid, care in preservation of the skin bridges by maintaining at all times a lighted anal retractor in the anal canal, and submucosal excision of any dilated or thickened varices beneath the skin ridges. Primary closure of the defect is then carried out using 3-0 chromic catgut. Closed hemorrhoidectomy is used routinely except for those patients who have a septic or necrotic hemorrhoidal condition. In patients with just one or two hemorrhoids, excision is done under local anesthesia. Any remaining minor hemorrhoids are treated with rubber band ligation. Pregnant patients with symptomatic hemorrhoids are treated using local anesthesia.

Victor W. Fazio

I have the following comments:

In my opinion, it is important to ask the patient to urinate before going to the operating room to prevent postoperative urinary retention.

I have no experience with laser hemorrhoidectomy.

I prefer partial lateral spbincterectomy to dilatation.

I routinely perform open hemorrhoidectomy and I have no further comment, as the technique has been wonderfully described.

I prefer caudal anesthesia for all anal procedures, and always with antibiotic cover.

Rolland Parc

Fissure in Ano

Victor W. Fazio

Open Sphincterotomy

Open sphincterotomy is the term applied to that treatment for anal fissure in which the caudad component of the internal sphincter is identified and divided under direct vision. The advantages (compared to closed sphincterotomy) are that the surgeon may be more certain of recognizing and dividing the appropriate sphincter; that one may gauge more accurately the amount of sphincter to be divided; and that hemostasis can be obtained more certainly. The disadvantage is the extent of the external skin incision, which is larger than that for the closed technique.

Preparation, Positioning, and Anesthesia

The procedure is performed on the same day as discharge (i.e., as a day case). My preference is for general anesthesia although there are many surgeons who prefer to use local anesthesia in an outpatient or office setting. Increasingly, surgeons (myself included) are using the latter technique on the basis of cost containment. For local anesthesia, we use 1 percent lidocaine with 1:100,000 epinephrine, infiltrating the fissure base as well as the incision site. If the patient is anxious, intravenous diazepam or midazolam is used and the patient is monitored with pulse oximetry. Because up to this point local anal pain has precluded an adequate anal examination, this is now done together with proctosigmoidoscopy if there has been no recent endoscopic study. Consequently, patients are given a rectal washout or enema prior to placement on the operating table.

For patients undergoing a general anesthetic one prefers to place the patient in a supine position with the legs in stirrups. In this way inhalation mask anesthesia can be used without the need for endotracheal intubation.

In situations where local anesthesia is used, I prefer the patient in the prone jack-knife position, as it is more comfortable for the surgeon and assistant. Antibiotics are not needed and intravenous fluids (in the case of general anesthesia) are used sparingly if at all to avoid urinary retention postoperatively.

Technique

The perineum is prepared with povidone-iodine and limited shaving of the perineum is done. The anal canal is dilated gently and a Ferguson retractor is inserted. The fissure, which is usually canoe shaped, may have varying features of chronicity, such as a pale base (exposed fibers of the internal sphincter), a hypertrophied anal papilla at its cephalad extent, and a sentinel tag at its caudal extent. Usually, the fissure will be posterior and midline, and occupy that part of the anal canal below the dentate line. Upon inspection or palpation, the intersphincteric groove can usually be identified (Fig. 5-15). A 1- to 5-cm incision is made about 5 mm *lateral* to the groove (Fig. 5-16A) to keep the incision from being drawn up into the anal canal, as it will for more medially placed incisions, when the patient is in the erect position. The incision is made posterolateral relative to the fissure and at a distance sufficient to avoid the risk of tunneling into the fissure bed itself (for anterior incisions an anterolateral incision is used). A hemostat is used to separate the skin wound to allow visualization of the internal sphincter. An Allis clamp is inserted into the wound and the lower border of the internal sphincer is grasped (Fig. 5-16B). Inadvertent grasping of the external sphincter may be minimized by placing the left index finger in the anal canal while advancing the open jaws of the Allis clamp slightly cephalad and medially until it is sensed that a bulk of muscle has been grasped. The spatial orientation provided by the left index finger also prevents the anal mucosa from being breached. The grasped muscle segment is then delivered through to the skin level (Fig. 5-16C). The internal sphincter muscle has pale, almost white fibers, whereas the external sphincter is reddish brown. More important as a means of distinguishing the two sphincters is the response of the muscle to contact with the diathermy (Bovie) tip. The external sphincter will contract vigorously, whereas the internal sphincter will not.

Figure 5-15.

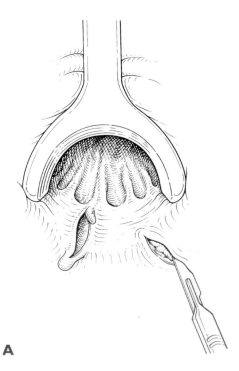

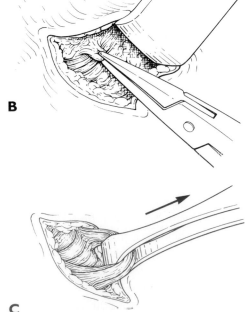

Figure 5-16.   **A**   **B**   **C**

At this point, having confirmed that the internal sphincter has been grasped, the surgeon must decide how much to divide. A general rule that is commonly followed is to divide an amount of the internal sphincter that corresponds to the length of the fissure. Most studies record high resting anal sphincter tone (contributed mostly by the internal sphincter), and we know that anal incontinence is quite uncommon (occurring in only 1 to 5 percent). For the average patient, therefore, one can divide what may seem to be a very generous amount (1.5 to 2 cm) of internal sphincter with safety. In patients for whom there are greater concerns about continence postoperatively (i.e., patients who have undergone previous sphincter division, e.g., sphincterotomy or fistulotomy, those with sphincter trauma from childbirth, multiparous patients, or female patients with an anterior fissure), one should be less radical and divide a smaller amount of internal sphincter (0.5 to 1.0 cm). The rationale here is that if one has a postoperative complication related to how much sphincter has been divided, it is better that it be a recurrent (or persistent) fissure than an incontinent patient.

The actual division of the sphincter is done in the following manner. A narrow-bladed right-angle clamp is placed through that part of the internal sphincter (in the grasp of the Allis clamp) that one judges necessary (Fig. 5-16D). Again, and with an assistant spreading the wound edges with a fine-bladed right-angle retractor, steady traction is applied to the Allis clamp while the right-angle clamp is manipulated. If there is any question of breaching the anal mucosa, the surgeon's left index finger should be inserted into the anal canal to act as a guide. The sphincter component that lies superficial to the right-angle clamp is then divided with diathermy after opening the blades of the right-angle clamp (Fig. 5-16E). Any bleeding vessels are cauterized as needed. If troublesome bleeding from the divided—and nonretracted—ends of the sphincter occurs, then further, deeper retraction and identification of the bleeding point is needed. This may or may not require further (lateral) extension of the skin incision. If the incision is longer than 1.5 cm, I prefer to place one or two absorbable sutures (e.g., Vicryl) to approximate the medial edges of the wound, leaving the lateral edges open for drainage.

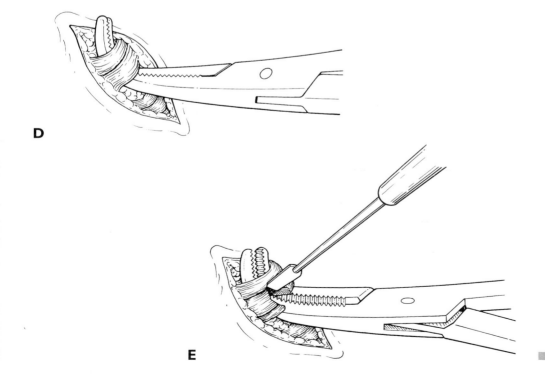

D

E

Figure 5-16.

Hypertrophied Papilla and Tag. The fissure is usually left alone; biopsy is appropriate if there is any question as to the nature of the fissure. In cases for which there is a high index of suspicion of other conditions (e.g., Crohn's disease, tuberculosis, or malignancy), biopsy is done without sphincterotomy. The hypertrophied anal papilla, if present, is excised and submitted for histologic examination. The question of excision of the skin tag or sentinel hemorrhoid is controversial. My preference is to excise the tag, especially if the tag is undermined and may hold up evacuation of collected fecal matter in the fissure itself. This tag excision may in fact be little more than a tapering of the caudal extent of the fissure to promote drainage of this area. A smooth contour of the verge is thus produced.

Associated Hemorrhoids. From the patient's history and intraoperative findings one has to make a judgment regarding the extent to which the hemorrhoids are symptomatic and contributing to the overall clinical picture. If judged to be significant (i.e., long-standing history of prolapse and pain), surgical treatment is appropriate. The closed hemorrhoidectomy using the Ferguson technique is performed *after* the sphincterotomy. In this way the hemorrhoid bundles may be grasped—and removed—in such a way that the sphincterotomy site is opposite an area of intact mucosal bridge. If this is not feasible because of the size and extent of the hemorrhoids, then the hemorrhoidectomy site nearest to the sphincterotomy is left open.

Associated Fistula in Ano. Occasionally one will find a pinpoint opening (external os) on the sentinel tag. The anal fissure itself—or its caudal extent—is the internal opening. In such cases we place a probe through the fistula tract (which is usually subcutaneous), divide the tissue superficial to the probe, and then excise or trim the edges. Unless there is pus present (a rare event), we then proceed with the sphincterotomy.

Suspected Crohn's Disease. The "typical" fissure of Crohn's disease is often laterally placed and indolent, being relatively painless and consisting of a large ulcer (extending to the dentate line or above) that requires no local surgery. However, the patient with Crohn's disease of the proximal intestinal tract may also have a painful small midline fissure of the type described earlier for his non-Crohn's counterpart. This presents a dilemma, as the potential for complications is higher. My approach has been to treat such patients medically for their Crohn's disease with psyllium compounds and antidiarrhea agents. If this treatment fails, then I use anal dilatation under anesthesia—two- to three-finger dilatation for 3 minutes—with follow-up self-dilatation. If this does not work, there may be a place for sphincterotomy—after careful disclosure to the patient of possible sequelae.

Aftercare

A small gauze pad is taped in place over the operative site and worn until the patient's first bowel movement. Bulking agents are given to prevent constipation, and sitz baths are an option in the management of pain. Perianal examination is done after 6 weeks to assess healing of the fissure and sphincterotomy site.

Closed Sphincterotomy

A bivalved speculum or Ferguson retractor placed in the anal canal is used to produce traction sufficient to permit palpation and identification of the internal sphincter by pressing on the intersphincteric groove. Using a narrow-bladed scalpel (e.g., a

Beaver blade or cataract knife), the perianal skin is <u>incised lateral to the fissure</u>. The incision is then advanced cranially to just above the dentate line (Fig. 5-17A). The plane of advancement is between the anoderm and the medial aspect of the internal sphincter, with the blunt and sharp edges of the knife lying parallel to these structures. In this way the risk of incising the anoderm is minimized. The blade is then rotated 90 degrees so that the cutting edge is adjacent to the internal sphincter (Fig. 5-17B). The caudad portion of the internal sphincter is then incised by drawing the blade caudally and laterally. Successful sphincterotomy can be recognized by a perceptible and sudden loss of internal sphincter tension. Digital anal examination is performed to assess completeness of the procedure. Finger pressure over the sphincterotomy site usually produces adequate tamponade and hemostasis.

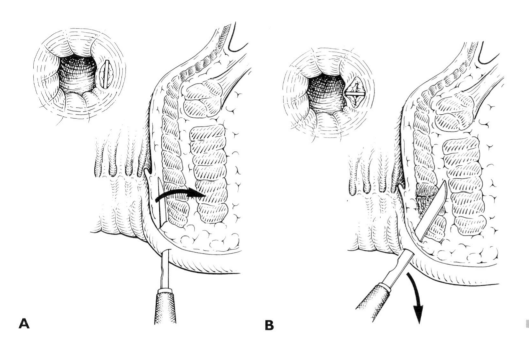

A   **B**   *Figure 5-17.*

Editorial Commentaries

I prefer the prone jackknife position when operating for fissure in ano, whether the procedure is performed under general or local anesthetic. I use a Park's retractor rather than a Ferguson retractor. I prefer an intra-anal incision to the laterally placed skin incision described because the intra-anal incision is not a skin wound. The only difficulty, however, is the need to dissect under the skin component in order to identify the lower extent of the anal sphincter. Using an anal incision there is far less risk of damage to the external anal sphincter because only the internal anal sphincter is identified from the incision onward. I also prefer to dissect the anal mucosa from the internal sphincter and to divide the internal sphincter partially with scissors. I close the intra-anal wound with running catgut.

Michael R. B. Keighley

(Continues)

My practice is essentially identical to Dr. Fazio's. Most of my patients undergoing a sphincterotomy have a chronic anal fissure, which is quite characteristic in appearance as opposed to acute anal fissures which, in our practice, are treated medically with an 80 percent chance of cure.

Most patients undergo lateral internal sphincterotomy under local anesthesia using lidocaine and epinephrine as described. Again, most patients undergo this procedure in the prone jackknife position.

Our incision is likewise made at the anal verge and the length of sphincterotomy is often as long as the length of the fissure itself. In women, especially those with a very unimpressive internal sphincter (small bulk and short length), the internal sphincterotomy performed is only about a half centimeter in length. As a general rule, we do not carry the sphincterotomy higher in the anal canal than the level of the dentate line. The entire wound is closed with a running, locking absorbable suture.

Patients with hypertrophied anal papillae undergo excision of the hypertrohied anal papillae, and if a sentinel pile is present, it too is removed. If patients have concomitant prolapsing internal hemorrhoids, these are removed using a closed technique.

Perhaps in contrast to Dr. Fazio, I do not treat any Crohn's ulcers of the anal canal surgically. If the anal canal is strictured, however, it will be dilated. I cannot comment on closed sphincterotomy, as the term "blind" seems quite appropriate.

John H. Pemberton

Fistula in Ano

John H. Pemberton

Nearly all anal fistulas are the result of an infection of the anal glands that traveled down the intersphincteric plane to form a draining perianal abscess. Although abscesses may drain in any direction and in any plane, about two-thirds of the fistulas are intersphincteric (Fig. 5-18). The external opening is not usually very close to the anal verge, and can be as much as 2 to 3 cm from the verge (Fig. 5-19).

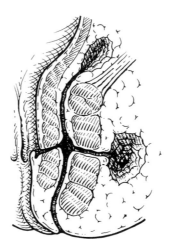

Figure 5-18.

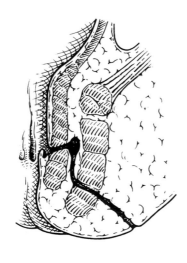

Figure 5-19.

This discussion presents the operative management of simple and more complex fistulas. Extremely complex fistulas are nearly always caused by the mishandling of a simple fistula by a surgeon who did not understand the anatomy of the area and misdiagnosed the type of abscess-fistula complex. Although one cannot determine how many of the most complex fistulas described in anal fistula classifications are actually caused by surgical mishandling of simpler anorectal fistulas, it is likely to be a fair number.

Figure 5-20 details Goodsall's rule: If a horizontal line is drawn across the anal sphincter, secondary openings in the perianal skin anterior to (ventral to) this line usually open in a direct line into the anal canal. Thus, a probe placed in the secondary site will exit at the dentate line in a direct line. However, if the secondary opening is posterior to (dorsal to) the horizontal line, the fistula nearly always tracts to the midline posteriorly, to the superficial or deep postanal space, and then to the dentate line. These posterior fistulas are more complex and need careful management.

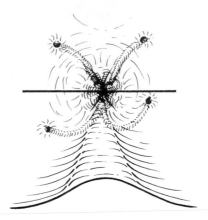

Figure 5-20.

Simple Fistulas

A simple fistula with a direct tract to the dentate line, as shown in Figure 5-21A, is usually very easy to feel, and by placing a probe into the secondary opening the entire tract may usually be defined (Fig. 5-21B). If necessary, a Kocher clamp may be applied at the secondary opening and pulled laterally in order to straighten the tract and allow the probe to drop into the anal canal. Figure 5-21C shows an incision of the subcutaneous tract with some internal sphincter and no external sphincter involvement. In this procedure, there is little chance of fecal incontinence, as only the distal half of the internal anal sphincter has been taken by the fistulotomy.

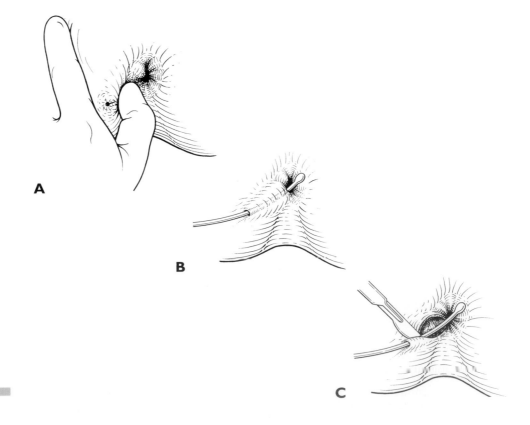

Figure 5-21.

Complex Fistulas

Intersphincteric fistulas, depending on which level of the external anal sphincter is involved, are more complex. A simple transsphincteric fistula with an associated ischiorectal abscess is shown in Figure 5-22. The level of internal and external anal sphincter that should be excised in order to manage this problem is also shown. In an older woman with a very short anal sphincter mechanism, incising half or more of the length of the external sphincter would probably be contraindicated, and placement of a cutting seton would be indicated instead. In Figure 5-23, a prodigious amount of external sphincter is shown distal to the fistula site. After the fistulous tract is identified from the secondary site, a probe is placed into the anal canal and a silk suture is tied to the end of the probe. The suture is pulled through and then tied to a small Penrose drain. The drain is pulled from the secondary site through the anal canal and tied tightly around the bulk of the anal sphincter mass (Fig. 5-23A). The skin overlying the tract between the primary and secondary sites is incised. Tightening of the seton causes little or no discomfort. Approximately 2 weeks after placement, the seton will cut through about half of the sphincter and will be quite loose (Fig. 5-23B). After further tightening the seton will cut its way through the rest of the sphincter during the ensuing 2-week period (Fig. 5-23C). When completed, the external anal sphincter will have retracted only very slightly and one can feel only a small defect in the muscle (Fig. 5-23C, inset). By not allowing the ends of the sphincter to retract, patients have a much greater chance of having excellent continence after fistulotomy.

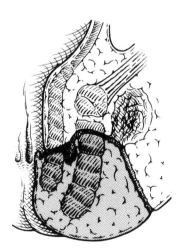

Figure 5-22.

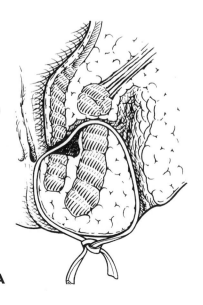

A

Figure 5-23.

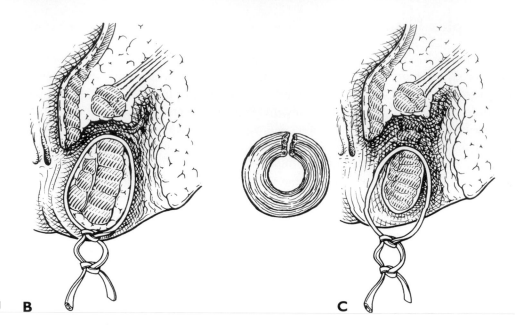

Figure 5-23.   **B**   **C**

Figure 5-24A details an intersphincteric fistula with a high blind tract. Although at one time I used to think this was uncommon, I have seen this more often recently. Whether this is caused by a poorly treated typical intersphincteric fistula with an external opening or not is unknown, but my feeling is that it often is. One deals with this fistula by intubating the primary site, tracing it proximally up the anal canal to the anorectal ring, and excising over the probe, thus performing, in effect, an endo anal canal internal sphincterotomy. It may not be necessary to continue the incision of the internal sphincter all the way to the anal verge. If there is a concomitant opening into the rectum, as shown in Figure 5-24B, then this is included in the line of incision of the internal sphincterotomy. If there is a high blind tract and an external opening, then the entire internal anal sphincter from the anal verge to the uppermost point of the high blind tract is taken using a seton.(Fig. 5-24C)

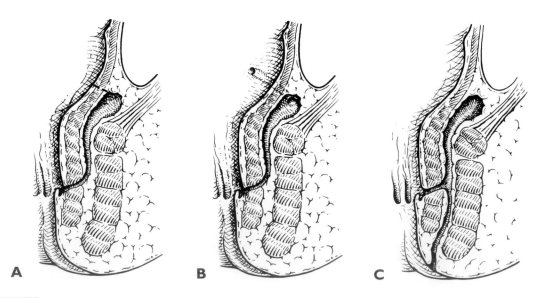

                   A   **B**   **C**

Figure 5-24

A final variation is a concomitant extrarectal extension of the high blind tract as an abscess (Fig. 5-25A). The intersphincteric and supralevator abscess is drained via the internal os using a small deRezza catheter (Fig. 5-25B). When sepsis has resolved one proceeds with internal anal sphincterotomy to the top of the high extension. If the fistulous tract is actually suprasphincteric and not transsphincteric, then a seton is placed around the entire muscle mass from the primary site to the secondary site and the deep abscess cavity counterdrained by a tube (Fig. 5-25C). Very rarely a fistula may be completely extrasphincteric; this situation is often caused by a surgical misadventure (Fig. 5-26A). In this situation, we counterdrain the fistulous tract, placing the drain at the level of the rectum, excise the tract in the rectum, and close it primarily, and then put a seton encircling the external anal sphincter mass from the primary through the secondary opening (Fig. 5-26B). The need for a diverting colostomy is a distinct possibility in this situation depending on the chronicity of the process.

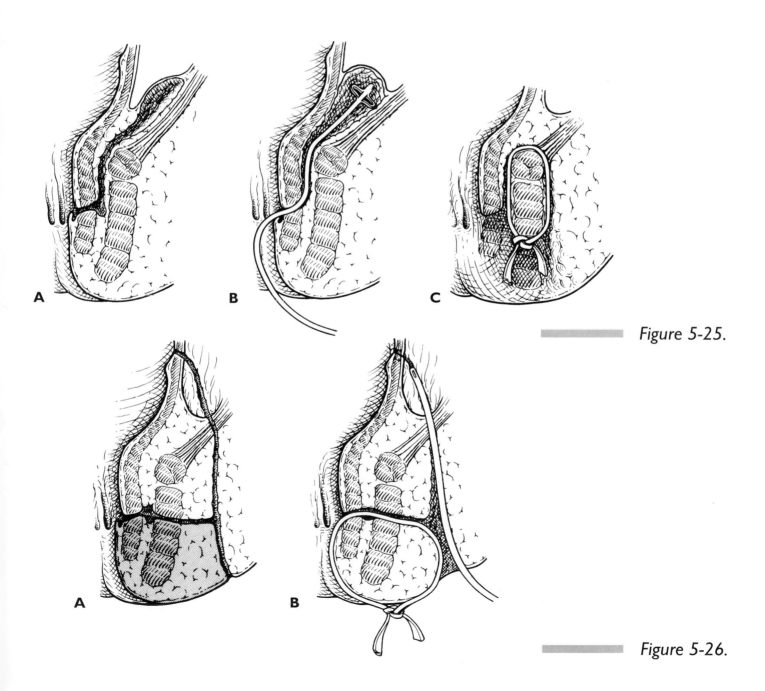

Figure 5-25.

Figure 5-26.

Horseshoe Fistula

Figure 5-27 represents our management approach to the particularly perplexing problem of the horseshoe fistula. Such a fistula would not have formed at all if the perineal septic process that predated the fistula had been treated correctly. Note, as shown in Fig. 5-27B, the fistulous tract does indeed communicate with the posterior dentate line, probably through the deep postanal space.

In this situation, we rarely open the skin overlying the fistula's tracts in the manner shown in Fig. 5-27A. More often, we use small incisions placed at intervals along the fistula tracts to avoid "floating" the anus, which can occur when long fistula tracts are unroofed in their entirety. We place a seton about the sphincter mass posteriorly between the primary site at the dentate line and the deep postanal space, and allow it to cut through slowly over a 4-week period (Fig. 5-27B).

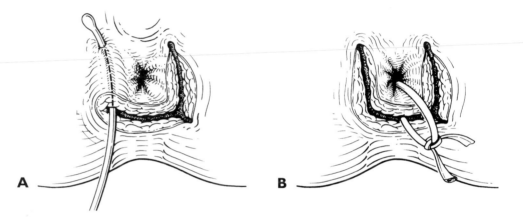

Figure 5-27.   ▬▬▬   A   B

On Whether or Not to Perform a Park's Fistuloctomy

In particularly difficult situations where incising any of the internal/external sphincter mass might lead to fecal incontinence (as in multiparous women, and in patients who suffered from fecal incontinence intermittently preoperatively), it is reasonable to consider a Park's fistulotomy. This is shown in Figure 5-28. Here, the lower half of the internal anal sphincter is divided to eradicate the causative anal gland and the peripheral fistula is managed by coring it out by curettage alone or incision and curettage. The major advantage is preservation of the external sphincter. Indeed, we would agree that this is an interesting approach and is useful in some situations, perhaps in perianal Crohn's disease. However, placement of a seton would accomplish this as well.

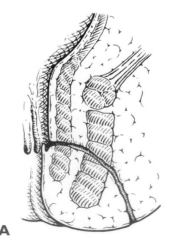 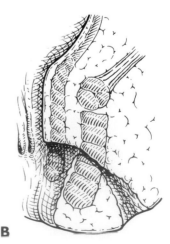

Figure 5-28.   ▬▬▬   A   B

A variation on the Park procedure is the rectal advancement flap for complex fistula with a secondary opening in the rectal vault. This has a place in treating certain high transsphincteric fistulas, but is used—unnecessarily—for low intersphincteric fistulas when the only piece of muscle to be divided is the internal sphincter at the dentate line. A rectal mucosal and muscle flap is fashioned with a broad base proximally and elevated in the anal canal (so it is indeed full thickness) (Fig. 5-29A). The internal opening is excised with the base of the flap and the granulation tissue curetted out where the tract transverses the internal/external sphincter. The opening through the muscle is usually sutured with 2-0 Vicryl. The flap is then pulled down and sutured high in the anal canal using interrupted sutures of 2-0 Vicryl (Fig. 5-29B). The tract is left open to drain (Fig. 5-29C). Infection or breakdown of the flap is not at all uncommon; therefore, this procedure should not be used for simple low fistulous tracts that may be near the primary openings or at the dentate line. I must add that the few advancement flaps I have performed all broke down—perhaps the base of the flap was too narrow; nevertheless I am not entirely sold on this technique.

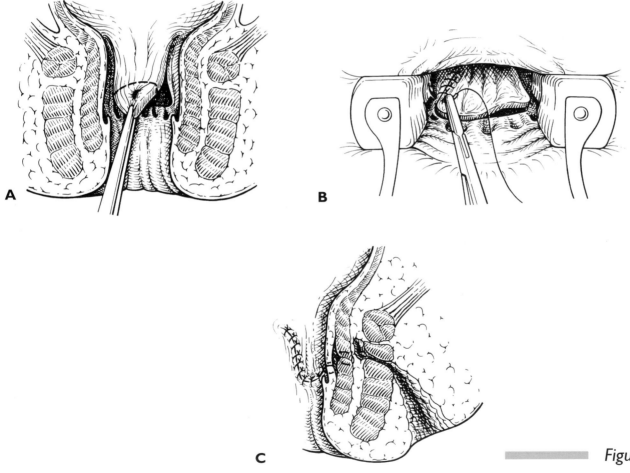

A

B

C

Figure 5-29.

A very, very uncommon finding is a diverticular abscess that has perforated into the pelvis through the levators and out through the ischiorectal fossa (Fig. 5-30). This sounds like a disaster, but it is easily treated (from what I am told) by merely resecting the area of sigmoid diverticular disease and counterdraining the fistulous tract. Beware the symptoms of diverticular disease: an acute flare and drainage of feculent material via the perineum.

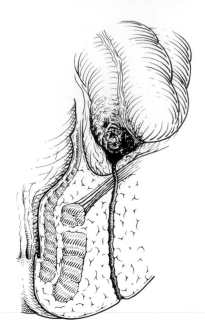

Figure 5-30.

Editorial Commentary

I wish to make a few practical remarks:

√ I believe that <u>examination under anesthesia</u> to define the area of induration or fibrosis gives a great deal of information regarding the anatomic tract of an anorectal fistula.

√ I tend to probe from the <u>inside out</u>. In this manner one is far less likely to create a false passage.

√ I like the idea of placing forceps adjacent to the external opening to straighten the tract.

√ I think that the use of a weak methylene blue solution, or even hydrogen peroxide, may occasionally help to delineate the path of the fistula.

√ If in doubt about the anatomy of the fistula, I leave it alone and arrange for reexamination under anesthesia at a later date.

If the patient no longer has a discharge from the external opening when electively investigated under anesthetic, I tend to leave the fistula alone. Meddlesome exploration of a closed external opening in a patient who has been asymptomatic for 3 to 4 weeks may do more harm than good.

Finally, I would say if a fistula in ano is associated with anorectal stenosis the functional outcome is often very poor. Furthermore, it may be quite difficult to define the true anatomic site of the fistula in such a circumstance. Stenosis is often the result of severe perirectal inflammation of unresolved sepsis or from repeated anorectal operations. Great care must be taken not to make matters worse by further surgery in these patients.

Michael R. B. Keighley

Anorectal Sepsis

John H. Pemberton

The diagnosis of anorectal sepsis is usually obvious; generally there is a painful lump near the anal canal, the history is short, and the pain is severe. There is perianal swelling, usually associated with erythema, and the area is very tender. In some patients, however, the diagnosis is not so obvious. In these patients, there are complaints of pain, but no swelling or edema, and the rectal examination is very uncomfortable. The unwary may ignore the patient's symptoms or consider the possibility of a fissure, but may miss the true diagnosis of deep sepsis. Any patient who complains of persistent anal pain of short duration in whom no fissure can be found should undergo an examination under anesthesia complete with needle aspiration, with the presumptive diagnosis of deep perianal or intersphincteric sepsis.

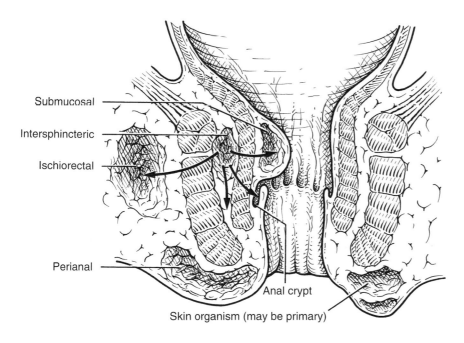

Submucosal

Intersphincteric

Ischiorectal

Perianal

Anal crypt

Skin organism (may be primary)

Figure 5-31.

Figure 5-31 shows the different manifestations of perianal sepsis. Perineal, intersphincteric, ischiorectal, or submucosal infections are usually linked to a primarily infected anal crypt. These are likewise almost always associated with a fistula; however, in only 50 percent of cases can such a fistula be found when the patient presents with acute perianal sepsis. The fistula can be demonstrated by applying pressure to the abscess, which will cause pus to be expressed at the dentate line (Fig. 5-32).

Technique

The examination is best performed under general anesthesia in order to determine the extent of the sepsis (Fig. 5-33). Figure 5-34 shows a typical perianal mass that is swollen, red, and very tender. The only reasonable way to manage such an obvious perianal abscess is to incise and drain it. A cruciate incision is made over the mass and a curved instrument is used to explore the abscess that lies underneath. If the abscess is superficial, any fistulous tract will generally be subcutaneous. In a deep ischiorectal abscess, however, the fistulous tract usually will be transsphincteric. It

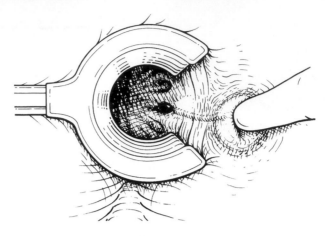

Figure 5-32. ━━━━━━

will communicate directly with the abscess site if it is located anterior to Goodsall's line (see discussion earlier in this chapter) (Fig. 5-35A); if it is posterior to Goodsall's line, it will run to the deep postanal space (Fig. 5-35B). In acute sepsis, the relationship of any fistulous tract to the sphincter muscle itself may be extremely difficult to establish. This is especially problematic anteriorly, where the sphincter is very difficult to find because of edema and induration. If the internal opening has been found, a probe can then be passed from the depth of the abscess cavity into the primary opening at the level of the dentate line. If it cannot be found readily, placing a Kocher clamp at the site of the incision and pulling laterally can often define the tract easily (Fig. 5-36). Another trick is to inject milk or hydrogen peroxide into the abscess cavity to see if it leaks out through the primary site at the dentate line. Methylene blue, although very messy, can also be helpful if sufficiently diluted. It cannot be overemphasized that overzealous probing of the depth of the abscess cavity can lead to the formation of a false tract.

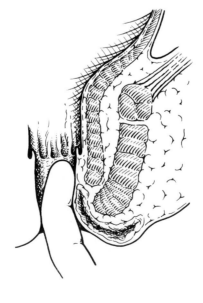

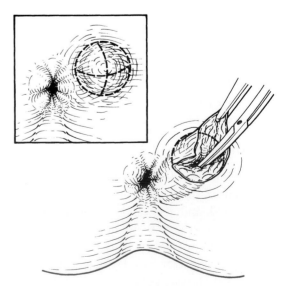

Figure 5-33. ━━━━━━

Figure 5-34. ━━━━━━

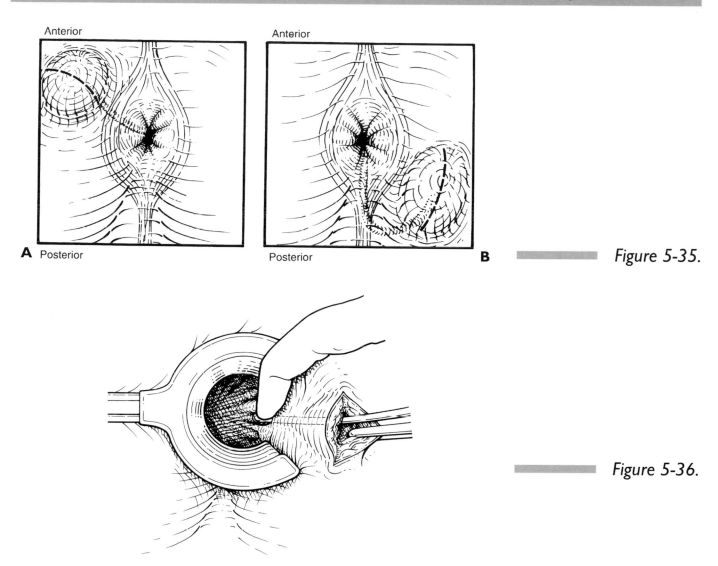

Anterior

A Posterior

Anterior

B Posterior

Figure 5-35.

Figure 5-36.

The management of the fistula depends on its relationship to the external anal sphincter. A low fistula is easily laid open at the time of abscess drainage. A more complex tract, however, is best managed by the placement of a seton (Fig. 5-37).

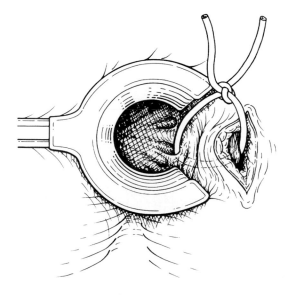

Figure 5-37.

A cigarette-sized Penrose drain is placed through the internal opening and into the abscess cavity, the underlying skin edge excised, and the seton tightened slightly. When the edema and inflammation dissipate, a better idea of the level of involvement of the external anal sphincter by the fistulous tract may be gained.

When no fistulous tract can be identified using the maneuvers noted above, it is quite possible that the fistulous tract was obliterated before presentation of the abscess and will never be found. In such cases incision and drainage will be enough to cure the sepsis.

When anorectal sepsis is present bilaterally (Fig. 5-38), the abscess cavity is nearly always connected via the superficial or deep postanal space. It is extremely important that this situation be managed adequately at the first operation. In bilateral sepsis,

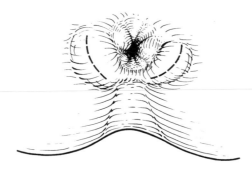

Figure 5-38.

the cryptoglandular process burrows directly into the postanal space, and thence to the ischiorectal fossa bilaterally. Thus, it is imperative that the fistulous tracking between the primary site at the dentate line and the deep postanal space be found. Expression of the dentate line will help to identify the primary site.

Drainage is complex, requiring incisions on either side of the midline and into the postanal space. An incision is made directly posteriorly, approximately 2 cm from the anal verge, and deepened directly into the postanal space. In a large man, this can require very deep probing. Once into the deep postanal space, the other sites of abscess on either side of the midline are incised and their connections to the deep postanal space identified. Loose Penrose drains are then placed through the fistulous tracts between the perineal skin incisions on either side of the midline and the deep postanal space. The fistula between the dentate line and the deep postanal space burrows through the internal and external sphincter. Because of its position posteriorly, a cigarette-sized Penrose seton is placed through this fistulous tract and tightened in

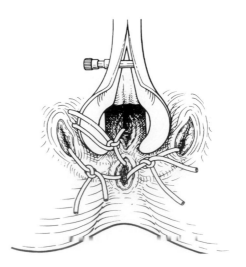

Figure 5-39.

order to allow progressive division of the external and internal anal sphincters over the succeeding 2- to 4-week period (Fig. 5-39). The other Penrose drains that were placed to keep the secondary fistulous tracts open and draining are removed after 2 weeks to allow complete reepithelialization of the more superficial abscesses.

Editorial Commentary

In essence I agree with all that Dr. Pemberton advises, particularly the importance of examination under anesthesia in any patient with undiagnosed anal pain so as to exclude undisclosed anorectal sepsis. Severe damage resulting in irreversible functional morbidity may result from untreated intersphincteric sepsis or sepsis in the deep postanal space.

Personally, I tend to be even more conservative in the management of an abscess with a coexisting fistula. I believe that the emergency treatment should be merely to identify the sepsis and to drain it effectively. In our experience, only 40 percent of patients with anorectal sepsis go on to develop an anorectal fistula. Therefore, in our opinion, intervention at the time of acute sepsis is meddlesome. If a fistula occurs at a later stage, we explore it in the manner described in the previous part of this chapter.

Michael R. B. Keighley

Anal Warts
Michael R. B. Keighley

If anal warts cannot be adequately controlled using topical agents such as podophyllum, or if immunotherapy and vaccination have failed, surgical treatment is generally indicated. Patients must be counseled and told that warts are often sexually transmitted, hence treatment of contacts is important for eradication. Furthermore, they should be told that persistent sexual activity is likely to result in reinoculation with the virus. It should be explained that the virus can lie dormant in the epidermis for many years, and that recurrence is common. As there is a small risk of dysplasia and carcinoma associated with the human papilloma virus, it is important to tell patients that excision will also provide an opportunity for histologic scrutiny.

There are two main methods of surgical ablation. One is by careful scissor excision of all perianal, perineal, and intra-anal warts. The alternative method is by some physical method of eradication using either diathermy or laser.

Scissor Excision

The technique of scissor excision requires meticulous attention to detail and is time consuming. A weak solution of epinephrine in saline (1:300,000) is used to elevate each warty excrescence from the skin so that only the epidermal attachment is removed (Fig. 5-40). The principle of this technique is that it causes minimal scarring and far less tissue destruction than diathermy or laser treatment (Fig. 5-41). For warts inside the anal canal, as well as for those on the perineum and perianal regions, an intra-anal bivalved speculum should be used (Fig. 5-42). There is no clinical evidence that this method is superior to the simpler diathermy and laser techniques.

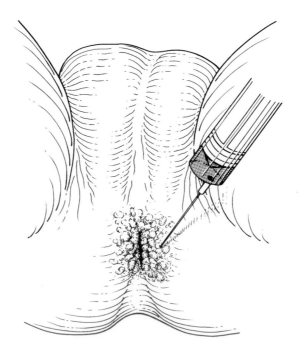

Figure 5-40.

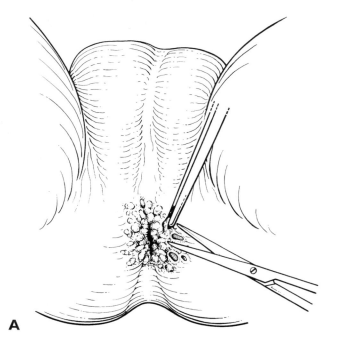

A

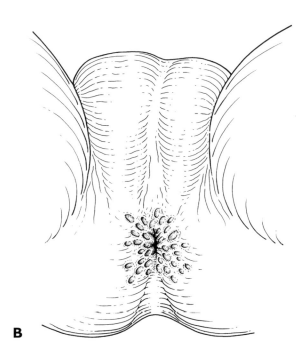

B

Figure 5-41.

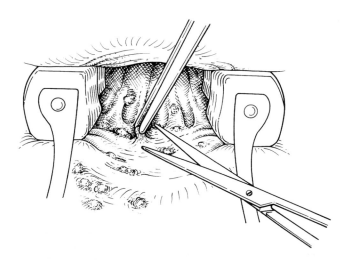

Figure 5-42.

Diathermy and Laser Excision

The key to diathermy eradication is the use of an extremely fine diathermy point, preferably with some optical magnification so that the diathermy is applied only to the base of each wart. The technique is much quicker than scissor excision. It is crucial to minimize the amount of diathermy used in order to avoid excessive scarring (Fig. 5-43). I see no advantage of laser over diathermy.

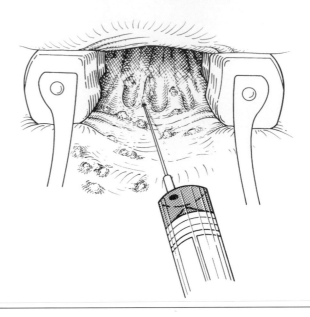

Figure 5-43.

Editorial Commentaries

I must differ with Dr. Keighley here. If there is one thing that the carbon dioxide laser is good for, it is in the management of anal and perineal warts.

The patient is placed in the lithotomy position and all warts vaporized. Destruction of normal tissue is indeed extraordinarily minimal. Care is taken to eradicate the core of the wart, which appears sometimes to lie beneath the skin surface itself. Anal canal warts can be treated with either laser or electrocoagulation. Bleeding, however, cannot be controlled with the laser, as the hemoglobin absorbs the laser energy; thus electrocautery should be available. The recovery is impressively speedy (some patients do not complain at all). The total stay in the hospital is overnight or one full day. In follow-up, scarring is almost nonexistent.

May I emphasize again that medical lasers do only a few things better than standard therapy; the treatment of warts is one of them.

John H. Pemberton

The treatment that I use for perianal as well as intra-anal canal warts is identical to that of Dr. Keighley. After completing the scissor excision (after previous infiltration with epinephrine), I will usually cauterize the small defects that remain. This is adding a thermal injury to the excisional treatment, but it also deals with problematic bleeding from the wound once the effect of the epinephrine has worn off. It should be emphasized that recurrence is the rule and that I will try to bring the patient back at 2- to 3-month intervals and use similar treatment while "recurrence" is still fairly limited. One further technical point is that I prefer to use iris scissors in dealing with these warts rather than the larger-appearing scissors in the figures shown.

I have no experience with laser therapy for this condition. I am unimpressed with the use of topical agents, immunotherapy, and vaccination.

Victor W. Fazio

I use diathermy routinely; I have no further comment.

Rolland Parc

Pilonidal Disease

John H. Pemberton

Pilonidal disease comprises a variety of problems, including abscess and the development of a chronic, recurrent, or nonhealing sinus cavity. The term *pilonidal disease* is thus more precise than *pilonidal cyst*. Conservative treatment is better than aggressive surgery in most cases, as aggressive surgery nearly invariably results in a large, non-healing wound that continues to get larger.

Interestingly, we rarely encounter pilonidal disease in patients older than about 35 or 40 years. Why people get it in the first place is still largely unknown.

Acute Disease (Abscess)

A simple problem calls for a simple solution. If the abscess cavity is off the midline, simple drainage of the abscess by means of a cruciate incision (using a # 11 blade) with the patient under local (lidocaine) anesthesia is adequate (Fig. 5-44). If the abscess is in the midline, the incision should be off the midline. The wound is packed with plain gauze for a few days, after which the patient is instructed to soak in the tub twice daily and keep a dressing in place.

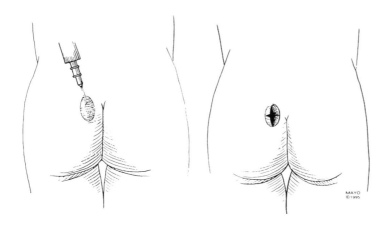

Figure 5-44.

Chronic Pilonidal Cavity and Sinus

It is important to remember that abscess drainage is only the first half of the procedure; a week or so later, when the midline pits and sinuses should be quite obvious, the procedure is completed. The off-midline incision is then lengthened and deepened into the midline cavity. The hair follicles, which are likely responsible for starting the disease in the first place (although this is a matter of controversy), can be seen in the midline. Granulation tissue and hair are aggressively curetted from the sinus cavity, and the cavity is irrigated (Fig. 5-45A). The pits and sinuses are then removed (Fig. 5-45B). The wound is packed open for several days, after which the patient is told to soak in the tub twice daily and to keep a dressing in place. Patients usually can resume sitting and return to work right away. We also inform the patient of the need to keep midline free of hair, and recommend having a partner or family member assist in shaving the area regularly. This minimal surgical approach works most of the time.

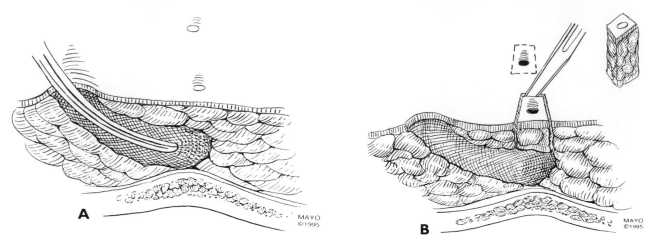

Figure 5-45.

Incision and Marsupialization

Midline sinus tracts and complex chronic abscess cavities with multiple deep tracts require incision (and/or excision) and marsupialization. The tracts are opened in the midline or the complex cavity is excised completely and the granulation tissue is curetted. Continuous absorbable 2-0 locking sutures are then placed between the skin edge and the fibrous tissue in the depths of the wound (Fig. 5-46). Marsupializing wounds decreases their size 50 to 60 percent, but they still take 6 weeks to heal.

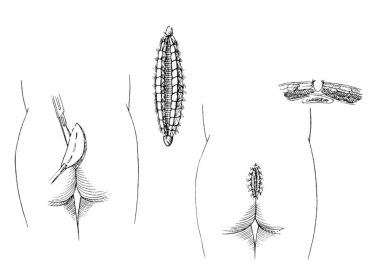

Figure 5-46.

Operations other than the above-described procedures, such as Z-plasties, primary closure, and flap advancement procedures for primary disease, are needlessly aggressive and thus are not recommended.

Persistent Disease

Poor healing, often caused iatrogenically, is usually responsible for persistent disease. Complex cavities, some of multiple years' duration, and sinuses with abundant hair and granulation tissue challenge the surgeon's ingenuity. Here aggressive surgery *is* required.

In our approach to this problem, the cleft between the buttocks is flattened and the complex lesion is excised in its entirety (Fig. 5-47A). Next, a V-shaped incision is made on both sides of the wound down to the gluteal fascia (Fig. 5-47B). On both sides myocutaneous flaps consisting of gluteal muscle and fascia are then moved to the midline and sutured in place using 0 or 2-0 Vicryl (Fig. 5-47C). The cleft is thus obliterated. A suction drain is left in place for 7 to 10 days. Our results with this procedure have been extraordinarily good.

Z-plasty and Bascom's "cleft closure" technique achieve the same result, but I have no experience with either procedure.

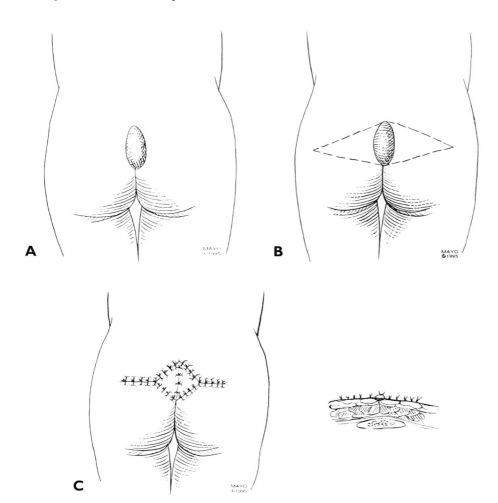

A   B   C

Figure 5-47.

Editorial Commentary

Dr. Pemberton correctly advises a conservative approach to the primary presentation of pilonidal disease. In some patients with noninfective disease I merely advise shaving the area and curettage of the sinus with a fine wire brush. Dr. Pemberton correctly stresses the importance of avoiding midline incisions. Sometimes the surgical management of this disease is worse than the disease itself.

Michael R. B. Keighley

6

Sphincter and Pelvic Floor Reconstruction

John H. Pemberton

The general surgical approach to the patient with fecal incontinence is first to identify any anatomic abnormality that may be present. This abnormality usually consists of a defect in the sphincter mechanism caused by childbirth injury or a surgical misadventure.

Our preferred approach to anterior sphincter defects generally is to perform an anterior repair, accessing the rectovaginal septum via an incision between the anal verge and the vaginal introitus. For lateral and posterior defects, the approach is straightforward: elevation of the perineal skin, identification of the severed ends of the external anal sphincter, and snug reapproximation.

The surgical approach to patients with neurogenic fecal incontinence is altogether different. The surgical options include postanal repair, anterior levatorplasty, total pelvic repair (anterior repair *and* levatorplasty), and gracilis muscle transfer. Because gracilis muscle transfer and electrically stimulated gracilis muscle transfer are performed very rarely, and then only by experienced operators, these will not be discussed in this chapter.

Anal Incontinence Caused By Childbirth or Surgical Trauma

Reconstruction of the Perineal Body and External Anal Sphincter Mechanism

A thinned rectovaginal septum with loss of the perineal body is absolutely characteristic of a torn anterior anal sphincter mechanism. Such a defect resulting from childbirth injury, causes loss of the pressure vector anteriorly. Simple overlapping sphincteroplasty will result in a completely inadequate high-pressure zone. Rather, complete repair of the anterior sphincter complex, including the levator muscles (puborectalis), is indicated.

The patient is placed in the lithotomy position. General anesthesia is used. In the case illustrated, the anal sphincter muscles are retracted to the 10- and 2-o'clock positions. A curvilinear incision is made from the 9- to the 12- to the 3-o'clock position through the skin of the perineum. A midline incision is then made in the vagina (Fig.

6-1A). The incisions are deepened and the posterior wall of the vagina is dissected off the thinned anorectal-vaginal septum (Fig. 6-1B). A muscle stimulator is used to find the retracted ends of the sphincter muscles (Fig. 6-2). These muscles can be found as far laterally as the 4 to 5 o'clock positions on the patient's left and the 7- to 8-o'clock positions on the patient's right, necessitating that the incisions on both sides of the anal verge be extended and brought posteriorly enough to find the muscle ends.

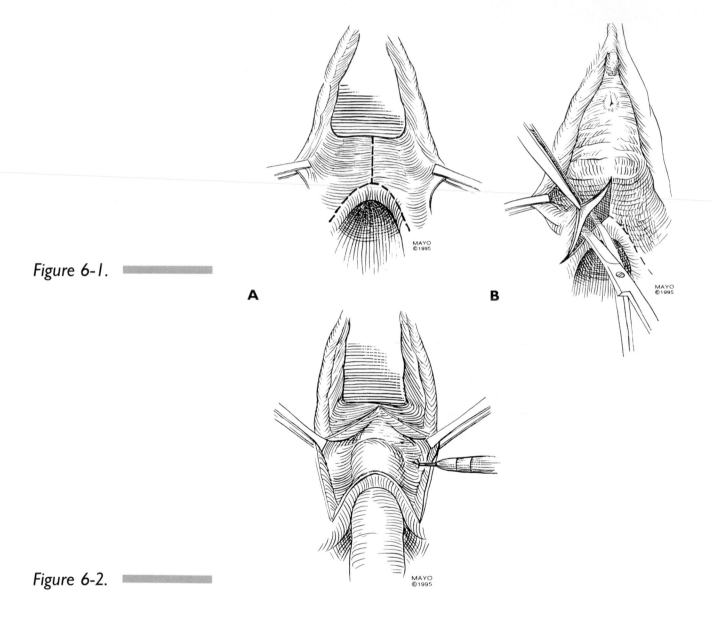

Figure 6-1.

A   **B**

Figure 6-2.

Once identified, the sphincter muscles are reapproximated using interrupted 0 monofilament delayed absorbable sutures. The initial suture is placed at the superior end of the incision at the highest point that can be reached; this and each additional suture are used to reestablish muscle continuity (Fig. 6-3). The 0 monofilament suture incorporates the retracted levator plateau (including the puborectalis muscle) superiorly and the external anal sphincter inferiorly, with intervening bites of the anterior anorectal wall. The approach thus incorporates a portion of the internal anal sphincter, and an equally deep bite on both sides of the anal canal incorporates the external anal sphincter (Fig. 6-3, inset). One needs to be especially careful that, when tied, the sutures do not narrow the vaginal introitus and form what is commonly termed a *posterior bar*. This is to be avoided assiduously as it can result in dyspareunia. When the surgeon is sure that a posterior bar will not be created, additional sutures are placed, each incorporating a full and deep bite of levator muscles superiorly and external sphincter muscle inferiorly, with intervening bites of the anterior anorectal wall. Usually between six and eight sutures are placed over a distance of 4 to 5 cm. Knowing that the anal sphincter mechanism in women is only 2 to 3 cm in length, 2 to 3 cm of this repair should also incorporate the levator muscles. After these sutures are tied, the anal canal will be severely narrowed. The highest suture is checked again to ensure that it would not cause dyspareunia. After the external sphincter and puborectalis muscles have been reapproximated, a second layer of tissue is sutured (Fig. 6-4). The completed repair thus reconstructs the anterior sphincter over a distance of 4 to 5 cm and restores the perineal body to its normal robustness (Fig. 6-5). No drains are used.

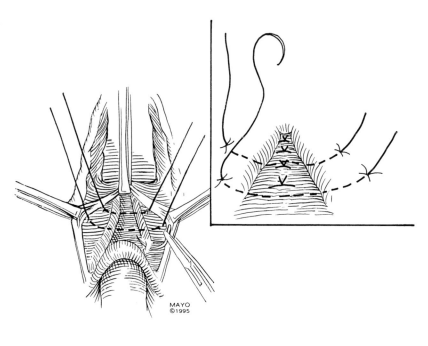

Figure 6-3.

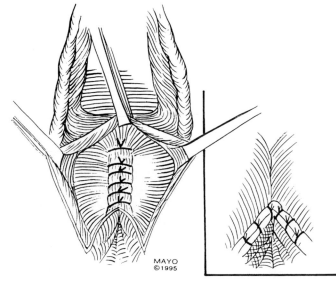

Figure 6-4.

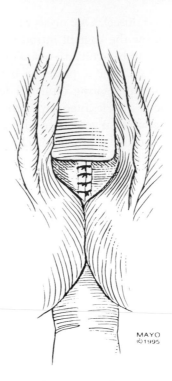

MAYO
©1995

Figure 6-5.

As soon as bowel function has returned to normal, the patient is encouraged to incorporate some bulk-forming agent (e.g., Metamucil) into the diet from day one. If pudendal nerve terminal motor latencies (PNTMLs) are normal, the results of such an anterior sphincter repair and reestablishment of the perineal body are excellent. On the other hand, if innervation of the external anal sphincter has been compromised (PNTMLs are increased), results are not nearly as predictable. However, some improvement can still be achieved if a rigorous program of sphincter augmentation and sensation training (biofeedback) is undertaken.

Simple Lateral Sphincter Repair

Lateral sphincter damage occurs as the result of a surgical misadventure. Such injury may occur during a hemorrhoidectomy if the surgeon does not fully understand the relationship between the hemorrhoidal groups, the internal anal sphincter, and the external anal sphincter, or during fistulotomy if, as discussed in Chapter 5, the surgeon cuts the external anal sphincter muscle instead of using a seton to achieve the fistulotomy.

The operation is performed using general anesthesia with the patient in the prone jackknife position. A wide incision centered on the scar tissue is made to encompass about half the circumference of the anal canal (Figs. 6-6 and 6-7). Next, the outer edge of the sphincter complex is identified by locating the ischiorectal fat (Fig. 6-8). It is important to ensure that the sphincter is exposed adequately in its depth. The sphincter muscle, which in a man is about 4 to 5 cm deep, should be repaired in its entirety. The nerves supplying the external anal sphincter (pudendal nerves) enter the sphincter complex at the 10- and 12-o'clock positions. They should be well out of the way of dissection. The scar should next be divided vertically down its entire length so as to permit reapproximation of the ends of the external anal sphincter. It is not practical to separate the internal from the external anal sphincter. Next, the inner aspect of the sphincter should be mobilized from the underlying mucosa for approximately half the circumference of the anal canal and to the same depth (Fig. 6-9). If there is scarring within the anal canal, it should be excised and the wound

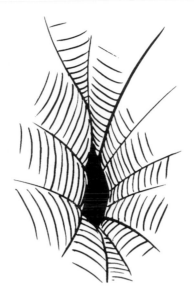

Figure 6-6.

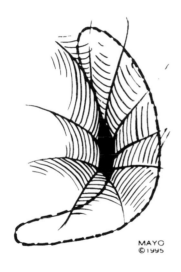

Figure 6-7.

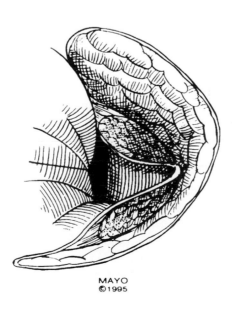

Figure 6-8.

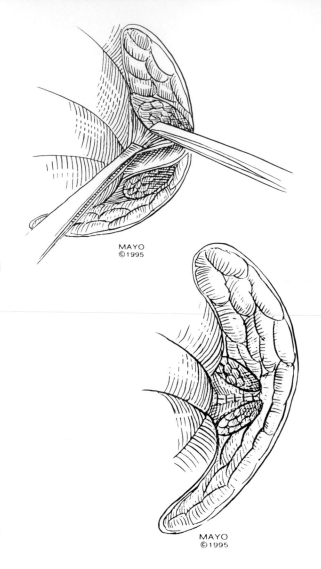

Figure 6-9.

Figure 6-10.

repaired with interrupted absorbable sutures (Fig. 6-10). Usually, an overlapping sphincter repair is performed over the entire length of the sphincter. One starts with the deepest part of the repair, placing four PDS or 2-0 Vicryl horizontal mattress sutures in a row about 1 cm apart (Fig. 6-11). The first bite, taken in the overlapped sphincter about 2 to 3 cm from its cut edge, passes through the scar, which has been left on the leading edge of the muscle. The skin is closed over the incision and the anal canal mucosa tacked to the repair (Fig. 6-12). In rare cases the overlapping repair is quite bulky and prevents primary closure of the skin.

Neurogenic Fecal Incontinence

Postanal Repair

Postanal repair is controversial. The patient is placed in the lithotomy position, prepped, and draped. A V-shaped incision is made approximately 6 cm behind the anal canal (Fig. 6-13). The incision must be far away from the anal verge because after closure the skin is drawn up toward the anal verge; if the incision is too close, it will be pulled into the anal canal. Next, the posterior fibers of the external anal sphincter and lower part of the internal anal sphincter are exposed (Fig. 6-14). The plane between the two is relatively bloodless. The internal and external anal sphinc-

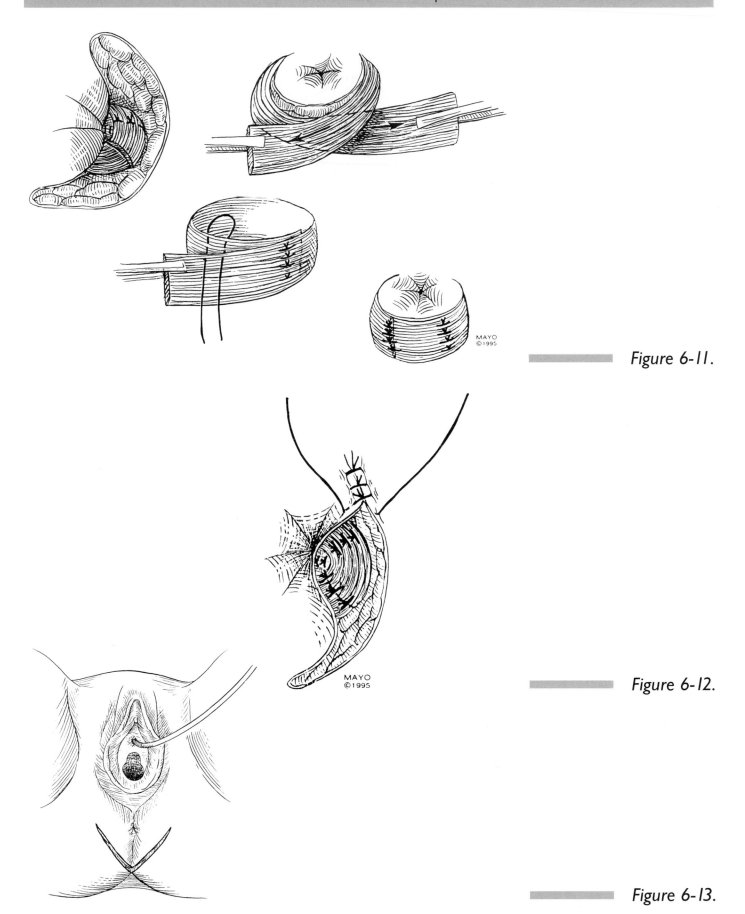

Figure 6-11.

Figure 6-12.

Figure 6-13.

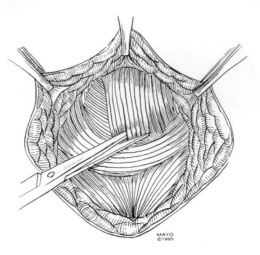

Figure 6-14.

ters can usually be easily identified: the external sphincter is usually red, whereas the internal sphincter is white. If the external anal sphincter has degenerated, the distinction can be quite difficult; however, using stimulation from the cautery, the external sphincter will be seen to contract.

By gentle dissection, the internal sphincter is displaced from the lower portion of the external anal sphincter. The rectum is lifted off the external anal sphincter, the dissection progressing onward and upward until the puborectalis muscle is reached (Fig. 6-15). One must be very careful not to deviate from this plane; it is easy to enter the rectum and even easier to dissect posteriorly into ischiorectal fat (Fig. 6-15, inset). Throughout the dissection, the separation between the two layers is carried as far forward on each lateral aspect of the anal canal as possible. Sometimes the anococcygeal ligament is encountered above the puborectal muscle and is divided, exposing the mesorectal fat. A deep retractor is then placed to hold the rectum upward and forward so that the origin of the levator ani muscles on both sides can be seen. Sutures of 2-0 Prolene are placed in a latticelike pattern across the muscle (Fig. 6-16). The highest and most lateral point of the levatorplasty is identified close to the ischial spine. A bite is taken into the fairly large bundle of levator on one side and then again on the other side. About three sutures are placed at this high level; they are tied without tension, forming a latticework behind the rectum. The next layer of sutures is placed more superficially into the upper part of the pubococcygeal muscle and again tied to form another latticework.

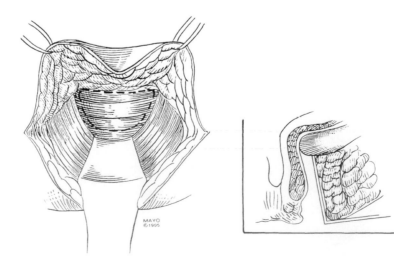

Figure 6-15.

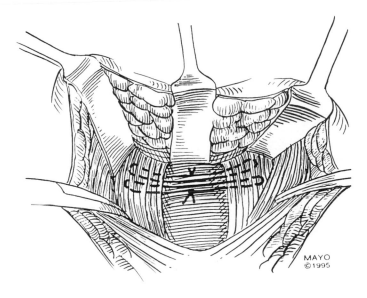

Figure 6-16.

The puborectalis muscle is the most important muscle for reconstruction; this is the strongest and thickest and is easiest to see. This muscle should be reapproximated very close to the rectum, leaving a small space for any swelling that may occur (Fig. 6-17). A final layer of sutures is placed on the external anal sphincter below the puborectalis muscle (Fig. 6-18). Subcuticular Vicryl is used to close the skin and the superficial subcutaneous tissues. A drain is sometimes placed in the subcutaneous tissues, but not in the deep tissues (Fig. 6-19). The drain is removed within 24 hours.

Total Pelvic Floor Repair

Total pelvic floor repair is a combination of a postanal repair with an anterior levatorplasty. One incision is made in exactly the same position as for the postanal repair and the other, a curvilinear incision, between the introitus and the anal verge. These incisions are deepened until, as in the postanal repair, the puborectalis muscle and levator plate are identified both anteriorly and posteriorly. A posterior repair is con-

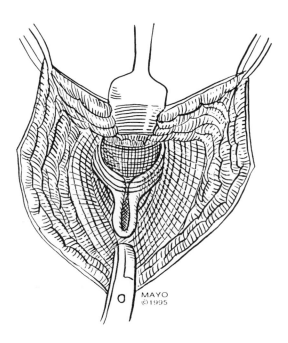

Figure 6-17.

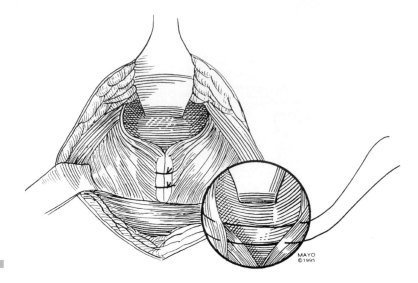

Figure 6-18.

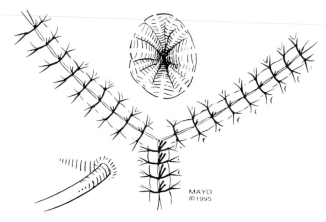

Figure 6-19.

ducted in the manner described in the previous section (see Figs. 6-13 to 6-19) and the anterior repair is performed as described earlier in this chapter (see Figs. 6-1 to 6-5). Once again, Prolene sutures are used to approximate the levator muscles across the midline posteriorly.

Results have been variable but in some hands quite acceptable. Again, the basic underlying principle here is elongation of the anal canal.

Benign Anal Stricture Causing Fecal Incontinence

Very rarely, anal strictures can cause a partial obstruction to the outflow of stool and thus overflow diarrhea and complaints of fecal incontinence. There are two straightforward methods for dealing with a simple anal stricture. The first is a V-Y anoplasty, in which a flap of perineal skin is used to reline the anal canal in order to correct the stenosis. The technique is very useful in thick and muscular men. The procedure is performed with the patient in the prone jackknife position. Local anesthesia with complete perineal and anal canal block is performed to supplement general anesthesia. The V-shaped flap is outlined as shown in Fig. 6-20. The apex of the incision is situated at the exterior excision line of the scar, and the incision is continued laterally to form a V shape. It is important that the base of the flap be very broad. Excision of the scar may sometimes be difficult, as the stenosis can be so severe that the use of a standard speculum is impossible; in that instance, a nasal speculum can be used. The flap is incised deeply to ensure that the subcutaneous fat is elevated with it

(Fig. 6-21). The flap is raised for a distance sufficient to enable the skin and subcutaneous fat to be advanced without tension to the dentate line or even just above it. Excellent hemostasis is critical. When good viability is assured, the apex of the mobilized flap is anchored to the anal canal wound at or above the dentate line using 3-0 sutures of Vicryl (Fig. 6-22).

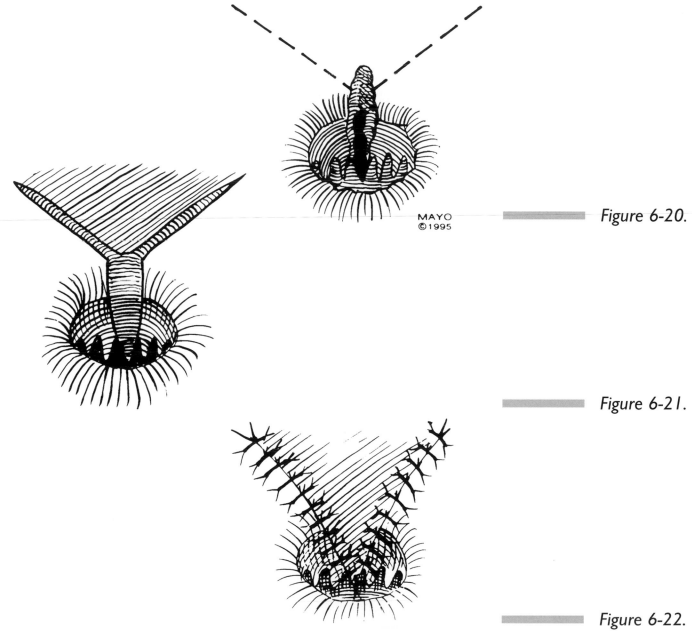

MAYO
©1995

Figure 6-20.

Figure 6-21.

Figure 6-22.

Soft perineal skin for a flap is obtained by creating a diamond advancement flap. Again, the patient is placed in the prone jackknife position and appropriate general anesthesia is used. The stricture is excised. The flap is an "island" of perianal skin with its subcutaneous fat (Fig. 6-23A). This technique can be used anywhere in the circumference of the anal canal, although it is best performed laterally. For very severe strictures, bilateral flaps are used. The technique can also be used in individuals with thin perineal skin. The incision is deepened into the subcutaneous fat (Fig. 6-23B); the perineal skin is advanced for a distance of several centimeters into the anal canal and is sutured just as in the V-Y anoplasty using absorbable 3-0 Vicryl (Fig. 6-23C & D). The results of this operation are quite satisfactory, and is actually a better technique than the V-Y plasty.

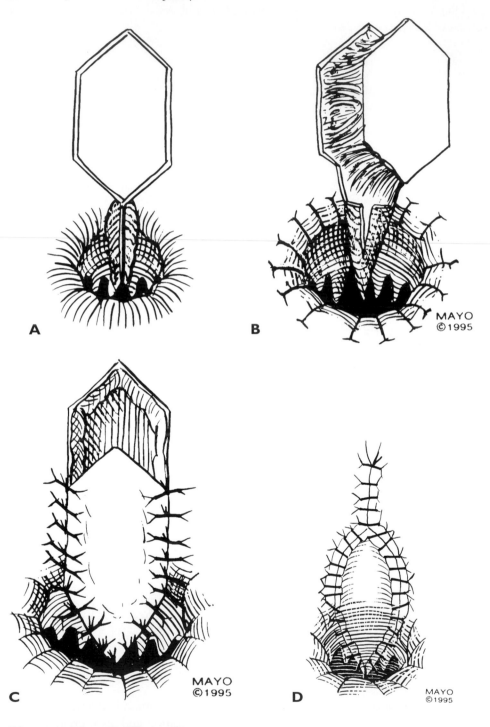

Figure 6-23.

Gluteal Muscle Transfer

In patients who have lost significant muscle mass about the anal canal as a result of trauma or congenital abnormality, several operations have been suggested to rebuild the sphincter mechanism. One is the gracilis muscle transfer, which has an uneven record of success. A newer approach is electrically stimulated gracilis muscle transfer, which holds great promise. Another strategy is gluteal muscle transfer. Here, the gluteal muscles are used to encircle the anal canal. For obvious reasons, the gluteal muscles would be more logical to use than the gracilis muscle.

The patient is placed in the prone jackknife position under general anesthesia, prepped, and draped. Bilateral parasacral incisions are made and carried deep to the level of the gluteal muscle. The lower edge of the gluteal muscle is identified and followed laterally outward bilaterally. Approximately 6 cm of muscle is incised from the origin of the muscle on the sacrum bilaterally, taking care not to interrupt the blood supply or nerve supply to the muscle during the mobilization. It is then split into two bilaterally, forming four ends of muscle. These ends are then wrapped around the anus. Separate incisions are made about the anus. A circumferential space is made at the deep level of the postanal space. The ends of muscle are then passed around the anus (Fig. 6-24). The cephalad ends of the split muscle are passed anteriorly and the more caudal ends posteriorly. This enables a scissorslike action to occur upon squeezing the gluteal muscles. The muscle ends are overlapped and sutured with nonabsorbable 2-0 sutures. Suction drains are placed in the bed of the resected muscle. The parasacral wounds are closed using 2-0 Vicryl, and those in the skin with nylon sutures. Subcuticular stitches are used to close the perianal incisions. Although this is an old operation, it has been rediscovered.

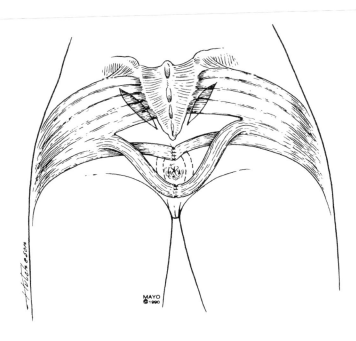

Figure 6-24.

Editorial Commentary

Dr. Pemberton correctly differentiates anterior sphincter defects from lateral and posterior defects. I entirely agree with his view that anterior sphincter defects inevitably are associated with a deficiency in the anterior component of the pelvic floor. Often there is a deficiency in the perineal body and the anus lies in close proximity to the posterior margin of the introitus. I believe that correction of these defects involves not only a flapover repair of the exter-

(Continues)

nal anal sphincter and a full anterior levatorplasty, as described by Dr. Pemberton, but also correction of the skin defect as well using a Z-plasty. Another technical point is that in order to achieve a full anterior levatorplasty, mobilization of the whole of the rectovaginal septum up to the peritoneum is absolutely essential. I also believe that a covering stoma is advisable, particularly if the end result consists of any narrowing at the anorectum. One of the real disasters of anterior levatorplasty and sphincter repair is for the patient to develop a bolus obstruction above a successful, but rather tight, repair. Attempts to clear this bolus obstruction postoperatively with enemas are extremely traumatic, and often result in a breakdown of the entire repair and sepsis in the skin. Thus, for a full anorectal reconstruction, I generally advise a covering stoma (preferably a loop ileostomy if the patient has had a full mechanical bowel preparation prior to the surgical procedure). I also adopt the jackknife position for the repair of anterior defects.

I fully agree with Dr. Pemberton that generally lateral and posterior defects simply involve full mobilization of the sphincter ring and a standard Mayo flap over the repair.

I also agree with Dr. Pemberton's comment regarding postanal repair. A technical point is the importance of dividing Waldeyer's fascia after the intersphincteric plane has been completely developed. This is essential if the rectum is to be fully mobilized off the sacral hollow, which in our experience is the only way to satisfactorily demonstrate the levator ani and the puborectalis. We tend not to use the lattice repair described by Dr. Pemberton. We use a mass closure technique to approximate both the levator ani and the puborectalis sling in the midline. This can easily be achieved if the sutures are placed and clipped but not tied until the retractor on the rectum is removed.

Total pelvic floor repair is now our operation of choice for women with postobstetric neuropathic fecal incontinence in whom the external anal sphincter is intact. Our 5-year results now suggest that only 35 percent of patients are fully continent to liquids and solids, but 70 percent of patients are substantially improved.

Although we have absolutely little experience with the gluteus muscle transfer, we have some experience with gracilis muscle transposition. I believe one of the reasons why the gracilis wrap has not been particularly successful in the past is the tendency of surgeons to wrap tendon rather than muscle belly around the anorectum. Using extensive mobilization of the gracilis muscle and employing an alpha loop, it is, in our experience, perfectly possible to wrap the anal canal with muscle rather than tendon. For the reasons stated by Dr. Pemberton I will not describe graciloplasty. However, the gracilis muscle transposition not only may play a useful role in the management of fecal incontinence where other treatments have failed, but also may be used to fill dead space on the perineum, particularly in patients with persistent perineal sinus.

At the time this was written, the stimulated gracilis neosphincter operation was in my view still experimental, and only time will tell whether the operation will join the armamentarium of the colorectal surgeon.

Michael R. B. Keighley

7

Rectal Prolapse

John H. Pemberton

Rectal prolapse is an uncommon, disabling condition that has long fascinated surgeons. Few clinical disorders have generated such a large number of surgical procedures, with varying degrees of successful outcomes, as has rectal prolapse. Only in the last few decades has our still incomplete understanding of the pathophysiology of rectal prolapse improved somewhat. That coupled with some reasonably rational surgical techniques has led to improved long-term rates of success.

Confusing terminology is a major problem in the study of rectal prolapse. The terms that must be distinguished are *mucosal prolapse, internal intussusception* (occult rectal prolapse), and *complete rectal prolapse* (procidentia). *Mucosal prolapse* is caused by a looseness or breaking down of the connective tissue between the submucosa of the rectum and anal canal and the underlying muscle. This usually starts in the anal canal and, in its earliest form, is represented by prolapsing hemorrhoids. With progression, more anal canal mucosa (hemorrhoids) and distal rectal mucosa protrude, leading to the characteristic picture of linear mucosal furrows and absence of the perianal sulcus. Mucosal prolapse does not progress to complete rectal prolapse and is best considered part of the spectrum of hemorrhoidal disease.

Internal intussusception of the rectum (occult rectal prolapse) is a distinct clinical entity that may represent the precursor of complete rectal prolapse. It can only be diagnosed reliably by obtaining a defecating proctogram. (Patients with internal intussusception should not undergo operation; the basic underlying abnormalities in pelvic floor function cannot be addressed by surgery.) *Complete rectal prolapse*, then, is defined as protrusion of the full thickness of the rectal wall through the anal orifice. It is this entity to which the various procedures described below are directed.

The goal of surgery for rectal prolapse is to correct the prolapse, avoid fecal incontinence and constipation, and do so with little or no mortality and morbidity. The operations for rectal prolapse are divided into two large categories, abdominal and perineal; each has its vocal supporters and detractors.

Although everyone seems to think they have "just the ticket" to cure prolapse, the best we can do is to choose one or two operations that seem to provide long-term relief with acceptable mortality and morbidity and that in turn do not create more problems then they solve.

This chapter describes several abdominal and perineal approaches to rectal prolapse repair. The operations I do most often are anterior resection and perineal rectosigmoidectomy; anterior resection in healthy young patients and perineal rectosigmoidectomy under opposite circumstances.

Abdominal Repair

Anterior Resection

There are many abdominal procedures for rectal prolapse. I believe the common thread winding between all such operations is the ultimate reliance upon presacral fibrosis to cure the prolapse.

Following a mechanical and antibiotic bowel preparation, and with the patient in the combined position, a midline laparotomy is performed. A nerve-preserving, relatively bloodless, nonperforating, rapid, and safe mobilization of the rectum can be accomplished if (1) the retrorectal space is sharply developed just behind the superior hemorrhoidal artery, (2) the retrosacral ligament is sharply incised, (3) the anterior dissection is carried out deep to Denonvilliers fascia, and (4) anterior and posterior dissections are completed before defining and ligating the lateral ligaments.

After freeing the sigmoid colon from any developmental lateral abdominal wall attachments, the "white line" is incised and the gonadal vessels and underlying left ureter are swept laterally (Fig. 7-1). Then, by firmly elevating the sigmoid loop, the inferior mesentery artery is stretched, making identification of the superior hemorrhoidal artery easier (Fig. 7-2). With the forceps, the tissue clinging to the superior hemorrhoidal artery is swept directly posteriorly, opening a window in the sigmoid mesentery immediately below the superior hemorrhoidal artery at the level of the aortic bifurcation. The tissue separated from the superior hemorrhoidal artery by this maneuver contains the aortic plexus and the origin of the presacral nerve and its left hypogastric nerve branch (Fig. 7-2).

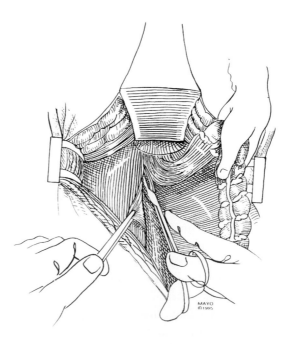

Figure 7-1.

The arch of the superior hemorrhoidal artery is followed forward toward the rectum, which, by strong upward traction, is oriented in an anterior and posterior direction. Again, using the forceps or scissors, the tissue behind the superior hemorrhoidal artery is pushed downward and once across the promontory, the presacral space is easily entered. Using the scissors, this space is developed sharply downward to about S3 and then downward and forward to the rectosacral fascia Waldeyer, at the level of S4. If easily seen, this fascia is then sharply incised. If not, the posterior dissection is carried laterally by sweeping hand motions that loosen the perirectal areolar tissue. Transecting the rectosacral fascia then allows safe, blunt finger dissection to the level of the levator raphe (Fig. 7-3). By using this technique to enter the pelvis behind the rectum, the hypogastric nerves and the hypogastric plexus are protected throughout their course.

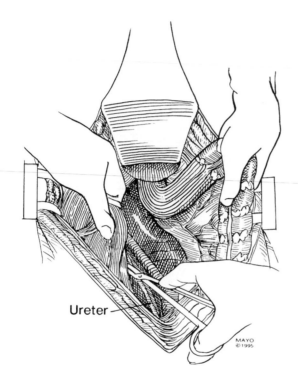

Ureter

Figure 7-2.

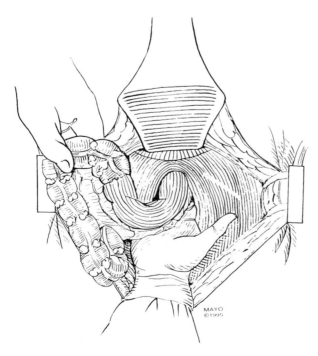

Figure 7-3.

The peritoneum on both sides of the rectum is then incised such that the incisions meet in the midline, over the rectum, in the rectovesical or vaginal pouch (Fig. 7-4). Then, sweeping hand motions from posterior to lateral are made on each side of the rectum, loosening and elevating the perirectal tissue. There are no nerves or vessels in this plane, as they lie on the pelvic sidewalls near the ureters. By elevating the rectum out of the pelvis, the lateral ligaments can be better identified.

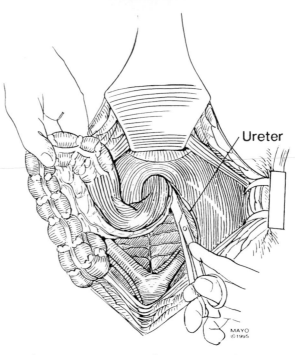

Figure 7-4.

After incising the peritoneum over the rectovesical or rectovaginal pouch (Fig. 7-5), sharp dissection is carried posteriorly toward the rectum, thus incising Denonvilliers fascia. The dissection proceeds sharply between the rectum and Denonvilliers fascia to the level of the low prostate or middle vagina. The periprostatic plexus is adjacent to this dissection, but its fibers supplying the genitalia and prostate lie deep to Denonvilliers fascia; they should, therefore, be protected by staying close to the rectum (Figs. 7-6 and 7-7).

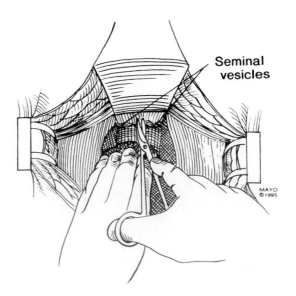

Figure 7-5.

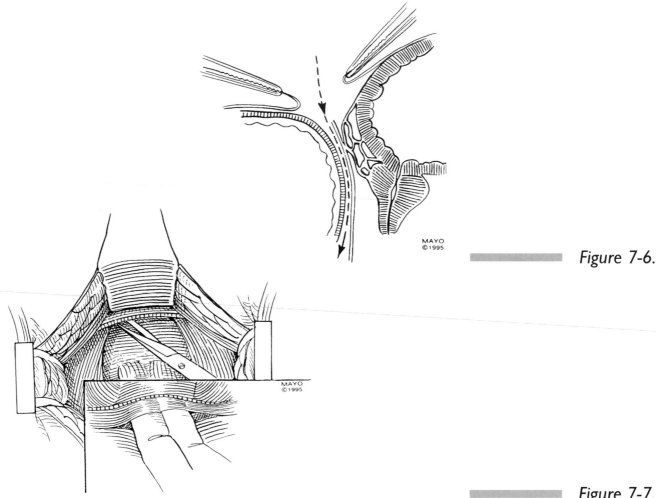

Figure 7-6.

Figure 7-7.

Only after anterior and posterior dissections are complete can the lateral ligaments be adequately defined and mobilized (Fig. 7-8). This is because traction of the rectum does not tent the ligaments if the posterior and anterior rectal attachments are present. The ligaments are defined by finger dissection and loosened *but not transected.* Complete rectal mobilization for repair of rectal prolapse, then, entails anterior mobilization to the midprostate and vagina anteriorly, and to the coccyx posteriorly and only loosening of the lateral ligaments, especially in men. It is important to remember that the pelvic plexus of nerves is quite lateral, being adjacent to the pelvic sidewalls, and that even relatively aggressive mobilization of the lateral ligaments, particularly this close to the rectum, should not result in nerve damage. At this point, the superior hemorrhoid artery and vein are clamped and ligated, taking care to confirm that the left ureter is below and lateral to the clamps (Fig. 7-9).

The anastomosis should be performed at the level of the abdominal wall. This is accomplished by tenting the rectum firmly out of the pelvis and transecting it flush with the abdominal wall (Fig. 7-10). The point of transection of the sigmoid/descending colon is likewise determined by pulling the colon out of the abdomen firmly and transecting it flush with the abdominal wall. In this way, the redundant sigmoid colon is resected. The anastomosis is then performed, usually using a hand suture technique (see Ch. 2) (Fig. 7-11). Because the levels of transection of the upper rectum and lower descending colon were determined as stated, when the anastomosis is dropped back to the pelvis, the rectum will lie in the natural curve of the pelvis without tension (Fig. 7-12). This type of anastomosis is thus a "high" anterior resection. Postoperative fibrosis in the pelvis and at the site of the anastomosis will fix the rectum to the sacrum. Finally, the deep pelvis is drained by two closed suction catheters (Fig. 7-12). I prefer to drain the pelvis until bowel function returns.

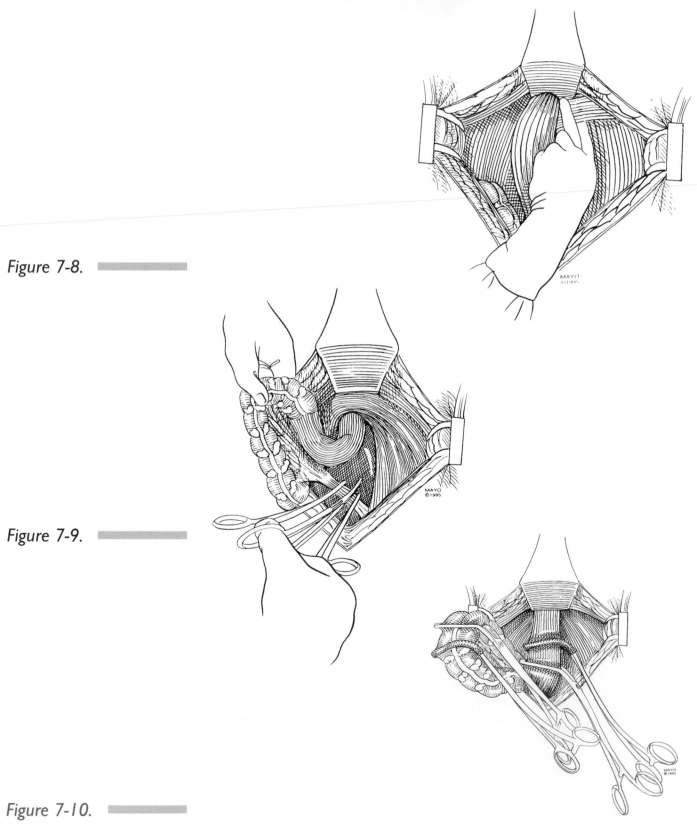

Figure 7-8.

Figure 7-9.

Figure 7-10.

Lerepai
levat
risk o
is too

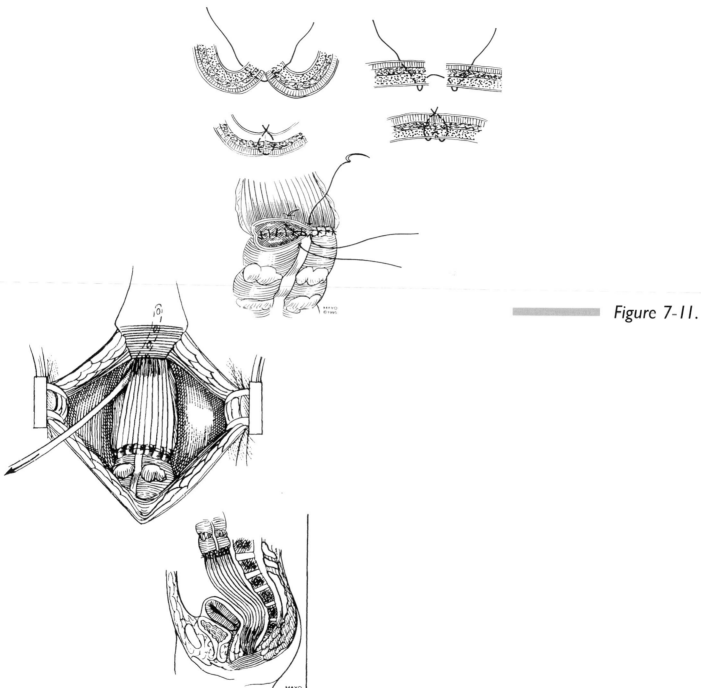

Figure 7-11.

Figure 7-12.

Note: In patients identified as having idiopathic slow-transit constipation by preoperative colon transit studies, abdominal colectomy and ileorectostomy should be considered for treatment of their complete rectal prolapse. Correcting the prolapse by anterior resection will not alleviate the problem of slow colonic transit; in fact, it may cause it to worsen postoperatively. Rather, by removing the entire colon and performing an ileorectostomy, both the prolapse and constipation are treated effectively simultaneously.

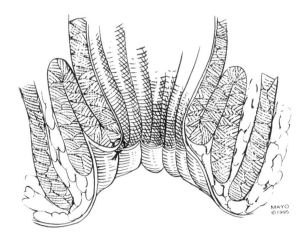

Figure 7-22.

Thiersch Procedure

The major advantage of the Thiersch procedure is that it is done with the patient under local anesthesia. Incisions are made with the patient in the lithotomy or in the prone jackknife position. Usually, two incisions are made, anterior and posterior to the anus, at the level of the anal verge. Encircling material, either silk fascia, tendon, nylon, Teflon, or Dacron or Dacron-reinforced Silastic (pictured) is passed through the ischiorectal fossa bilaterally and through the superficial or deep postanal space (Fig. 7-23) and stapled or tied over the surgeon's finger as shown in Figure 7-24. The

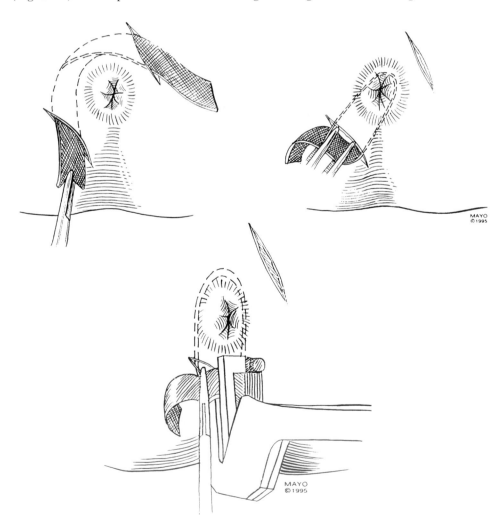

Figure 7-23.

Figure 7-24.

artificial material rests around the entire sphincter apparatus, as shown in Figure 7-25. The incisions are then closed.

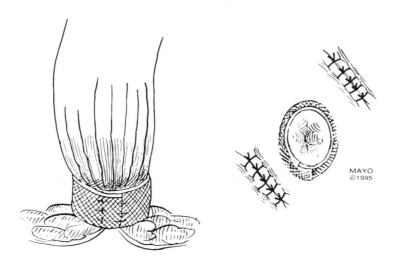

Figure 7-25.

There is little doubt that the Thiersch operation has fallen into disfavor: The material erodes and the patient becomes hopelessly obstructed. The procedure is included for historic purposes only. Today with the perineal rectosigmoidectomy procedure readily performed, there is little reason to do the Thiersch operation.

Placement of Artificial Material

The Ivalon sponge wrap and the Ripstein procedure are basically the same, although they use different materials to attempt to anchor the rectum and to cause the intense scarring in the presacral space that prevents future prolapse. The rectum and the sigmoid colon are mobilized in the usual fashion to the coccyx posteriorly and to the midvagina or midprostate anteriorly, and the lateral stalks are mobilized completely as described. Then, a sheet of Ivalon sponge (used in Europe only) or Marlex mesh material (approximately 5 cm wide and 12 to 15 cm in length) is affixed to the sacrum using interrupted sutures of 2-0 Prolene (Figs. 7-26 and 7-27).

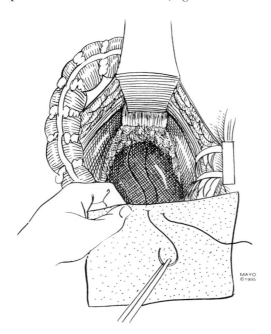

Figure 7-26.

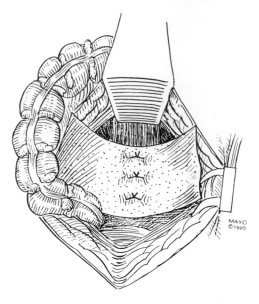

Figure 7-27. ▬▬▬▬

Perhaps the most important part of the operation is the attachment of mesh to the rectum. Complete encircling of the rectum with artificial material is a technical error and should not be performed because it causes a stricture. The "wings" of the artificial material are positioned such that they do not wrap completely around the rectum and are attached to the sides of the rectum (Fig. 7-28). The peritoneum is reconstructed after each procedure.

The position of the mobilized rectum in the pelvis after the Ripstein procedure is shown in Figure 7-28. There are many variations of rectopexy, but as the Ripstein procedure classically does not include resection of the sigmoid colon, we do not perform this operation at all, believing that resection and rectopexy (sutured or not) is the procedure of choice.

Coloanal Anastomosis for Solitary Rectal Ulcer

The standard approaches for repair of rectal prolapse are not always appropriate for patients with solitary rectal ulcer, as the ulcer causes intense inflammation about the perirectal tissues. This area needs to be resected, particularly if there is bleeding or

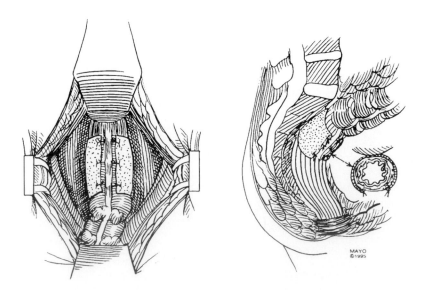

Figure 7-28. ▬▬▬▬

stenosis, and not merely mobilized; thus, coloanal anastomosis is indicated, although it is a bit aggressive.

Mobilization of the rectum past the coccyx posteriorly, and the low vagina or prostate anteriorly, is performed in a manner no different from that described for ulcerative colitis (see Ch. 12). A mucosal resection is performed utilizing the Lone Star or Gelpi retractor beginning at approximately 1 to 2 cm above the dentate line and proceeding for a distance of approximately 5 to 6 cm (Fig. 7-29). Figure 7-30 shows the area of solitary rectal ulcer, low in the rectum.

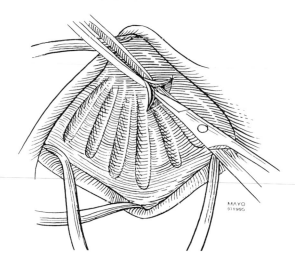

Figure 7-29.

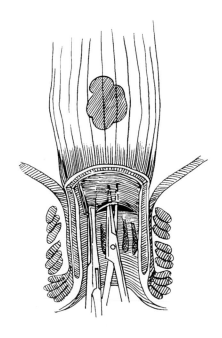

Figure 7-30.

The use of a colonic J-pouch depends on whether the bowel brought to the dentate line is sigmoid colon or descending colon. If it is sigmoid colon, then a J-pouch should be performed in the relatively straightforward maneuver, depicted in Figure 7-31: a single apically fired GIA-70 staple is used to form the very short (6 to 7 cm) limbed colon pouch. The coloanal anastomosis is usually performed by hand in the anal canal (Fig. 7-32). The anatomy at completion is shown in Figure 7-33. Alternatively, a circular stapled technique (Fig. 7-34) may be used. After coloanal anastomosis by either method, transabdominal suction drainage and diverting loop ileostomy are performed.

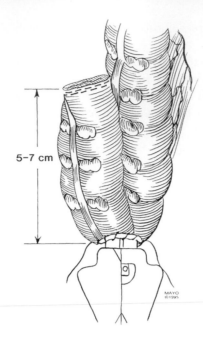

Figure 7-31.

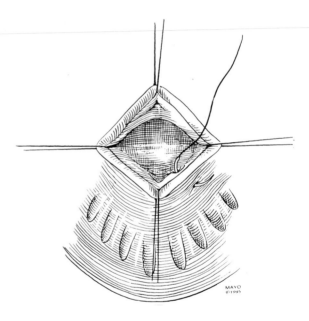

Figure 7-32.

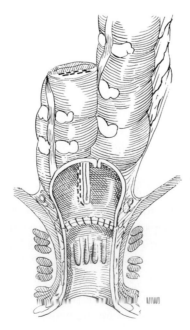

Figure 7-33.

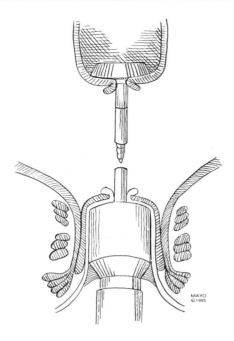

Figure 7-34.

Editorial Commentaries

I like Dr. Pemberton's classification of rectal prolapse (intermucosal, internal intussusception, and complete). I do, however, believe the complete rectal prolapse should be subdivided into short complete and full complete. Short complete rectal prolapse does not include the rectovaginal peritoneal pouch within the prolapse and as such, the operation of the perineal rectosigmoidectomy is actually quite difficult because the sigmoid colon is never encountered. By contrast, full complete rectal prolapse has an anterior bulge to it, signifying that the rectovaginal pouch has come right out through the anorectum. Once this sign is evident one can be fairly certain that the perineal rectosigmoidectomy will go well, the peritoneal pouch easily opened, and the sigmoid colon delivered.

I certainly agree that an internal intussusception is no indication for surgical intervention.

It is also worth reminding our readers that complete rectal prolapse is always associated with a patulous anus. Hence, sphincter function is always compromised. Thus, a decision concerning the most appropriate operation must take into consideration the fact that although some recovery of sphincter function may occur after an operation for rectal prolapse, continence may still be compromised.

I do believe that there are some very elderly frail patients in whom operations for rectal prolapse can be quite satisfactorily performed under spinal or epidural anesthetic.

Anterior resection is, I think, a bad name for the operation that Dr. Pemberton describes. In effect, Dr. Pemberton is describing a full rectopexy without suturing the rectum to the presacral fascia and with a complete sigmoidectomy. The main objection to resection for the treatment of rectal

(Continues)

prolapse is, of course, the risk of an anastomotic dehiscence, which although very low is still a real threat in the elderly, infirm patient.

Resection rectopexy is, in my opinion, the operation of choice for all patients in whom there is a history of coexisting constipation. In our experience it is unnecessary to perform a full anterior resection. If the rectum is mobilized down to the tip of the coccyx and the lateral ligaments are divided close to the rectum, the whole of the rectum can be pulled up without disturbing the rectovaginal pouch or engaging in rectoprostatic dissection. We have moved away from using foreign materials such as Ivalon and Marlex and now entirely rely on sutures placed between the presacral fascia in the midline and the mesorectum after the rectum has been forcibly pulled upward and out of the pelvis.

In our institution, perineal rectosigmoidectomy is nearly always performed with the patient in the prone jackknife position. Instead of using Babcock tissue forceps as described by Dr. Pemberton, we tend to place sutures through the rectal prolapse as a form of traction because we found it causes less damage to the tissues. We use a liberal supply of bupivacaine with epinephrine (1:200,000) because this cuts down the amount of bleeding and provides some postoperative analgesia. The infiltration of bupivacaine with epinephrine is not merely confined to the mucosa and submucosa beyond the dentate line but also is used to infiltrate the pelvic floor as well. We divide the mesorectum between the curved artery forceps and fully divide the bowel until an anterior and posterior levatorplasty is performed. Great care must be exercised in ensuring that the levatorplasty is not too tight, and this should be tested with a finger inside the bowel before the rectum and sigmoid are amputated prior to coloanal anastomosis. In our experience the main functional problem of perineal rectosigmoidectomy is that the patient is left without any form of rectal reservoir. The luminal diameter of the upper sigmoid colon, which is usually used for coloanal anastomosis, is quite small and many of these patients do suffer from urgency.

We have very little experience with the Delormé operation and have been discouraged from adopting it by the high recurrence rate now reported.

The Theirsch procedure is, I believe, now a totally outmoded operation. Either the material around the anus is too tight and the patient becomes constipated or the material around the anus erodes through, extrudes, and becomes infected. Alternatively, it is not tight enough, and the prolapse recurs.

In our experience, great care should be undertaken in selecting the right operation for patients with rectal prolapse. I believe this is one operation where the surgical procedure must be tailored to physiologic needs, thus evaluation of pudendal nerve latency, anorectal sensation, rectal emptying, perineal descent, and colonic transit is essential. If the prolapse patient is incontinent, then, I think, a perineal rectosigmoidectomy is optimum so that some form of levatorplasty may be undertaken at the time of removing the prolapse. If, on the other hand, the patient is constipated and if there is objective evidence of impaired colonic transit then some form of abdominal approach is essential. Under these circumstances, we usually perform a resection rectopexy, but if the degree of colonic inertia is extensive then an extended left hemicolectomy or even subtotal colectomy may be performed.

The role of laparoscopy should be addressed in the management of rectal prolapse. There is no doubt that a retrorectal dissection may be effectively performed, thus a laparoscopic rectopexy does appear feasible. Only time will tell whether the recurrence rates are unacceptably high, as I suspect they may be. The one major problem with the laparoscopic approach to rectopexy is that the degree of upward traction on the mobilized rectum achieved laparoscopically at the time of fixation of the rectum to the presacral fascia may be inadequate.

I welcome the rather aggressive approach to solitary rectal ulcer described by Dr. Pemberton. In our experience the results of rectopexy are awful in patients with solitary rectal ulcer and we agree that resection is certainly indicated if the ulcer is complicated by stenosis or bleeding. Thus, rectal excision and coloanal anastomosis in our experience is the procedure of first choice in complicated solitary rectal ulcer and if it is possible we construct a colonic reservoir because a pouch coloanal anastomosis does provide the best functional result.

Michael R. B. Keighley

Our routine operation for total rectal prolapse is the Loygue operation. The following description is taken, with modification, from *Robin Smith's Operative Surgery*, 5th edition, edited by L.P. Fielding and S.M. Goldberg (Butterworth and Heinemann, Oxford, UK, 1994, pp. 718–720).

With the patient supine, the surgeon stands on the left side and the first assistant stands on the right. A midline incision extending from the pubic symphysis to the epigastric region is made, after which the patient is tilted into a moderate head-down position. A self-retaining retractor is placed and the small bowel is packed into the upper abdomen.

The sigmoid colon and mesocolon are mobilized from the posterior parietal peritoneum. The rectum is then mobilized as far down as possible anteriorly and posteriorly by dissection in its sheath. The rectal peritoneum is first incised along its line of reflection from the pelvic wall to the rectum. The incision is in the shape of an inverted U. The peritoneal incision begins on the right side of the base of the mesosigmoid immediately lateral to the inferior mesenteric artery, continues, close to the right side of the rectum, to the pouch of Douglas, and then comes back up on the left side. The presacral connective tissue is opened just in front of the presacral fascia on the right side at the beginning of the peritoneal incision immediately behind the inferior mesenteric vessels, which are carefully preserved. The presacral nerve remains posteriorly. The rectum is then mobilized posteriorly down to the levator ani muscle, taking care not to tear the presacral veins. Anteriorly, dissection exposes the posterior vaginal wall or the fascia of Denonvilliers. Laterally, the lateral ligaments can usually be preserved. If any vascular ligatures are necessary to ease the mobilization of the rectum, they should be carried out close to the bowel wall so as not to injure the parasympathetic nerves. Dissection can be more difficult in patients with a previous hysterectomy.

(Continues)

A 1-cm-wide nylon strip is then sutured as far down as possible on each side of the rectum using a double row of four or five nonabsorbable stitches over a length of 5 cm. Sutures are placed directly into the muscularis of the rectum and not into the perirectal fat. Gentle traction on the rectum must be able to pull up the anterior reflection line of the peritoneum up to the level of the sacral promontory. The two nylon strips are then sutured, under moderate tension and as far from the midline as possible, to the prevertebral fascia, but not to the intervertebral disc itself. Four nonresorbable stitches are used. Care must be taken not to tear the iliac vein during this step of the procedure.

The posterior peritoneum of the uterus in women and of the bladder in men is resected and the pouch of Douglas is obliterated by suturing the peritoneal edges together. One or two closed suction drains are left in place in the retroperitoneal space for 2 to 3 days. The posterior peritoneum is closed, covering the nylon strips, and then the abdominal wall is closed.

Rolland Parc

8

Constipation

Rolland Parc

Principles

Hirschsprung's Disease (Congenital Megacolon)

Diagnosis. Hirschsprung's disease is an autosomal dominant condition characterized by a marked dilatation of the colon proximal to a narrowed segment in which ganglion cells are absent. Although rare, it offers one of the clearest indications for operative management of constipation. Most individuals have a history of constipation and enema use. In some cases, fecalomas may lead to sigmoid volvulus or may require manual evacuation. The diagnosis of Hirschsprung's disease is usually easy in the adult patient. In its most common form, the aganglionic segment starts at the junction of the rectum and anus, but it can extend as far as the midsigmoid (Fig. 8-1). On barium enema examination the diseased segment appears of normal caliber; however, the bowel proximal to the diseased segment appears very large and contains a large amount of fecal residue. Long-term misdiagnosis may occur if lateral views are omitted from the barium examination, because in the anteroposterior view the nondilated diseased segment may lie hidden behind an enlarged upper sigmoid colon, filling the pouch of Douglas.

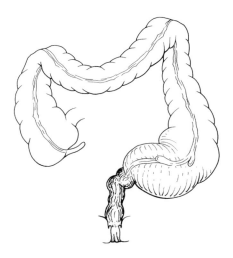

Figure 8-1.

165

Anorectal physiologic studies demonstrate an absence of the rectoanal inhibitory reflex in Hirschsprung's disease. This sign, while diagnostic of Hirschsprung's disease, may be present in other disorders as well. A full-thickness rectal biopsy has traditionally been a useful method of diagnosis, but it is not necessary in all adult cases, especially if barium enema examination and anorectal manometry are diagnostic.

Surgical Treatment Options. *Swenson, Soave, and Duhamel Operations.* The Swenson operation, excision of the rectum followed by a straight coloanal anastomosis, was the first procedure used to treat Hirschsprung's disease. Total resection of the noninnervated rectum is not theoretically necessary if this nonfunctional part of the gut can be bypassed.

The Soave procedure, or internal bypass of the aganglionic zone, consists of resecting the upper rectum and performing a mucosectomy of the distal rectum to the dentate line. Normal innervated colon is thus brought down through the rectal muscular cuff.

The Duhamel procedure, or retrorectal bypass, consists of resection of the upper rectum and closure of the lower rectal stump at the level of the pouch of Douglas. A retrorectal presacral plane is developed and the proximal innervated colon is brought down to the level of the levator ani just above the sphincter ring. A colorectal anastomosis is thus created on the posterior wall of the rectum.

In all of these procedures the normal colon is anastomosed to the anus. The Swenson procedure is not commonly performed in adults because of the risk of pelvic autonomic nerve damage, which is minimized by the Soave and Duhamel procedures. The choice between the Soave and Duhamel operations is influenced by the fact that it is easier to avoid a covering stoma after the Duhamel procedure than after the Soave coloanal sleeve anastomosis. Another point in favor of the Duhamel procedure is the absence of urgency due to the preservation of a rectal reservoir, which is not the case after the Soave operation.

The Soave operation is also useful in the treatment of postirradiation rectovaginal fistula, rectal stenosis, and bleeding from rectal hemangiomas, and in patients with a very short rectal stump after the Hartmann operation. It could also be the sphincter-saving procedure of choice in cases of stenosis of a colorectal anastomosis with or without a vaginal fistula.

Anorectal Myectomy. Anorectal myectomy involves excising the internal anal sphincter and the rectal circular muscle. It is used both as a method of histopathologic diagnosis of Hirschsprung's disease and also as therapy of ultra-short-segment Hirschsprung's disease. However, in most of our patients the results have been disappointing and recurrent constipation is common.

Preoperative Bowel Preparation. Good mechanical bowel preparation is important irrespective of the type of procedure to be undertaken. Fecalomas should be evacuated preoperatively. The bowel must be rigorously cleared of residue proximal to the aganglionic segment so that the size of the colon to be brought down to the anus is of normal caliber. We use a low-residue diet and daily administration of polyethylene glycol solution, as well as daily water enemas given by a tube of sufficient length to reach the sigmoid. This tube is left in place for at least half an hour in order to achieve satisfactory evacuation. It is sometimes necessary for the tube to be left in situ for many weeks before the size of the colon becomes normal. A temporary colostomy is needed when a fecaloma is too bulky to be fragmented or when an emergency operation is necessary, as, for instance, in a patient presenting with sigmoid volvulus. The best plan, if a stoma is necessary, is to construct it at the most distal portion of the distended (innervated) colon. Sometimes it is necessary to resect the sigmoid colon if it is completely distended by fecalomas.

Idiopathic Megacolon/Megarectum

The Swenson, Soave, and Duhamel operations are also usually suitable for the relatively rare group of patients whose constipation is caused by idiopathic megacolon/megarectum. These causes must be distinguished from the more common varieties of constipation, such as slow-transit constipation (without dilatation) and outlet obstruction (amismus), since in the nondilated colon total colectomy with ileorectal anastomosis is frequently followed by recurrence of constipation, abdominal pain, and small bowel distension. Many of these patients have a motility disorder of the small as well as the large intestine, and some patients have incapacitating diarrhea after major colonic resection. In megarectum a variable amount of proximal colon is hugely dilated with fecalomas (Fig. 8-2); there is no narrow aganglionic section as in Hirschsprung's disease. For isolated megarectum the Swenson or Duhamel operation, or even the Soave procedure, appears to be satisfactory, but it is not easy to avoid damage to the presacral nerves in megarectum, particularly if the Swenson operation is to be performed. We personally prefer the Duhamel procedure, as the rectum is preserved and the risk of impotence is significantly reduced. If the dilated proximal segment involves the whole of the colon, a more extensive resection is necessary; in these cases, the proximal colon must be delivered down behind the rectal stump, or else the ileum must be used for the anastomosis.

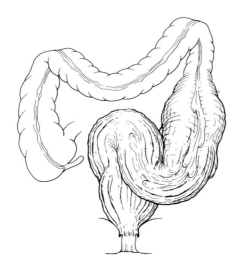

Figure 8-2.

Slow-Transit Constipation

Resection of part of the colon and rectum may be justified in carefully selected patients with long-standing constipation provided there is no evidence of impaired gastric emptying or delayed small bowel transit and provided the patient is well adjusted and psychologically stable. All of these patients undergo careful investigation, including motility and transit studies, anorectal physiologic studies, and assessment of rectal emptying. A simple psychological screening process is also advised.

If there is normal rectal emptying and the delay in transit is confined to a segment of or the whole colon, either segmental colectomy and anastomosis or subtotal colectomy and ileorectal anastomosis may be advised. If, as often occurs after hysterectomy or other pelvic operations, the delay is confined to the sigmoid and rectum and rectal evacuation is impaired, the rectum, sigmoid, and part of the left colon may be resected and a coloanal anastomosis constructed with or without a colonic pouch, and we then prefer the Duhamel procedure, as a pouch is then not necessary. Some of these patients have evidence of intermittent sigmoid volvulus and some present with repeated episodes of pseudo-obstruction, which may indicate the need for a more aggressive surgical approach.

We do not think that there is any role for resection or rectopexy in patients with impaired rectal evacuation and incomplete intussusception. Also, we do not advise repair of a rectocele alone in an attempt to correct rectal inertia in constipated patients.

Surgical Techniques

Duhamel Operation

Preoperative Bowel Preparation. For idiopathic megacolon/megarectum as well as for Hirschsprung's disease it is wise to take plenty of time to achieve a satisfactory mechanical bowel preparation. Usually the patient is given 2 L polyethylene glycol solution daily for 3 or 4 days before the operation. In some cases it may be necessary to break up a fecaloma manually or by use of a rectal tube. Repeated attempts at manual evacuation should be avoided, however, as they may cause damage to the anal sphincter and pelvic floor. On the evening before the operation the abdomen and perineum are shaved and the patient is asked to shower with povidone-iodine solution.

Positioning. The patient is placed in the lithotomy position with the hips abducted through 30 degrees of flexion for the abdominal phase of the operation. Flexion to 100 degrees is required for the perineal phase. A nasogastric tube is introduced into the stomach and a Foley catheter is placed into the bladder and strapped to the right thigh. The skin of the abdomen and perineum is prepared with povidone-iodine and the area draped to exclude the genital organs from the operative field.

Incision and Laparotomy. The surgeon stands on the patient's right side, the first assistant on the left, and the second assistant between the patient's legs. A long midline incision is made from the midepigastric region to the symphysis pubis. Any peritoneal adhesions from previous operations are gently and meticulously divided. In Hirschsprung's disease it is usually easy to identify the involved segment; a normal-sized sigmoid and extraperitoneal rectum will be observed, whereas a normally innervated and rather distended left colon will be seen lying proximal. In idiopathic megacolon/megarectum the whole rectum and a variable length of proximal colon may be seen to be enormously dilated; indeed, the anal canal itself will be dilated along with the rectum. There will be no normal-caliber distal rectum; in these cases the normally innervated bowel is the nondilated proximal colon.

Mobilization of the Left Colon. The splenic flexure must be thoroughly mobilized to provide sufficient length to the proximal colon so that there is absolutely no tension on the future coloanal anastomosis.

Mobilization of the left colon starts with incision of the peritoneum in the left paracolic gutter, dividing all anatomic adhesions (Fig. 8-3A). Great care should be taken to visualize the left ureter, not only to make sure of its position but to avoid mobilizing it. The avascular plane between the mesocolon and the perinephric fat is usually easy to define. Frequently in Hirschsprung's disease, as in idiopathic megacolon, the mesosigmoid is very long and may even be attached up to the level of the splenic flexure. If mobilization of the left colon has been performed as part of a previous surgical procedure, great care has to be taken so as not to damage the blood supply to the proximal colon. The colon is retracted to the right and using blunt and sharp dissection mobilization of the colon is continued toward the spleen. The splenic flexure is easier to free after the left side of the transverse colon is dissected from the greater omentum because this opens the lesser sac (Fig. 8-3B). Attention must be paid to Riolan's arcade and the middle colic artery. The surgeon then holds the two limbs of the splenic flexure and completes the division of all remaining adhesions. The mesentery of the left transverse colon must be mobilized to the lower border of the tail of the pancreas in order to allow easy ligation of the junction of the inferior mesenteric vein and the splenic vein under the pancreas (Fig. 8-3B, inset). This high ligation of the inferior mesenteric vein is the key maneuver for ensuring the mesocolon is of adequate length to permit the splenic flexure and the descending colon to be brought down to the pelvis without tension. There is no need to ligate the inferior mesenteric artery at its origin; its branches are divided and ligated in such a way as to preserve the arcade. The mesocolon between the branches of the inferior mesenteric vessels is divided toward the arcade. These mesenteric windows are a means of lengthening the mesocolon. If a sigmoid colostomy has been previously constructed it is taken down and temporarily closed either with staples or sutures. The small bowel is placed in the right upper part of the abdomen, covered with drapes, and kept away from the field using self-retaining retractors, leaving the colon free for subsequent rerouting.

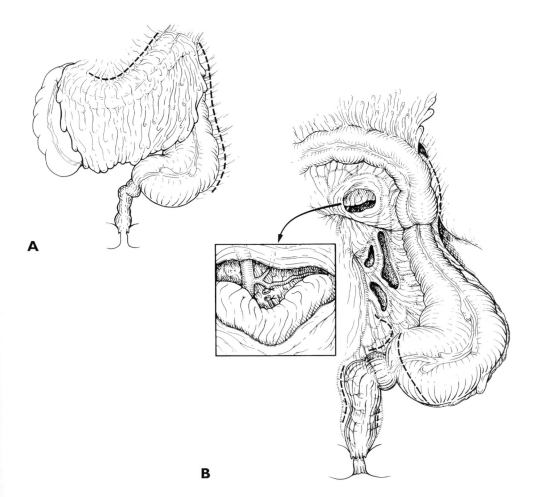

A

B

Figure 8-3.

Pelvic Dissection and Division of the Rectum (Creation of the Retrorectal Route for the Colon). The surgeon moves to the patient's left side and the first assistant to the right. The table is tilted into the Trendelenburg position. The sigmoid vessels are ligated and divided. When the rectosigmoid junction is reached, dissection is continued close to the rectal wall (Fig. 8-3B). This maneuver minimizes the risk of damage to the hypogastric nerves. By progressive division of the sigmoid vessels it is possible to stay between the two branches of the superior hemorrhoidal artery. Just behind the rectum and below the sacral promontory there is an avascular plane; with the scissors it is very easy to continue down this plane to the level of the levator ani. The mesorectum is clamped and divided at the level of the bottom of the pouch of Douglas. The peritoneum on the anterior aspect of the rectum is circumferentially divided at this level (Fig. 8-4). It is very important at this juncture to establish a wide retrorectal route for the colon by means of scissor dissection and electrocautery behind the rectum and in front of the sacrum.

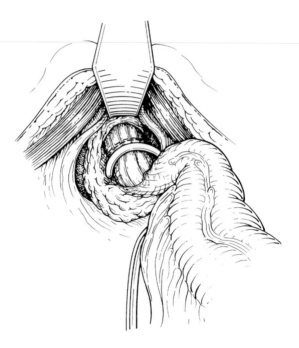

Figure 8-4.

The rectal stump below the level of the crushing clamp is washed out through the anus with povidone-iodine solution. Division of the rectum is achieved with application of a transverse stapling device (TA 55) distal to the crushing clamp. After disection of the rectum, hemostasis in the pelvis is carefully checked.

The choice of a suitable site for division of the colon is dependent on both the size of the colon and the quality of its proximal blood supply. We usually divide a small mesenteric vessel adjacent to the colon in order to visualize the blood flow within the divided vessel. If the proximal colon is not too dilated, as in Hirschsprung's disease, we usually retain the upper half of the descending colon. If the end of the colon can reach 10 cm below the front of the symphysis pubis without tension, there will be no problem with colonic length and subsequent coloanal anastomosis (Fig. 8-5). The colon is then divided, with a further transverse stapling device applied proximal to the crushing clamp on the descending colon. In Hirschsprung's disease the proximal end of the specimen should be checked histologically to ensure that there is no evidence of aganglionosis.

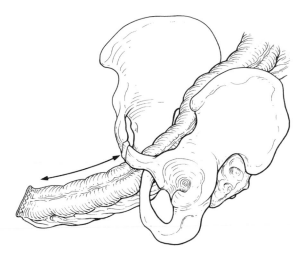

Figure 8-5.

Retrorectal Dissection, Construction of the Retrorectal Tunnel, and Exteriorization of the Colon. The surgeon next moves to the perineum after flexing the patient's hips to 100 degrees. Two Gelpi retractors are applied at 90 degrees to one another on the anal margin. The dentate line is thus clearly identified. Saline containing a weak epinephrine solution (1:10,000) is injected into the submucosa to float the mucosa off the muscularis propria on the posterior half of the anus. Using scissors, the mucosa is then divided at the level of the dentate line on the posterior hemicircumference of the anus. By sharp scissor dissection, the mucosa is freed from the internal sphincter to the upper limit of the sphincter ring (Fig. 8-6). A 25-mm-diameter tunnel is necessary.

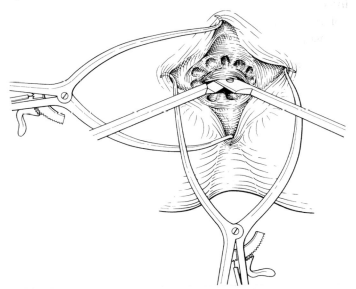

Figure 8-6.

An assistant working at the abdomen then passes a pair of scissors down to the levator ani inside the puborectalis within the retrorectal space. By performing this maneuver it is very easy for the surgeon to repair the upper limit of the sphincter ring and to join the retrorectal and retroanal spaces by opening the posterior wall of the rectum through the anus (Fig. 8-7). This is safely achieved by pushing a pair of scissors through the anus or by cutting the rectal muscular layer on the surface of the abdominal scissors. Once the plane is established, long scissors are used to open the defect in the posterior rectal wall further and obtain a wide rectal muscular orifice.

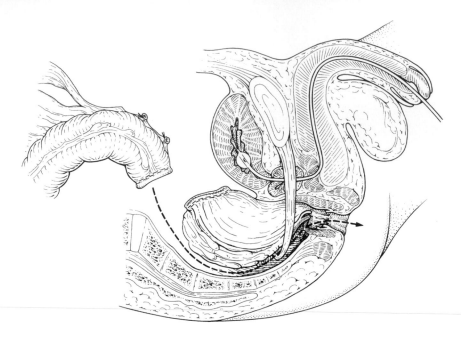

Figure 8-7.

A pair of forceps is introduced through the anus, the posterior rectal wall, and the retrorectal space so as to reach the abdomen and grasp the stapled colon, which is then delivered down and exteriorized 10 cm outside the anus. A finger introduced into the anus and directed toward the retrorectal space is sometimes helpful in exteriorizing the colon.

In order to avoid the risks of dehiscence of the anastomosis and subsequent pelvic infection, and also to avoid a covering stoma, the anastomosis is postponed and the colon is left out of the anus for 14 days. The stapled distal end of the colon, once opened, thus works as a perineal colostomy.

Postoperative Care. Antimicrobial prophylaxis is given perioperatively and for a day after the operation. Intravenous infusion and nasogastric aspiration are maintained until normal bowel function returns. Due to the tone of the anal sphincter and edema of the exteriorized colon, it is often necessary to pass a tube into the descending colon in order for the perineal colostomy to function. We usually remove the pelvic suction drains after 2 days, and the urinary catheter when the patient is mobile.

Completion of the Operation. The patient is returned to the operating room 14 days later for construction of the side-to-side colorectal anastomosis and the coloanal anastomosis. The spur between the anterior descending colon and the rectum is divided and stapled using a linear staple cutter (e.g., PLC, Ethicon; GIA, Autosuture). One of the stapler forks is introduced into the posterior aspect of the anorectum while the second fork is introduced through a small enterotomy made in the distal exteriorized retrorectal colon (Fig. 8-8). The stapler is fired and the anastomosis is checked by palpation. The residual redundant colon is excised and the end sutured to the defect in the posterior rectum using an intra-anal suture technique (partial coloanal anastomosis), as described in Chapter 2. It is often unnecessary to suture the colon to the anus, as further adhesions may have developed between the colon and the anus while the colon was exteriorized. Drainage is not mandatory.

The patient should be allowed a normal diet the first postoperative day. Full continence and normal bowel function are to be expected a couple of weeks later. Any modification in frequency of bowel movements mandates a digital examination of the anastomosis. Any stretching can be easily checked by an application of the linear staple cutter.

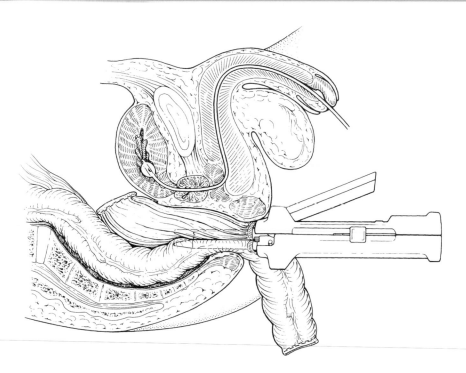

Figure 8-8.

Soave Operation

Many steps of the Soave procedure are similar to those of the Duhamel operation. The pelvic phase is specific, especially when this operation is used after a failed colorectal anastomosis.

The Patient with No Previous Rectal Resection. The principal indications for the Soave operation are postirradiation rectal damage (i.e., stenosis, rectovaginal fistula, or hemorrhage), and benign rectal diseases (e.g., hemangiomas). The colonic dissection is conducted in the same way as for the Duhamel operation. Resection of the rectum is limited to its intraperitoneal aspect and the vessels are divided in close proximity to the muscular layer of the rectum.

Frequently the infraperitoneal part of the rectum is surrounded by fibrosis, especially in postirradiation proctitis, and it is not easy to establish a plane of dissection between the rectum and ureters and between the rectum and the presacral veins. In hemangiomas of the rectum, the bowel is surrounded by huge veins and the perirectal space is very bloody. For these reasons, when the distal limit of the pouch of Douglas is reached during the abdominal resection, a crushing clamp is applied to the rectum at this point. The distal part of the rectum is then washed out transanally using a solution of povidone-iodine. The muscular layer of the rectum is then circumferentially divided below the clamp (Fig. 8-9). Every effort is made to stay in the submucosal plane when removing the rectal mucosa from the distal rectal stump. In hemangiomas of the rectum, however, this space is occupied by huge vessels and so it is safer to make the dissection in the intermuscular plane between the longitudinal and circular fibers of the rectum, where the veins are less prominent.

Mucosectomy of the distal rectum, with or without the internal part of the muscular cuff, is commenced by the abdominal route and carried down as far as possible toward the anus. The mucosa is divided at the endpoint of the dissection and the specimen is delivered through the abdomen. The level of the colonic section for application of the stapler for coloanal anastomosis is chosen as described for the Duhamel procedure. The remaining steps are performed transanally and are described later.

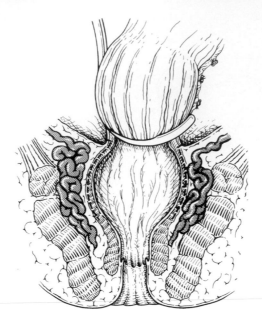

Figure 8-9.

The Patient with a Previous Rectal Resection. The Soave procedure can be very helpful as a method of restoring intestinal continuity in cases of stricture at a previous colorectal anastomosis. The operation may also be useful in the treatment of rectovaginal fistula, provided, of course, that there is no evidence of recurrence or residual tumor.

The first maneuver is to mobilize the colon down to the level of the previous anastomosis, bearing in mind that the vascular pedicle will be running beside the colon. When the dissection reaches the level of the anastomosis the bowel is merely divided at this point and the colon delivered from the pelvis into the wound without any attempt to dissect around the rectal stump.

In our experience it is very dangerous to attempt dissection of the rectal stump low in the pelvis because it is invariably encased in fibrotic tissues and the ureters are at risk of being damaged. To open the stenosed anastomotic site and commence the mucosectomy, we usually stretch the stricture by introducing a pair of long scissors into the rectum from above. By forcing the scissors open it is possible to create an opening large enough to admit three fingers (Fig. 8-10). If this cannot be done, it will be impossible to deliver the proximal colon through the rectal stump. If necessary, a vertical midline incision can be made in the posterior rectal wall.

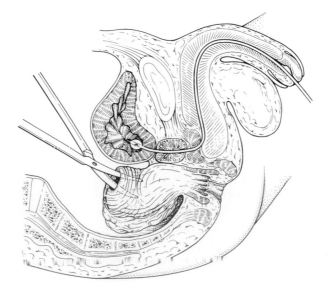

Figure 8-10.

The mucosectomy is then started from above through the abdomen and is carried down as described above. In the case of a rectovaginal fistula, no attempt is made to close the defect in the vagina.

In the case of reoperation for restoration of digestive continuity after a very low Hartmann procedure (especially a salvage procedure for sepsis) or after a very low colorectal anastomosis, it might be difficult and dangerous to find the rectal stump. In most male patients and also in hysterectomized women, the bladder covers the rectal stump. In such cases it is helpful to place a bougie in the rectal stump transanally; by exerting pressure on the apex an incision can be made over the bougie, thereby avoiding damage to the bladder (Fig. 8-11). Thereafter, a pair of long scissors can be introduced to stretch the apex of the short rectal stump, as already described. If there is extensive fibrosis and the bladder is densely adherent, we some-times deliberately open the bladder through the space of Retzius to ascertain the position of the trigone.

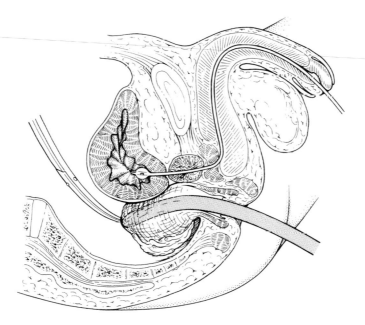

Figure 8-11.

The Patient with a Previous Colonic Resection. In some patients the sigmoid and descending colon may have been resected previously or there may be damage from previous irradiation that requires excision at the time of the Soave procedure. It is possible to bring the transverse colon down to the anus by dividing all attach-ments of the omentum to the transverse mesocolon so that a straight length of bowel, supplied by the right colic artery, to the arcade of Riolan is available for anastomosis. The shortest route for the colon is through a hole in the mesentery (Fig. 8-12). A window large enough for the colon and its mesentery is then made in front of the midjejunum. If the colon is very short it may be necessary to divide the right colic artery to enable the proximal colon to be brought down to the anus. If the right colic artery is divided the arcades in the mesentery must be preserved so that the end of the colon can be adequately supplied through the ileocolic arteries. The ascending colon and hepatic flexure will thus remain well vascularized. After being fully mobilized the right colon is then delivered over the right pelvic brim and taken through the rectal stump to reach the anus (Fig. 8-13). Despite this quite extensive resection, the functional results of this type of coloanal anastomo-sis are often quite satisfactory.

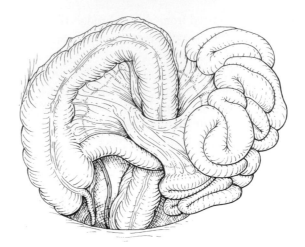

Figure 8-12. ▬▬▬▬▬

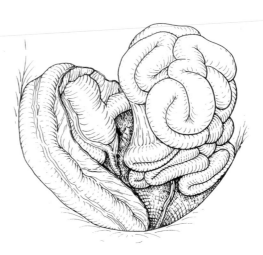

Figure 8-13. ▬▬▬▬▬

Distal Rectal Mucosectomy and Straight Coloanal Anastomosis. The patient's hips are flexed and two Gelpi retractors are then applied to the anal margin. A weak epinephrine solution (1:300,000) is injected into the submucosa around the full circumference of the anus. The mucosa of the anorectum is then circumferentially removed from just above the dentate line using sharp scissor dissection. The mucosectomy continues upward until the abdominal mucosectomy is reached. The denuded rectal stump should allow passage of three fingers from the anus to the top of the stump. If this is not achieved, the maneuvers described previously are repeated. Once the wide rectal muscular tube has been created, a Duval forceps introduced through the anus is used to grasp the distal end of the colon and bring it down to the dentate line. An interrupted hand-sewn coloanal anastomosis is performed between the full thickness of the colon and the anal mucosa, taking bites of the muscular layer and using absorbable sutures (see Ch. 2). Four sutures are initially placed at the 3-, 6-, 9-, and 12-o'clock positions; subsequently, sutures are added to each of the four quadrants (Fig. 8-14). A soft drainage tube is placed from above into the rectal sleeve down to the level of the anastomosis and is left on suction for 1 to 2 days.

Drainage and Temporary Ileostomy. Where possible, two suction drains are placed between the colon and the rectal cuff. If this is not possible, the drains should be placed as deeply as possible in the pelvis and brought out through the iliac fossa opposite the temporary ileostomy site.

If the mesocolon is very loose its free border should be sutured to the posterior peritoneal wall, especially around the duodenojejunal flexure so as to avoid postoper-

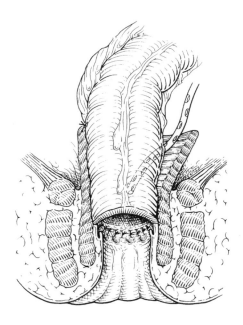

Figure 8-14.

ative obstruction by entrapment of the jejunum behind the mesocolon. Similarly, the colon should be fixed to the posterior abdominal wall where it descends through the small bowel mesentery.

Anorectal Myectomy

Anorectal myectomy entails removal of a strip of internal sphincter and rectal circular muscle, which is then sent for histologic examination to exclude Hirschsprung's disease. It is not used therapeutically.

The procedure should not be attempted unless the rectum has been emptied. A small transverse incision is made at the dentate line and the lower margin of the anal skin is retracted downward, exposing the lower fibers of the internal anal sphincter (Fig. 8-15). The submucosal plane is then developed for about 10 cm using scissors; if necessary, the third blade of the intra-anal retractor can be placed underneath the mucosa so as to expose the circular muscular fibers. The intersphincteric plane is then opened for a similar length so as to allow a noncrushing clamp to be applied to the visceral muscle. The muscle is then retracted with scissors and the distal end of the strip is marked with a suture (Fig. 8-16). Finally, hemostasis is achieved and the transverse anal incision is closed with a running absorbable suture.

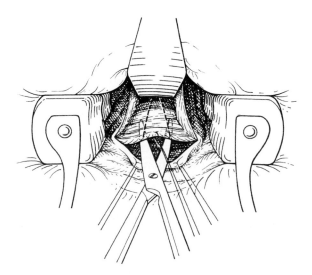

Figure 8-15.

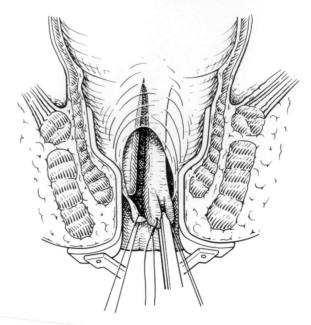

Figure 8-16.

Subtotal Colectomy and Ileorectal Anastomosis or Segmental Colectomy

Segmental colectomy may occasionally be indicated for localized colonic stasis. However, in our limited experience, results are more predictable following subtotal colectomy and ileorectal anastomosis, as described in Chapter 10. Colonic resection may be the operation of choice for megacolon with a normal-caliber rectum, and is also used for slow-transit constipation when rectal evacuation is normal.

Extended Proctosigmoidectomy and Coloanal Anastomosis With or Without a Pouch

This option, which is described for low rectal carcinoma in Chapter 10, may be indicated for megarectum and for a normal-caliber colon. The operation might also be indicated for delayed transit confined to the rectum and sigmoid colon.

Editorial Commentaries

I agree with most of Professor Parc's account of the management of Hirschsprung's disease. The absence of ganglia in the lower segment of an anorectal myectomy specimen as an indicator of Hirschsprung's disease should be viewed with caution because ganglia at this site are normally sparse. Some of us are quite skeptical about the label "ultra-short-segment Hirschsprung's disease" and wonder if it really is a disease entity. Although we have no experience with the Duhamel operation we do use the Soave procedure, usually taking the rectum lower than in the above description. Low transection makes mucosectomy much easier and enables a colonic pouch to be accommodated above the coloanal anastomosis. We always advise the creation of a colonic reservoir and frequently perform an anal transection with the linear stapler and a stapled coloanal anastomosis, which avoids a mucosectomy altogether. However, the double-staple technique is only feasible in Hirschsprung's disease because the tissues are too thick for stapling in acquired megarectum.

Adult megacolon and megarectum is quite different from Hirschsprung's disease. We agree that it is frequently a panenteric autonomic neuropathy sometimes associated with dilated ureters and a large atonic bladder. Many patients with megabowel in our experience have coexisting neurologic disorders. The presentation is one of chronic constipation, abdominal distension due to colonic impaction, and where there is megarectum, a huge fecaloma. The condition and its prognosis are quite different from slow-transit constipation. We find preoperative physiologic assessment impossible because of the presence of the fecaloma. We do not believe that the fecaloma should be extracted before operation for fear of damaging an already-compromised anal sphincter. Thus, we use no preoperative mechanical bowel preparation and merely milk the fecaloma back into the dilated bowel, which is then resected. Following resection, on-table lavage is used to clear fecal material from the proximal nondilated bowel. Great care must be taken during rectal mobilization because of the presence of huge pararectal veins, which will bleed extensively unless they are ligated prior to rectal transection. In megarectum there is no normal anal canal. The grossly dilated rectum terminates in a wide and very thick-walled anus. Stapling is impossible; we, therefore, prefer construction of a small (10-cm) colonic pouch and sutured coloanal anastomosis, often without a mucosectomy.

Patients with slow-transit constipation should be told that surgical treatment is rarely successful, apart from achieving more frequent spontaneous bowel movements. The symptoms of nausea, abdominal pain, and abdominal distension almost always persist after colectomy. Furthermore, most patients with slow-transit constipation have a major psychological disturbance, irritable bowel syndrome, impaired small bowel transit, and defective rectal emptying. In addition, most of these patients are articulate and manipulative, and pressure the surgeon to do something based on an unreliable history. In a very few patients, colectomy may be justified provided there are no underlying psychological factors, the motility disorder is confined to the colon, and the patient is prepared to accept a stoma if necessary. We have found segmental colectomy to give poor results even in patients with an isolated area of impaired transit and recommend subtotal colectomy and ileorectal anastomosis in those few patients in whom resection is considered justified.

Michael R. B. Keighley

In general, Professor Parc's descriptions of the different operative approaches for patients with Hirschsprung's disease and constipation are straightforward and provide few areas of disagreement. I do believe, however, that although the absence of a rectoanal inhibitory reflex is a helpful sign, confirmation of Hirschsprung's disease by biopsy should be done in all cases before an extensive operation is undertaken. I agree entirely that the proximal level of resection needs to be controlled by histologic confirmation of the presence of ganglion cells. Of course, the approach and specifics of anastomosis vary from surgeon to surgeon, and I feel that Professor Parc's approach is an excellent one.

(Continues)

I disagree that anything other than a colectomy and ileorectostomy is not indicated for patients with slow-transit constipation. As Professor Parc states toward the end of the chapter, better results are obtained with ileorectal anastomosis for this problem than with segmental colectomy, and I couldn't agree more. I agree, too, that there is no operation indicated for occult intussusception and that rectocele repair is not indicated if it alone is responsible for difficulty with evacuation. Often such difficulties with evacuation are physiologically and not anatomically based.

John H. Pemberton

9

Rectal Polyps

Rolland Parc

Many of the operations used to treat polyps are described elsewhere in this book; however, seven procedures will be briefly described herein. They include intrarectal polypectomy snare, intra-(trans-)anal excision, posterior rectotomy, transsphincteric excision, sleeve mucosectomy (intrarectal), sleeve mucosectomy (prolapse), and resection.

Minimally Invasive Surgery

Some midrectal polyps are now managed using water-filled or gas-filled endorectal excision; trasanal endoscopic microsurgery (TEM) although this technique has its advocates, we believe that most polyps can in fact be managed by perianal and conventional intrarectal procedures.

Laparoscopy

Laparoscopy has been advocated for resection of large polyps with high-grade dysplasia or even malignant change. The whole question of laparoscopic resection for carcinoma is currently hotly debated. Provided resections can be performed as entirely closed procedures where there is no risk of seeding malignant cells, laparoscopic resection certainly does offer an important therapeutic avenue. Laparoscopic techniques are discussed further in Chapter 3.

Intrarectal Polypectomy

The patient has a full mechanical bowel preparation. A diagnostic sigmoidoscopy is performed. Polypectomy is then undertaken with an insulated sigmoidoscope and a loop diathermy snare. Once the neck of the polyp has been grasped by the snare (Fig. 9-1), the current is applied and the polyp is excised and retrieved. After the procedure careful attention must be paid to the diathermized stalk to ensure that there is no bleeding and that the rectal wall has not been tented, a situation that might result in rectal perforation unless the base of the polyp is properly inspected.

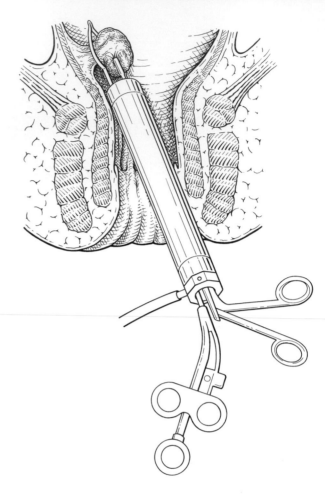

Figure 9-1.

Intra-(Trans-)Anal Excision

A bivalved intra-anal speculum, usually of the Park type, is introduced and the polyp is identified. The base of the polyp is infiltrated with a weak epinephrine solution (1:300,000) so that the mucosa is lifted off the submucosa. A 1-cm margin around the polyp is included in the excision, particularly for villous lesions, so that the entire mucosa and polypoidal lesion is excised, leaving bare rectal wall at the base (Fig. 9-2). A polyp that cannot be easily excised in this plane suggests malignant invasion, in which case the operation should be immediately converted to a full disc excision of the lesion, as described in Chapter 10.

Posterior Rectotomy

A full mechanical bowel preparation is undertaken. The patient is placed on the operating table on the left side with the hips and knees fully flexed. The tip of the coccyx is palpated. A longitudinal incision is made between the third sacral body and the perianal region (Fig. 9-3A). Segments 4 and 5 of the sacrum and the coccyx are excised using bone-cutting forceps. Hemostasis is achieved to the bone end. Great care is taken not to divide any vessels lying on the presacral fascia, which is preserved. The rectum is then divided through the retrorectal fat. A longitudinal rectotomy is made between pursestring sutures, leaving intact the external anal sphincter and the puborectalis muscle (Fig. 9-3B). The rectal polyp is then identified and excised in the usual way. After polypectomy the rectum is reconstructed using a running 3-0 PDS suture. A suction drain is left to the operation site and the skin is closed.

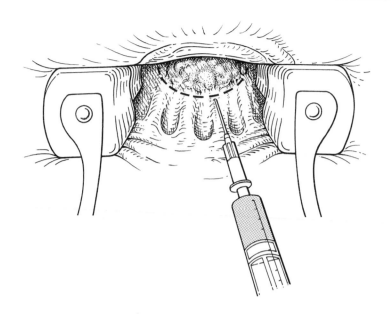

Figure 9-2.

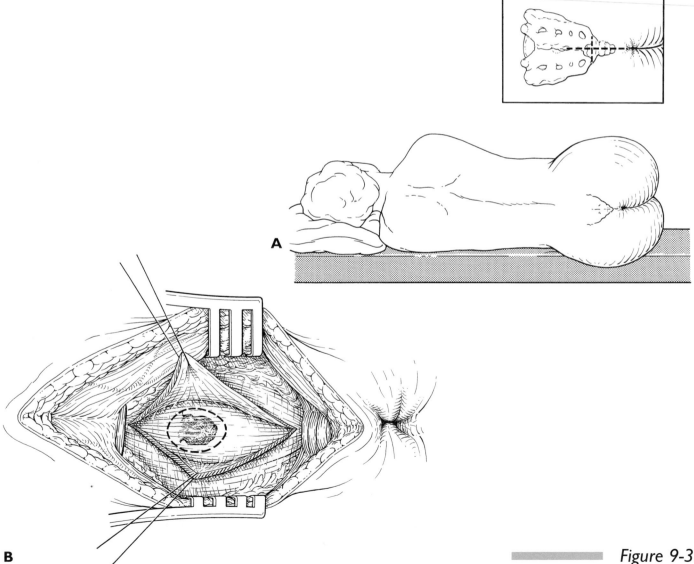

A

B

Figure 9-3.

Transsphincteric Excision

Transsphincteric resection is rarely performed today because peranal and posterior rectotomy achieve comparable exposure without the risk of division and resuture of the sphincters and pelvic floor.

The patient undergoes a full mechanical bowel preparation. The patient is placed in the prone jackknife position. An oblique incision is made over the buttock down through the anal margin. The external anal sphincter and puborectalis are identified. Stay sutures are placed on both muscles and the somatic muscle layers are divided longitudinally. The internal anal sphincter and the longitudinal rectal muscle are then divided longitudinally between stay sutures and the entire posterior wall of the rectum is opened longitudinally (Fig. 9-4). The intrarectal polyp and a disc of normal

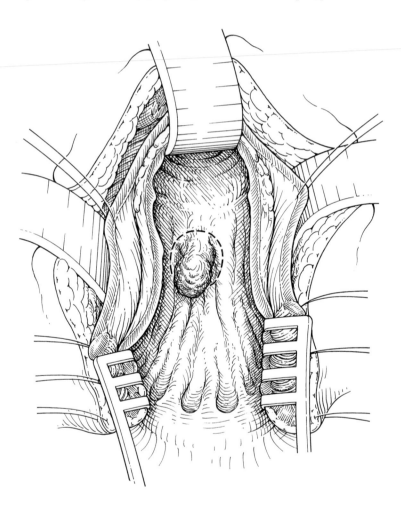

Figure 9-4.

healthy mucosa of at least 1 cm in diameter is dissected in the usual manner, either as a submucosal excision or as a full-thickness excision, depending on the degree of infiltration of the submucosal structures. Reconstruction after polypectomy is performed using a running 3-0 PDS running suture, first on the rectal wall, then on the visceral musculature (i.e., the internal anal sphincter and rectal longitudinal muscle). Finally, the somatic muscular structures (puborectalis and external anal sphincter) are opposed in the midline and the skin is closed over suction drains. See Chapter 10 for further details.

Sleeve Mucosectomies

Intrarectal Sleeve Mucosectomy

Occasionally, when a large polyp in the rectum is excised, the defect is so wide that an advancement flap is needed for reconstruction. The polyp is excised, taking a segment of mucosa wider proximally than distally in order to ensure an adequate blood supply to the flap to be created (Fig. 9-5A). Once the flap has been excised, the mucosa above it is mobilized fully and brought down over the defect and closed (Fig. 9-5B). The effect of the sleeve excision and reconstruction is a pleating of the rectal wall.

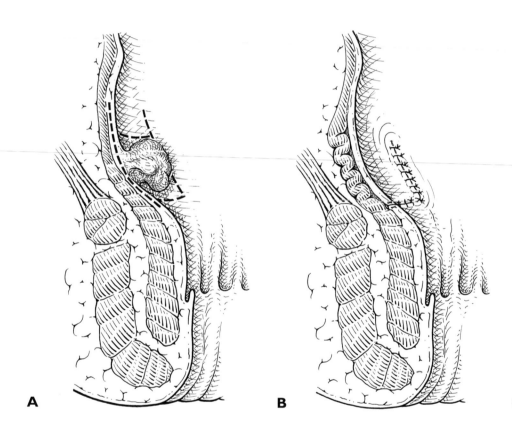

A   **B**   *Figure 9-5.*

Sleeve Mucosectomy as a Prolapse Procedure

Sometimes a large polyp may be inaccessible using the intrarectal approach. Under these circumstances, it may be possible to prolapse the entire rectum by placing stay sutures on the polyp and slowly delivering the rectum as an intussusception (Fig. 9-6A). Once the rectum has been turned inside out, the polyp can be locally excised (Fig. 9-6B) or a Delormé-type procedure may be performed, as described in Chapter 7.

Resection

Extremely large polyps demonstrating high-grade dysplasia or carcinoma in situ, or even a focus of malignant change, should be treated by resection, particularly if the polyp is sessile or where colonoscopic resection is not deemed wise or feasible. For polyps in the right colon a standard right hemicolectomy is performed (Fig. 9-7A). For polyps in the transverse colon, either a transverse colectomy (Fig. 9-7B) or an extended right hemicolectomy (Fig. 9-7C) may be performed. For polyps in the

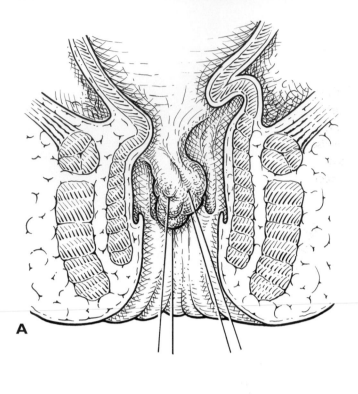

A

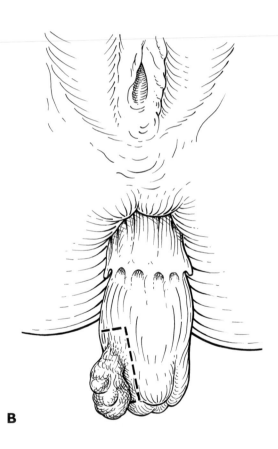

B

Figure 9-6.

descending colon, resection of the descending colon with the sigmoid is usually advised (Fig. 9-7D), whereas for polyps confined to the sigmoid colon, a segmental sigmoidectomy is probably sufficient (Fig. 9-7E). For high rectal lesions, an anterior resection (Fig. 9-7F) may be feasible, but for very low carpeted polypoidal lesions, total rectal incision with the sigmoid colon and reconstruction as a coloanal procedure may be advisable (Fig. 9-7G). For details of these resections, see Chapter 10.

For multiple polyps or in familial adenomatous polyposis, subtotal colectomy and an ileorectal anastomosis may be performed (Fig. 9-7H). In our opinion, however, it is preferable to undertake a totally ablative procedure, performing a restorative procto-colectomy with an anal mucosectomy and pouch anal anastomosis (Fig. 9-7I). For details of ileorectal anastomosis and pouch procedures with mucosectomy, see Chapter 13.

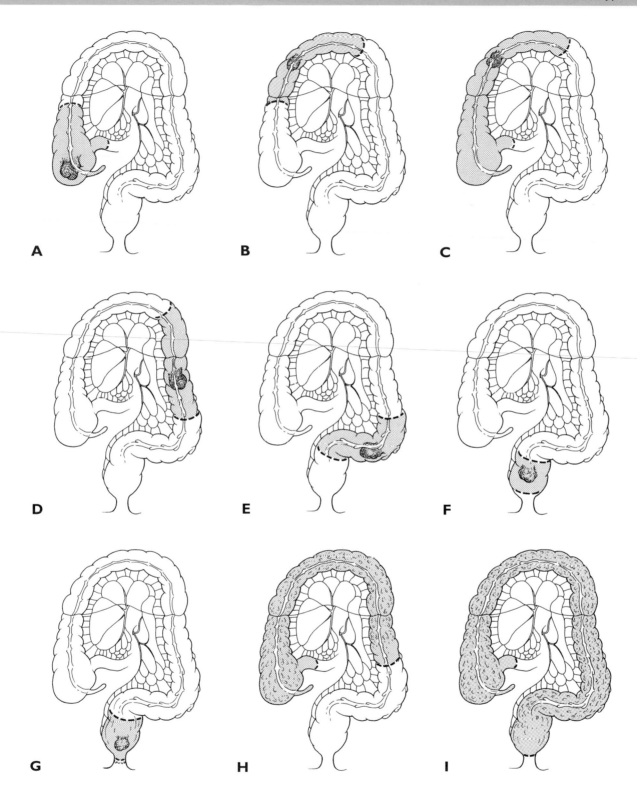

Figure 9-7.

Editorial Commentaries

I do not differ with the approach described by Dr. Parc. We favor restorative proctocolectomy with anal mucosectomy for familial adenomatosis polyposis because the risk of rectal cancer 25 years after ileorectal anastomosis in this unit is 22 percent. Although we accept that there is an even higher risk of noncolorectal neoplasms, nevertheless these patients may default from follow-up and the problems of later rectal excision, particularly after repeat rectal polyp fulguration, can be formidable.

Michael R. B. Keighley

I agree that polyps located in the low rectum are suitable for local excision using transanal techniques. Those located 8 cm or higher in the rectum can be addressed using anterior resection, whereas those 4 to 8 cm high can be excised using a York-Mason approach. Therefore, the water-filled endorectal excision technique is of extremely limited use and is, in fact, not used at our institution.

Posterior Rectotomy. I approach the posterior rectum in an entirely different way from Dr. Parc. I use the York-Mason approach: A parasacral incision is brought down to the midline at the level of the coccyx; it is then brought to the anal verge if the tumor or polyp is located that low, or is terminated above the anal sphincters if the polyp is higher. The anal sphincters can be reapproximated easily if they are tagged during their incision. We do not take the coccyx unless it is in the way. After removing the polyp, the posterior rectotomy is reconstructed in two layers using absorbable sutures. A drain is placed in all overlying tissues.

John H. Pemberton

10

Colorectal Cancer

Michael R. B. Keighley

Principles

Curative surgical treatment of colorectal cancer involves (1) the complete excision of the primary tumor, taking, if necessary, any adjacent structures provided they can be safely excised and (2) complete lymphatic clearance to the drainage area for the tumor. Hence, radical lymphatic clearance involves high vascular pedicle ligation without compromise to the remaining large intestine.

In order to plan appropriate surgical treatment, the tumor should be accurately staged preoperatively by a combination of clinical examination, chest roentgenography, computed tomography (CT) of the liver, and cross-sectional imaging of the tumor itself to evaluate the extent of tumor penetration through the bowel wall and to adjacent lymph glands. Unfortunately, presently most methods of tumor staging are imprecise. CT is probably the best modality for assessment of liver metastases and extent of tumor penetration, but both CT and magnetic resonance imaging provide disappointing data on lymphatic involvement. Improved preoperative staging might be achieved with endoscopically guided ultrasonography of the tumor, as well as with laparoscopically guided ultrasonography of the liver and the tumor (see Ch. 3). The entire large intestine should be visualized, colonoscopically if possible, in order to detect the presence of synchronous tumors, which may present in up to 10 percent of patients.

The staging process in rectal cancer is slightly different and the need for precise information on tumor involvement of adjacent organs is particularly important because of the size of the pelvis in relation to the tumor. Staging should identify involvement of critical structures, such as the major blood vessels, ureters, vagina, prostate seminal vesicles, and the sidewall of the pelvis. Furthermore, in rectal cancer, there is an opportunity in appropriate patients to consider preoperative radiation therapy and chemotherapy in order to downstage the tumor, thereby facilitating curative resection of a tumor that might otherwise have been fixed by malignant disease to adjacent structures that cannot be excised. Hence, for rectal tumors, cross-sectional imaging is particularly valuable, combined with intrarectal ultrasonography. Ultrasonography is important in potentially favorable T1 lesions in order to determine whether curative local resection is an option.

Preoperative Preparation

A full mechanical bowel preparation is used in patients with nonobstructing tumors. Those patients with tumors severely compromising the lumen of the colon may require a more prolonged period of mechanical preparation to clear fecal residue from the colon. In some, complete evacuation of fecal material proximal to the tumor may be impossible; under these circumstances, the technique of on-table colonic lavage is recommended (Fig. 10-1). The management of large bowel obstruction is discussed in Chapter 13. The methods of mechanical bowel preparation will differ according to the institution, but it is our practice to use two sachets of Picolax on the day before the operation, the first dose given at 7 A.M. and the second at 11 A.M. This method of purgation causes dehydration, hence the patient is admitted on the afternoon before the operation for an intravenous infusion once the bowel preparation is completed.

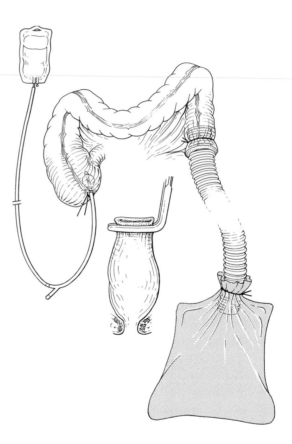

Figure 10-1.

Perioperative antibiotic prophylaxis with one or two doses only is used in all patients provided there is no gross contamination or coexisting sepsis at the time of operation; hence the duration of antibiotic cover is limited merely to the surgical procedure. In high-risk patients or where there is coexisting infection, antibiotic administration is continued for 3 to 5 days.

Resections for colorectal cancer are uniformly performed through a midline laparotomy. This gives the best possible access, it does not compromise potential stoma sites, and it can be extended if there is any difficulty with mobilization. Its main disadvantages are those of postoperative pain and a long, unsightly scar. However, with modern methods of postoperative pain control, particularly patient-controlled analgesia, the use of anti-inflammatory agents, epidural anesthesia, and local infiltration along the incision and postoperatively through fine cannulas (Fig. 10-2), the amount of postoperative pain following midline laparotomy has been greatly reduced.

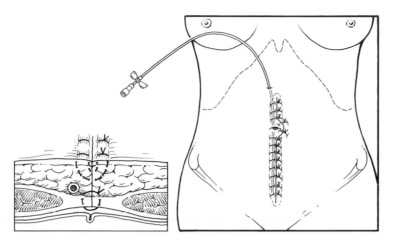

Figure 10-2.

Because the surgeon never knows when a defunctioning stoma may be needed, we ensure that potential stoma sites are marked on both sides of the abdomen preoperatively just in case an end ileostomy and a mucous fistulotomy are needed.

All colorectal tumor operations are performed with the patient in the modified lithotomy Trendelenburg position using Allen stirrups to support the heels and calves (Fig. 10-3). The use of the modified lithotomy Trendelenburg position leaves all options open, particularly if intraoperative colonoscopy or rectal washout with cytocidal agents is deemed necessary, and it provides access to the bowel if a stapled anastomosis needs to be tested. All patients are catheterized after anesthesia so as to allow monitoring of urine output intraoperatively, to decompress the bladder for adequate access to the pelvic organs, and to drain the bladder in the immediate postoperative period.

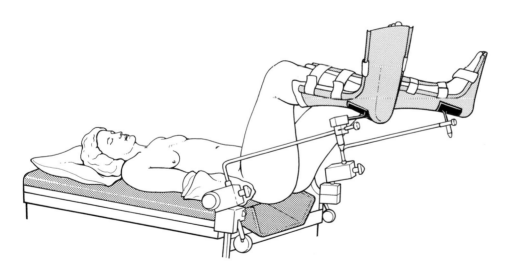

Figure 10-3.

Intraoperative Staging

Laparotomy for patients with large bowel cancer provides a further method of tumor staging and assessment. The liver should be inspected and surface hepatic ultrasonography performed to enhance detection of liver metastases (Fig. 10-4). The tumor is then assessed, particularly to determine involvement of adjacent organs and adherence to omentum and loops of small bowel as well as to the other pelvic organs. Sometimes tumors are adherent to the parietal structures, such as the psoas, quadratus lumborum, and transverse abdominus muscles, the anterior abdominal wall, and the rectus muscle (Fig. 10-5). There may be involvement of the kidney, the ureter, or the duodenum. In the pelvis, there may be fixity to the sacrum, the iliac vessels, the

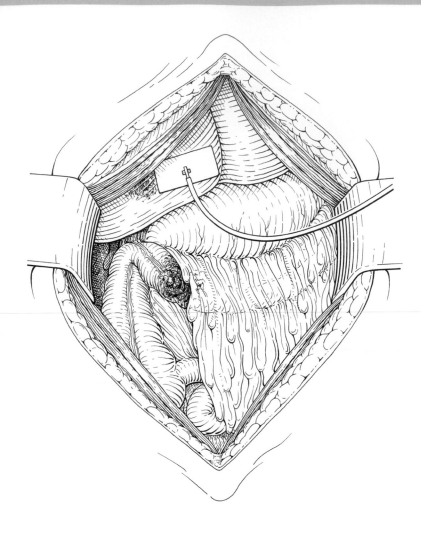

Figure 10-4.

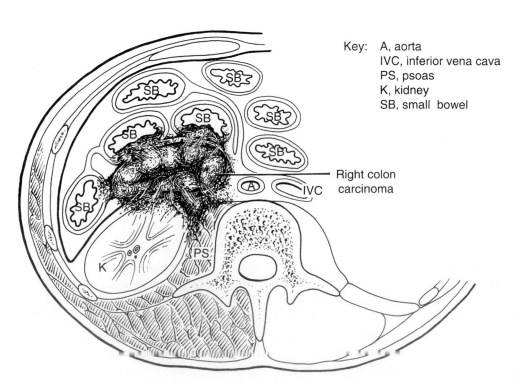

Key: A, aorta
        IVC, inferior vena cava
        PS, psoas
        K, kidney
        SB, small bowel

Right colon
carcinoma

Figure 10-5.

obturator internus, the levator ani, or the piriformis. Once local fixity has been assessed, lymphatic involvement should be verified. Involvement of pericolic and epicolic nodes may be relatively unimportant because they will be removed with the tumor. However, nodes in the intermediate and apical groups lying adjacent to the vascular supply should be noted. If there is obvious tumor involvement of the apical nodes around the inferior or superior mesenteric artery, or if para-aortic nodes are involved, the prognosis is poor and any resection is liable to be merely palliative. Hence, information concerning tumor involvement of the high lymphatic drainage areas provides important staging information.

Right Hemicolectomy

The right colon and ileocecal regions are first mobilized by dividing the peritoneum lateral to the cecum and ascending colon. During this maneuver the peritoneal attachment to the terminal ileum is also divided lateral to and below the appendix. At this point the right ureter can usually be identified. The hepatic flexure is also mobilized (Fig. 10-6A). Potentially sizable retroperitoneal veins may need to be secured by ligature or diathermy. Care must be taken here not to damage the duodenum, which lies underneath the hepatic flexure. If the tumor lies in the transverse colon, the entire omentum is taken with the colon, and the vessels running toward the omentum from the gastroepiploic arcade are separately ligated (Fig. 10-6B). In this way the middle colic artery is exposed and its origin from the superior mesenteric artery identified. It is now possible to lift the entire right colon and transverse colon with its vascular supply from the retroperitoneum and omentum, provided, of course, that the tumor is not adherent posteriorly to the psoas, iliacus, transversus abdominus, kidney, or duodenum (Fig. 10-6C). If it is adherent, the structures must be taken en bloc with the tumor without entering malignant tissue. Even if the kidney, ureter, and duodenum are involved, they can be resected in favorable cases where there is no evidence of disseminated disease. If there is renal involvement, nephroureterectomy is indicated. Furthermore, the duodenum can be reconstructed with a roux-en-Y procedure (Fig. 10-6D) and the ureter can be reanastomosed, sutured to a Boari flap or psoas hitch, taken across to the opposite ureter to construct an end-to-side anastomosis, or sutured to an ileal conduit (Fig. 10-6E). Occasionally, the stomach may be involved with a carcinoma of the transverse colon, in which case a partial gastrectomy may be indicated as well (Fig. 10-6F). Local adherence to the liver necessitates a wedge excision of the liver (Fig. 10-6G).

The next task is to assess the length of bowel to resect. This is largely determined by the position of the tumor. For cecal lesions or lesions in the right colon only, the right half of the transverse colon with the ascending colon will have to be removed. However, for lesions in the transverse colon, the entire transverse colon with the right colon should be excised, having taken down the splenic flexure (Fig. 10-6H).

At this point, we believe it is important to isolate the tumor-bearing segment of the colon. A window is thus constructed between the vascular arcades in the terminal ileum at the point of proposed division of the transverse colon (Fig. 10-6I). Tapes may be tied around the bowel to isolate it or, preferably, a linear staple cutter may be applied to completely seal off and divide the bowel at these points. We advise injecting a tumoricidal agent into the lumen of the gut prior to stapled transection of the colon and ileum so as to minimize the risk of anastomotic recurrence from implanted tumor (Fig. 10-6J).

Attention may now be directed toward high vascular pedicle ligation in order to achieve full lymphadenectomy. For lesions in the right colon, the origin of the ileocolic artery on the superior mesenteric artery must be identified. The artery should be ligated, preserving the ileal arcade and dividing the small bowel mesentery appropriately. For lesions in the transverse colon, it is necessary to ligate the middle colic artery and the ileocolic artery from their origin on the superior mesenteric artery. Hence, the blood supply to the distal colonic resection margin is dependent on the patency of the arcade of Riolan and the inferior mesenteric artery. If for any reason the arcade is not patent or the mesenteric artery is occluded, it may be necessary to totally mobilize the splenic flexure and anastomose the ileum to either viable descending colon or the proximal sigmoid. The tumor with its blood supply can now be removed and intestinal continuity restored using the author's preferred method of anastomosis (see Ch. 2).

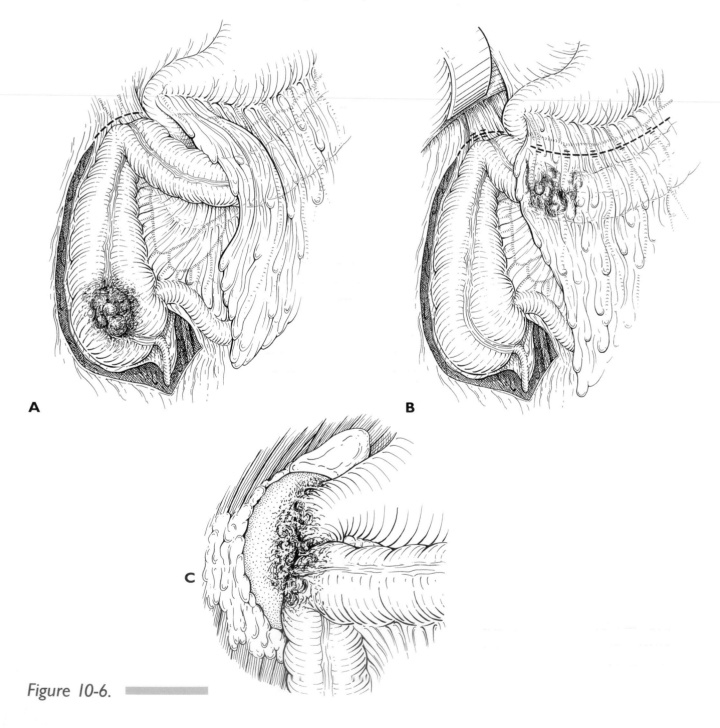

A

B

C

Figure 10-6.

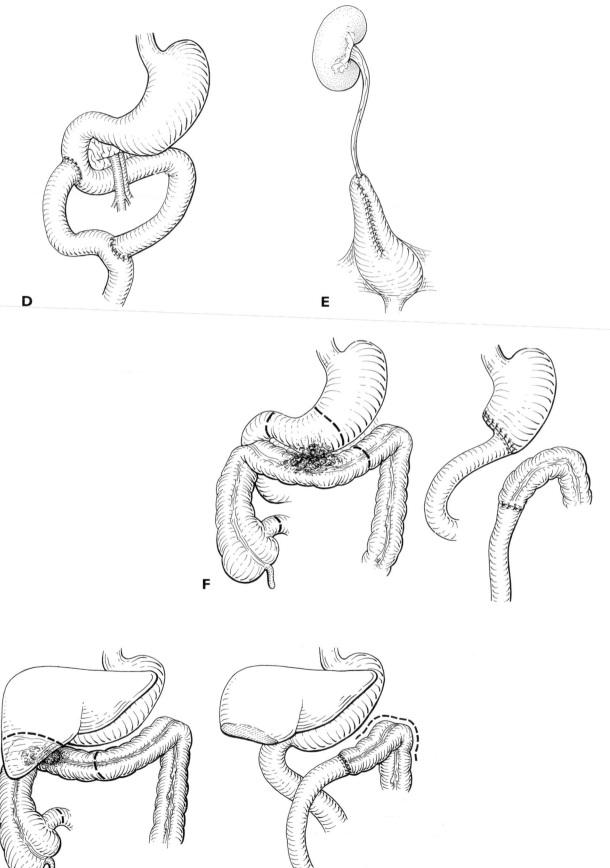

Figure 10-6.

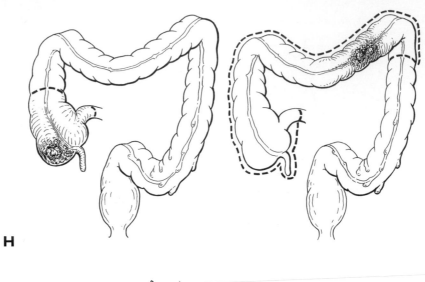

H

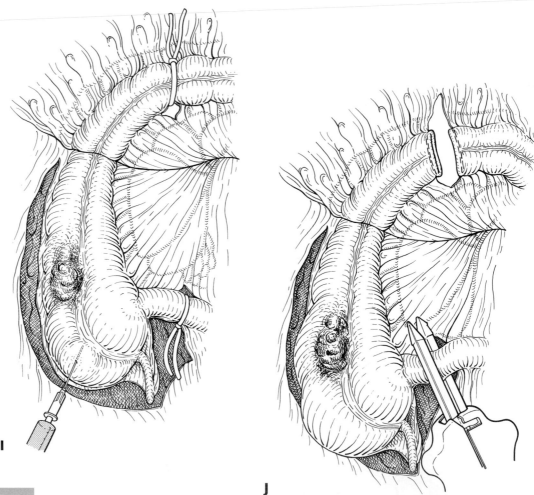

I

J

Figure 10-6. ━━━━━━

If there is any technical difficulty in fashioning the anastomosis or if there has been coexisting sepsis, it may be wise either to raise a loop ileostomy proximal to the anastomosis (Fig. 10-7A) or to bring out both ends of the bowel as an end ileostomy and mucous fistula. We generally bring two small suction drains out through a separate stab incision to drain any blood from the right retrocolic space. The abdomen is closed as described in Chapter 1.

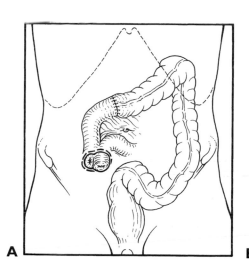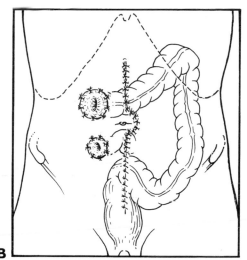

Figure 10-7.

Left Hemicolectomy and High Anterior Resection

Left hemicolectomy and high anterior resection will be described together because, in my view, tumors found in the left side of the transverse colon, splenic flexure, descending colon, or sigmoid are managed in precisely the same way. The operation involves en bloc removal of the left side of the transverse colon, splenic flexure, descending colon, and sigmoid, with rectal anastomosis between the transverse colon and the upper third of the rectum. In this way, high ligation of the inferior mesenteric artery can be achieved and the blood supply to the proximal colon derived from the middle colic artery through the marginal artery of Riolan (Fig. 10-8).

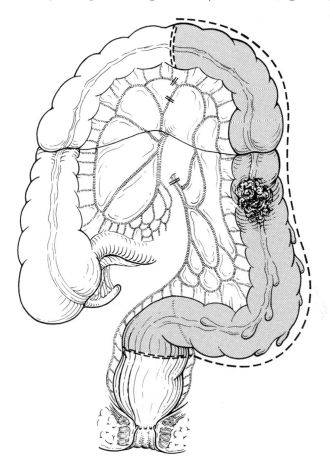

Figure 10-8.

The operation commences with division of the peritoneum over the aorta and right posterolateral aspect of the pelvis. This allows the origin of the inferior mesenteric artery to be identified and, if necessary, the vessel ligated at this point. The peritoneum over the lateral aspect of the descending colon is then divided and this incision is extended downward so as to divide the peritoneum lateral to the sigmoid colon and finally to the posterolateral aspect of the left side of the pelvis (Fig. 10-9A). The splenic flexure is then taken down with great care so as not to injure the marginal artery. The descending colon and sigmoid colon can then be gently mobilized medially on their vascular pedicle, carefully separating the left colonic vessels from the ureter, left ovarian or testicular vessels, and the kidney (Fig. 10-9B). Only in this way is it possible to appreciate that the inferior mesenteric vein diverges from the inferior mesenteric artery, which has already been ligated, and enters the splenic vein underneath the pancreas, where it can be safely divided (Fig. 10-9C). If care has been taken to develop this avascular plane, no damage will occur to the arcade of Riolan and the entire colon with a thin sheet of peritoneum containing its vessels can be delivered from the posterior abdominal wall. If, of course, there is any involvement by the tumor of the left psoas, iliacus, transversus abdominis, left ureter, or genital vessels, it will have to be excised widely so as not to enter the tumor. Defects in the ureter will be managed as previously described. If there is involvement of the kidney, nephroureterectomy would be indicated; similarly, a partial gastrectomy is performed if a tumor of the transverse colon invades the stomach. Involvement of the distal pancreas necessitates distal pancreatectomy en bloc with the tumor, whereas direct invasion of the liver is managed by hepatectomy. The tumor-bearing segment of the bowel is then isolated after having first injected a cytocidal agent into the bowel lumen (Fig. 10-9D). We use a solution of chlorhexadine; others prefer alcohol or sterile water, or even mercuric perchloride. Windows are developed

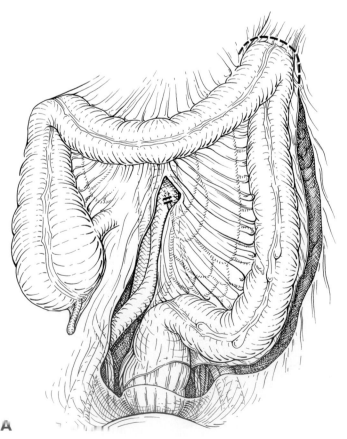

Figure 10-9. ━━━━━━   **A**

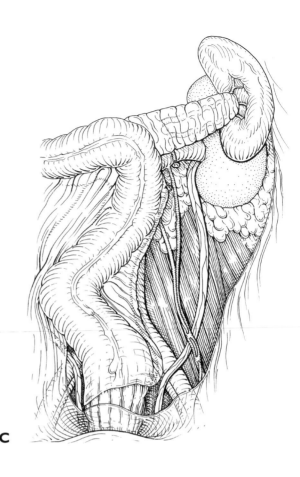

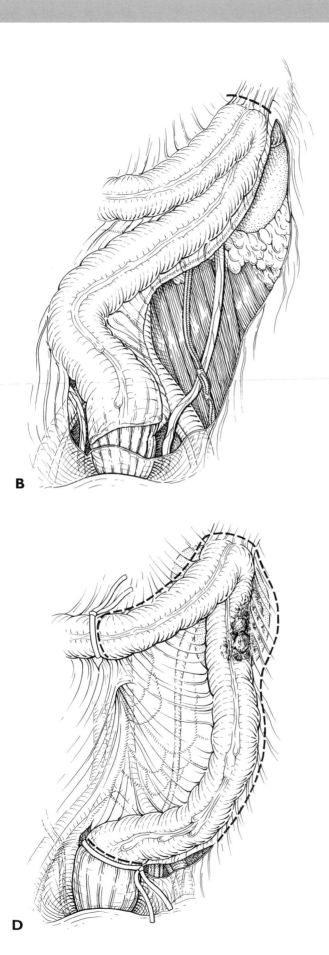

Figure 10-9.

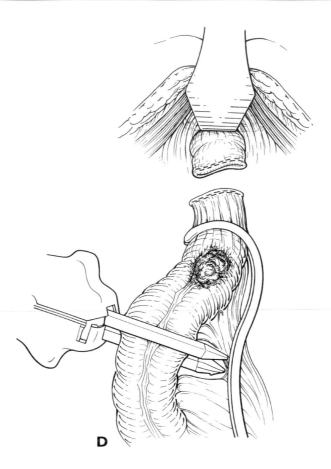

Figure 10-14.   **D**

If there have been any technical difficulties with the anastomosis or if there is coexisting sepsis, it may be wise to use a protecting stoma. We would advise either a right transverse colostomy (so as not to impair the blood supply of the marginal artery) or, preferably, a loop ileostomy (provided that the bowel has been adequately prepared and there is minimal fecal residue in the proximal colon). Two suction drains are placed down into the pelvis and the abdomen is closed as described in Chapter 1.

Extended Subtotal Colectomy for Synchronous Cancer

Occasionally it is necessary to remove all at-risk colonic epithelium so that only the rectum has to remain under surveillance. This option is pertinent for patients with more than one invasive carcinoma in the colon. It is also appropriate for those with high-grade dysplasia. If subtotal colectomy and ileorectal anastomosis is contemplated, the patient must be prepared to return for annual sigmoidoscopic assessment of the rectal stump. It is an inappropriate option if there is severe dysplasia in the rectum, and because under these circumstances total excision of the colon and rectum with ileoanal anastomosis would be advised, as in restorative proctocolectomy for familial adenomatous polyposis (Fig. 10-15). Alternatively, if an advanced low rectal cancer is associated with malignant disease in the colon as well, some might advocate a radical proctocolectomy and end ileostomy (described later), but the extent of the rectal excision depends on the size, site, and position of the tumor.

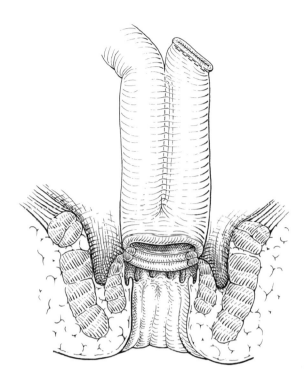

Figure 10-15.

The procedure of extended subtotal colectomy and ileorectal anastomosis may also be indicated for obstructing left-sided colon carcinoma (see Ch. 13). This option is preferred by some to that of on-table colonic lavage with limited left-sided resection and anastomosis, particularly in younger patients.

The extent of the resection should include the whole colon with or without the sigmoid, depending on the location of the tumors, as well as high ligation of the inferior mesenteric, middle colic, and ileocolic arteries, as described in earlier sections of this chapter (Fig. 10-16A). Intestinal continuity is then restored, either by constructing an ileosigmoid anastomosis (Fig. 10-16B), which may be sutured or stapled, or by the construction of an ileorectal anastomosis (Fig. 10-16C), using either sutures or staples, as described in Chapter 2.

Suction drains are needed only if there has been excessive bleeding. If there has been any technical difficulty with the anastomosis, or if there is coexisting sepsis at the time of operation, a proximal loop ileostomy should be raised, as described in Chapter 4. The abdomen is then closed as described in Chapter 1.

Synchronous Partial Cystectomy with Colorectal Anastomosis for Malignancy

Probably the most common situation in which a partial cystectomy is necessary is when a neoplasm of the sigmoid is adherent to the dome of the bladder. Generally this is a very favorable situation, because such tumors are often locally advanced but without widespread metastases. Under these circumstances, the colonic tumor is mobilized as described for left hemicolectomy and high anterior resection. However, the point at which the tumor is adherent to the bladder requires careful assessment. If the dome of the bladder only is involved, it is a simple matter to place stay sutures on either side of the adherent portion and, using a diathermy, to remove the wall of the bladder to which the tumor is adherent (Fig. 10-17A). The bladder is inspected to ensure that

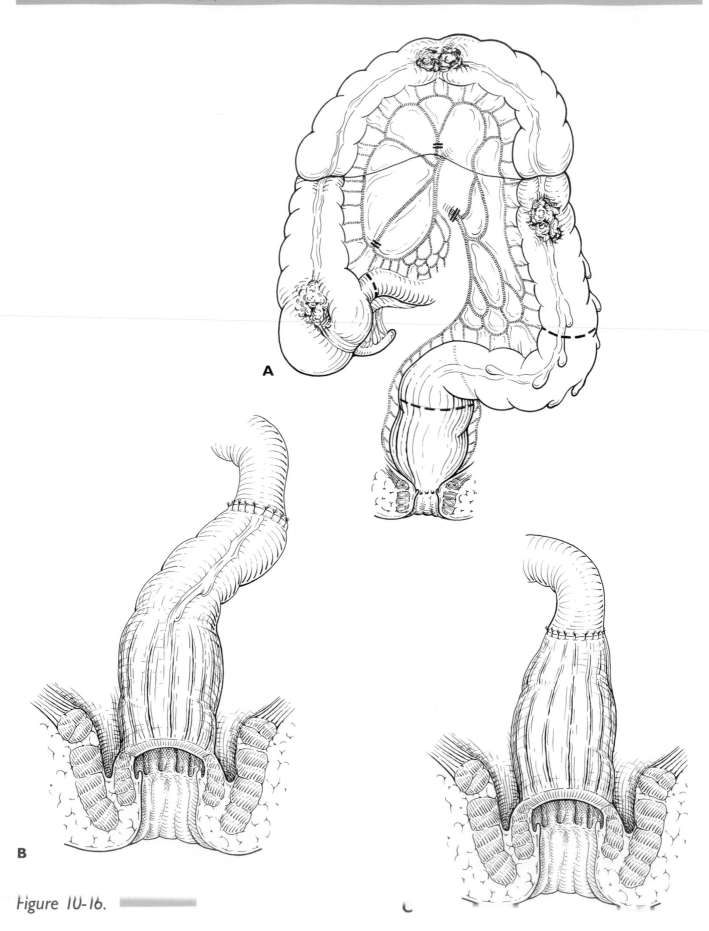

A

B

Figure 10-16.

there are no other deposits in the transitional cell epithelium and to ensure that local clearance has been adequate, whereupon the mucosa of the bladder is closed with continuous sutures of catgut, the detrusor muscle is closed with continuous sutures of either catgut or Vicryl, and the serosa of the bladder closed as a third layer (Fig. 10-17B). The bladder catheter is usually left in situ for at least a week. We usually check the integrity of the bladder closure by performing a cystogram prior to removal of the catheter.

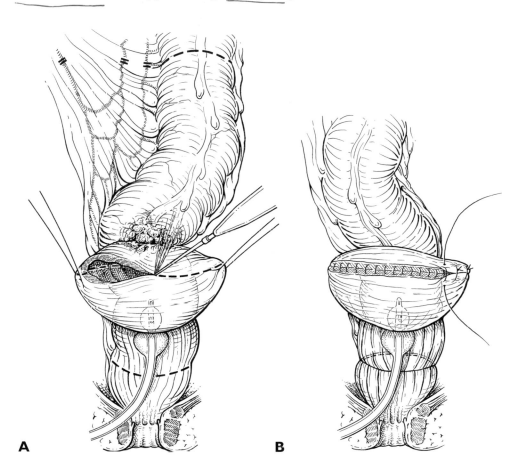

A   **B**   *Figure 10-17.*

If the rectosigmoid junction is involved with tumor and if it appears to encroach posteriorly beyond the dome of the bladder, we advise anterior cystotomy (Fig. 10-18). We prefer a transverse incision over the dome of the bladder for this purpose. This maneuver is done to assess under direct vision whether or not the tumor involves the ureteric orifices. If the ureteric orifices are involved, a urologic surgeon must assess the case, because partial or total cystectomy may be indicated. The details of partial or total cystectomy, including the construction of a Boari flap and ileal conduits, and augmentation cystoplasty, are not included here, and the reader is advised to consult an operative urology text.

If careful inspection of the bladder indicates that the ureteric orifices are not involved, a wide local excision should be performed. It is essential under these circumstances to identify both ureters and to trace them down to the bladder base. Some surgeons will advise insertion of ureteric catheters, but this is not always necessary. A monoblock excision of the tumor in the rectum and bladder should be performed under direct vision, controlling any bleeding points as they present themselves, and ensuring that complete tumor clearance is achieved, preferably without sacrifice of the ureters. The tumor-bearing segment of the colon and rectum is then removed, thereupon the surgeon will need to attend to closure of the large bladder defect. If there is any risk of compromise to the ureteric orifice or if closure of the bladder is likely to leave the patient with a narrow contracted viscus, urologic expertise should be sought. Usually, however, closure of the bladder presents no difficulty and a three-layer closure as already described can be performed.

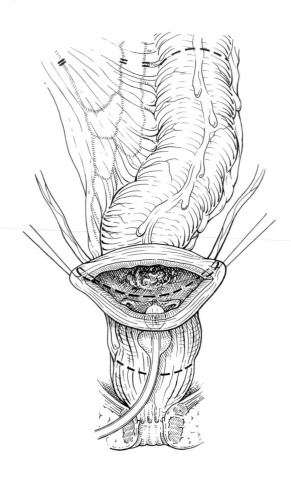

Figure 10-18.

Synchronous Hysterectomy with Colorectal Resection for Malignancy

Hysterectomy is occasionally needed for complete ablation of a rectal or sigmoid tumor. However, direct infiltration of the body of the uterus is remarkably uncommon in large bowel cancer. It is far more common for a tumor to invade directly into the vagina, necessitating concomitant excision, than into the uterus. Nevertheless, there are occasions when anterior rectal lesions and lesions in the rectosigmoid necessitate total abdominal hysterectomy in order to achieve full tumor clearance. The primary lesion will be in either the sigmoid or the upper rectum, hence the extent of colonic resection and the planes of dissection are those described for high or low anterior resection. When the tumor is adherent to the uterus, and if it is to be excised en bloc, then various modifications to the technique so far described are necessary.

The first step is to achieve full rectal mobilization so as to clear the mesorectum from the posterolateral aspects of the pelvis (Fig. 10-19A). The next phase is total abdominal hysterectomy. The lateral pelvic peritoneum is divided widely and the round ligaments on either side of the uterus are ligated. The next important landmark is the ureter, which must be identified on both sides and traced downward. The ovarian vessels should then be ligated and divided on either side. The next step involves division of the anterior peritoneum down to the level of the upper vagina. Lateral parauterine dissection must keep close to the course of the ureter (Fig. 10-19B). A series of crushing jaw-ended clamps provide the best means of ligating the uterine veins and artery and securing hemostasis by transfixion around the clamps (Fig. 10-19B, inset). The extent of the lateral uterine clearance can be verified by palpation of the cervix through the anterior border of the vagina. Once this level has been reached on either side, the vagina should be completely divided, leaving only the tumorous attachment of the rectum to the uterus.

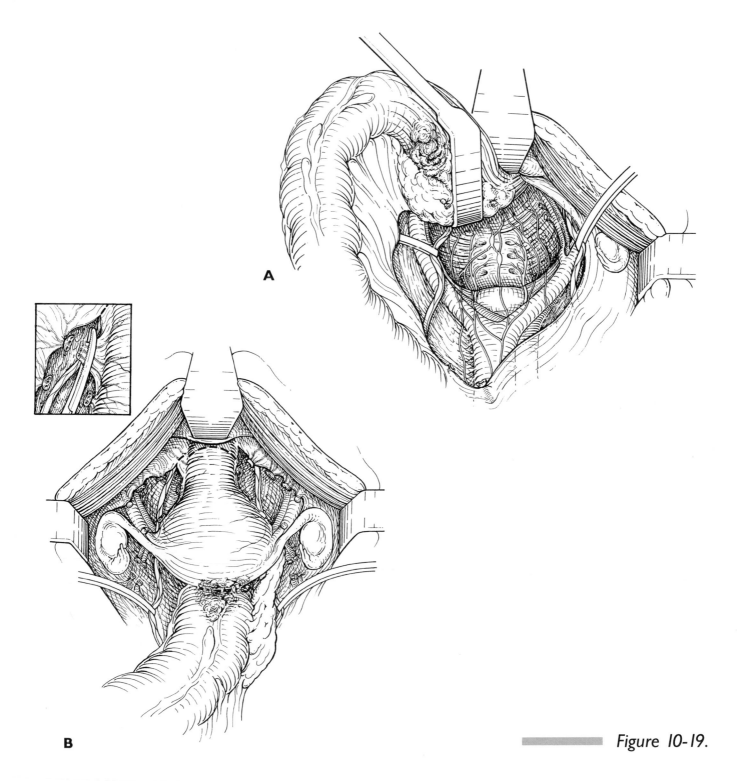

A

B

Figure 10-19.

Now, and only now, can the anterior aspect of the rectum be observed and dissected from the back of the vagina. It is preferable to achieve a 2- to 4-cm clearance beyond the site of the vaginal transection so that the colorectal anastomosis can be placed at a lower level than the vaginal closure line (Fig. 10-19C). The next move is to achieve complete lateral clearance of the rectal tumor by dividing the lateral ligaments and the middle rectal vessels between a Roberts clamp or by diathermy.

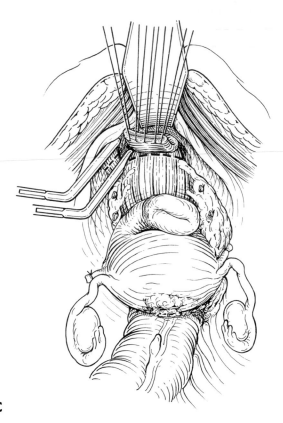

Figure 10-19.   C

At this point, having applied a noncrushing clamp across the rectum, a rectal washout can be performed. A stapled anastomosis is then achieved between the descending colon and the lower rectum using either a double-staple technique or two pursestring sutures, as described in Chapter 2. The tumor can then be removed once the lower pursestring has been applied or after staple transection of the rectum. A decision must then be made as to whether or not to close the vaginal stump. The vagina can either be left open to act as a pelvic drain or, if hemostasis is satisfactory and there is no coexisting pelvic sepsis, be oversewn with a running 0-0 chromic catgut suture on a cutting needle (Fig. 10-19D).

Occasionally, the tumor mass is so large that restorative resection is neither feasible nor desirable. Such a situation may occur in very bulky anterior rectal lesions involving the posterior fornix and the back of the uterus. Under these circumstances, a radical excision and hysterectomy is likely to involve abdominoperineal excision with hysterectomy and excision of the posterior vaginal wall. The conduct of the dissection is exactly as described for abdominoperineal excision, except that a wide excision of the tumor-bearing segment of the posterior vagina should be made in continuity with the hysterectomy. Usually the vagina is completely removed in conjunction with the perineal surgery. The low rectum is then completely removed as described for abdominoperineal excision of the rectum (Fig. 10-20).

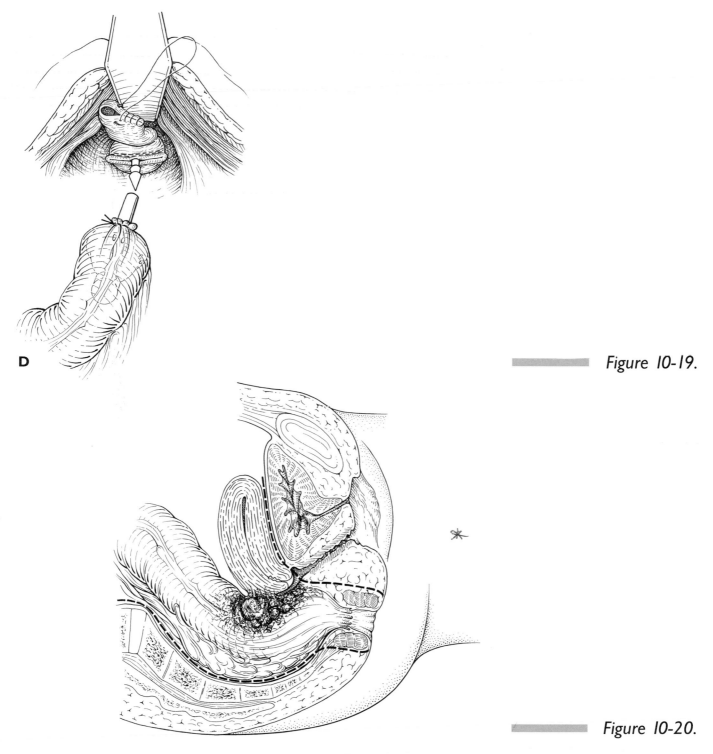

D

Figure 10-19.

Figure 10-20.

Total Rectal Excision and Coloanal Anastomosis

I use total rectal excision and coloanal anastomosis in most patients with a carcinoma in the lower two thirds of the rectum. As stapling procedures have become easier, and as experience with anal anastomosis as a consequence of restorative proctocolectomy has grown, this operation is now being used far more frequently for rectal cancer than was our experience 5 years ago. The operation of rectal excision and coloanal anasto-mosis ensures that the entire rectum is removed and involves the construction of an anastomosis between the descending colon and the anal canal, either a straight end-to-end anastomosis or, now more frequently, an end-to-side anastomosis, after construction of a colonic pouch. In some respects we believe it is a far safer operation than low anterior resection because there is no compromise to the blood supply to the anal stump despite radical excision of the mesorectum. Furthermore, it is almost easier technically to perform an end-to-side coloanal anastomosis than an end-to-end colorectal anastomosis, particularly in the narrow pelvis. It is also entirely feasible to combine the operation with hysterectomy or excision of the vagina.

The most important technical consideration in coloanal anastomosis, particularly if a pouch is to be constructed, is the viability of the descending colon based on the marginal artery supplied by the middle colic artery. It is crucial to ensure vigorous bleeding from both the marginal artery when it is divided and from the colon at the site of transection before the colonic pouch or straight coloanal anastomosis is constructed. In elderly patients with extensive atherosclerosis, or under circumstances where there may have been some damage at the splenic flexure resulting in trauma to the arcade of Riolan, problems of blood supply may be a real issue, and if the left colon becomes ischemic, it must be resected, the hepatic flexure taken down, and a straight coloanal anastomosis constructed based on the ileocolic artery (Fig. 10-21).

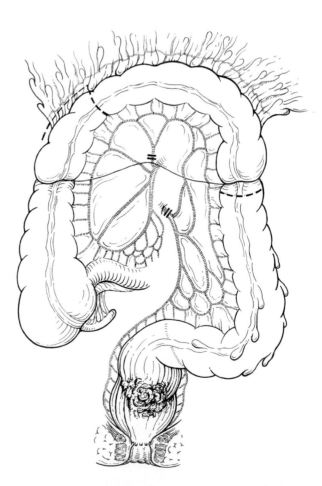

Figure 10-21.

Assessment and mobilization of the splenic flexure, descending colon, and sigmoid is precisely as described for left hemicolectomy and high anterior resection. The rectal dissection is essentially identical to that described for low anterior resection. The only difference relates to the extent of distal rectal clearance. In this operation the posterior dissection continues beyond the tip of the coccyx and involves division of Waldeyer's fascia behind the rectum so as to allow entry into the infralevator plane (Fig. 10-22A). This technique is particularly important for posteriorly situated tumors. Extreme care must be exercised during this maneuver in order to avoid damage to the anal canal, which at this juncture is supported only by longitudinal fibers and the internal anal sphincter. Lateral dissection should also clear the anal canal from the medial fibers of the puborectalis. Likewise, the anterior plane must be developed between the anal canal and the vagina in the female patient and between the anal canal and periprostatic tissues in the male. Obviously, this operation is not suitable for large, bulky tumors in the lower third of the rectum that have involved the full thickness of the anorectal wall, or tumors where there is fixity to adjacent structures, particularly the prostate, puborectalis sling, or vagina. Under these circumstances, an abdominoperineal excision would be advised.

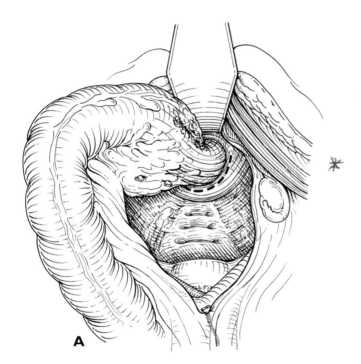

A

Figure 10-22.

The next maneuver is transection of the anal canal with staples. I prefer the RL30 stapler, but the 3M PT30 is equally efficient. Both have the advantage that there is an interlocking pin that allows the surgeon to advance or retract the transverse stapler to the optimum site for transection (Fig. 10-22B). At this point, the abdominal surgeon, standing on the patient's left, checks the height of the anal transection by reaching over the left groin and placing the index finger into the anal canal to ensure complete clearance of tumor and also to ascertain that the transection of the anal canal will not be too low, the consequence of which would be that a substantial portion of the anal sphincter would be excised, which may compromise continence (Fig. 10-22C). As in previously described procedures, a cytocidal washout is recommended; this is introduced into the anal canal immediately prior to application and closure of the transverse stapling device (Fig. 10-22D). The site of colonic transection depends on the length of bowel needed to achieve a safe coloanal anastomosis without tension, as well as on the viability of the colon after full mobilization. Because viability is the key determinant, it is our practice to perform the transection at a point on the colon where pulsation of the marginal artery can be palpated. The mobilized descending colon is then divided. The mesenteric attachment of the left colon is next divided and the marginal artery is transected to ensure that it bleeds satisfactorily before ligature. If there is any doubt about blood flow in the marginal artery, either the mesentery must be divided at a higher level or the bowel transected at this point to ensure that the submucosal vessels bleed briskly before application of the transverse stapler. Once a viable segment of descending colon has been transected, the tumor-bearing segment of the large bowel and rectum can be removed.

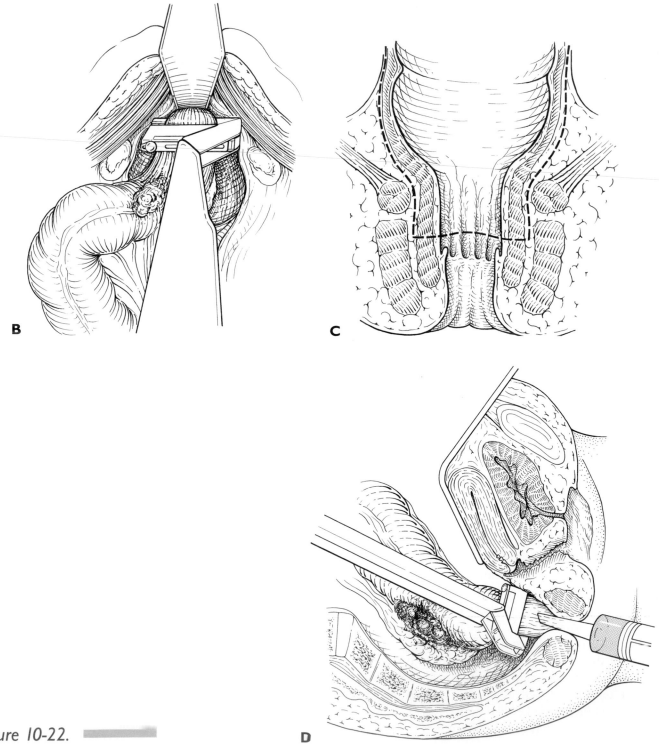

Figure 10-22.

Finally, it is essential to ensure absolute hemostasis in the pelvis. Use of a head-lamp greatly facilitates the whole surgical procedure and, with the attachment of a video camera, allows visualization of the depths of the pelvis by the assistants. This is a valuable teaching tool. Using a deep pelvic retractor, held in the left hand, to visualize the field, the surgeon identifies any bleeding points, and with the right hand picks up vessels with a long nontoothed forceps for diathermy (Fig. 10-22E).

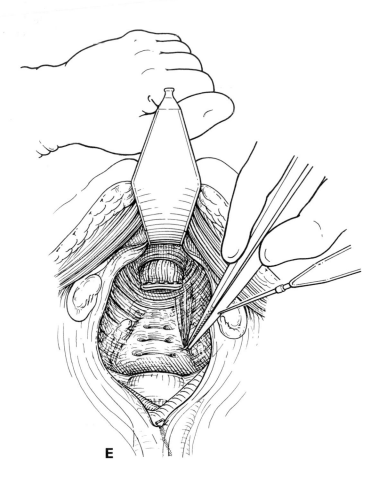

E

Figure 10-22.

Coloanal Anastomosis

Straight Stapled Coloanal Anastomosis

If the bowel is of insufficient length to construct a colonic reservoir, an end-to-end coloanal anastomosis will likely be satisfactory given that the descending colon (which has a wide diameter) is used for the reconstruction. Under these circumstances, the staple line is excised from the descending colon, an adequate blood supply is again ascertained, bleeding vessels in the submucosa are diathermized, and a pursestring suture is placed around the bowel end prior to the introduction of the anvil of the circular stapling device (usually a size 29 or 31). The central pin of the cartridge section of the circular stapling device is withdrawn inside the edges of the circular stapling device. The well-lubricated device is gently inserted through the anal sphincter by the assistant while the abdominal surgeon checks the position of the cartridge section in relation to the transected anal staple line. Again, it is often necessary for the abdominal surgeon to grasp the shaft of the circular stapling device with the left hand while holding the pelvic retractor with the right to ensure that the circular rim of the cartridge section is centered on the anal transection line. Once the surgeon is satisfied that the position is correct, the assistant rotates the wing nut or proximal wheel counterclockwise so as to advance the central pin through the center of the transected staple line. The central spindle is advanced to its full extent and the plastic spike is either withdrawn to accommodate the pin of the anvil section or, as is the case with the ILS instrument, the shaft of the anvil is advanced over the central spike of the cartridge section so that the two components are completely engaged. The wing nut or central wheel of the stapling device is then closed by clockwise rotation in order to approximate the anvil and cartridge sections.

During this procedure, it is most important to ensure that no structure becomes entrapped between the two bowel segments. This is particularly important in female patients, in whom vaginal entrapment may occur. This complication can be avoided either by the assistant placing a finger in the vagina and lifting it upward or by the abdominal surgeon controlling the deep pelvic retractor over the vagina to ensure that no tissue becomes entrapped during the closure of the stapling device. Once the staple gun is closed, the safety catch is released and the staple gun knife is advanced by closing the proximal screws or handles of the instrument. At this point the pursestring suture is divided by the circular knife. The wing nut or screw is released, and the circular stapling device rotated through 360 degrees and levered gently from the anal canal either by the assistant or, preferably, by the surgeon, who leans over the patient's left groin and withdraws the instrument with the left hand while steadying the proximal colon with the right hand to ensure that the instrument can be extracted freely without damage to the bowel. The assistant then opens the circular stapling device to ensure that two complete tissue rings have been recovered (Fig. 10-23A). The rings are reexamined after the knot on the pursestring has been cut. The surgeon then palpates the coloanal anastomosis with the index finger of the left hand to ensure that it feels satisfactory. The pelvis is then filled with saline and the assistant injects air through a 50-ml syringe via the anal canal while the surgeon occludes the proximal colon with a finger and thumb of the left hand. Distension of the colon beyond the anastomosis is observed and any air leakage noted (Fig. 10-23B). If there is no leakage demonstrated, the test is repeated two or three times to ensure that the anastomosis is secure. If the anastomosis is in any way unsatisfactory, a proximal stoma must be raised (if there is a

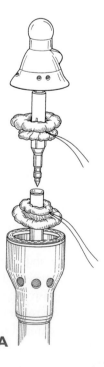

Figure 10-23.   A

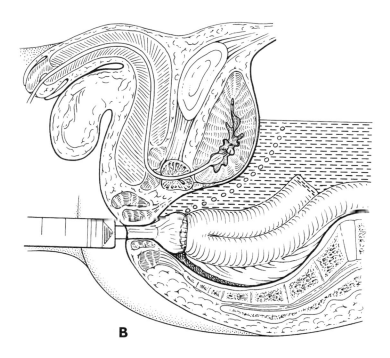

B

Figure 10-23.

minor leak) or the coloanal anastomosis must be taken down and a hand-sewn anastomosis fashioned (if there is a major leak) (see Ch. 2).

Hand-Sewn Coloanal Anastomosis

If a sutured coloanal anastomosis is called for, either because a stapled anastomosis has
failed or because of the preference of the surgeon (particularly with the fear of implantation of malignant cells at the stapled transection site), the proximal colon must be
delivered through the pelvic floor and the sphincters to the anal canal inside some form
of anal retractor (Fig. 10-24A). Various forms of anal retraction have been described. I
still prefer an intra-anal speculum of the Parks variety using small blades only. Admittedly, this results in a certain amount of dilation of the anal sphincters, but it does facilitate a deeper anastomosis at the level of the dentate line. An alternative method of
anal retraction is the use of one or two Gelpi retractors to efface the anal canal and provide reasonable access (Fig. 10-24B). The spikes of the Gelpi retractor, however, may
cause a certain amount of trauma. Another technique, now popular in the United
States, is to use the Lone Star retractor. Essentially, this consists of a series of hooks
applied around the anal canal and mounted on a rectangular stand surrounding the
anal canal. This apparatus is extremely simple, causes no tissue damage, and effaces the
anal canal to facilitate creation of the anastomosis.

   Whatever method of retraction is used, the colon must be delivered to the dentate
line without tension. We prefer to use two lateral stay sutures placed in the jaws of a
Roberts clamp that has been advanced into the pelvis through the anus. As they are
gently withdrawn toward the perineum the colon is delivered to the dentate line (Fig.
10-24A). The end of the colon and the mucosa and internal sphincter of the anal canal
are then sutured using interrupted full-thickness sutures (Fig. 10-24C). We use 2-0 Vicryl
on a 25-mm needle, as the needle tends not to bend within the anal canal. We also use a
Heeney needle holder, which allows the surgeon to grasp the needle in any position so as
to precisely coapt the colon and anal canal. We start the anastomosis in the midline
anteriorly. Each suture is clipped and either attached to the perineum with a towel clip
or to the Lone Star retractor mount. Two anterolateral sutures are then applied just
above the lateral blades of an intra-anal retractor (if one is used). The intervening
sutures are then inserted, leaving all sutures long until they have all been positioned.

Attention is then directed to the posterior suture line. Anastomosis commences in the midline posteriorly, then two posterolateral sutures are inserted; finally the posterior line is completed. The two lateral components of the anastomosis that are obscured by the retractor remain to be completed. The retractor is reoriented anteroposteriorly over the already completed suture line and the remaining lateral sutures placed under direct vision (Fig. 10-24D). Alternatively, the retractor need not be replaced; two stay sutures may be placed in the perineal skin on either side of the anal canal, and the remaining sutures completed. With the use of Gelpi retractors or the Lone Star retractor, these additional maneuvers are unnecessary because all sutures can be placed under direct vision (Fig. 10-24E).

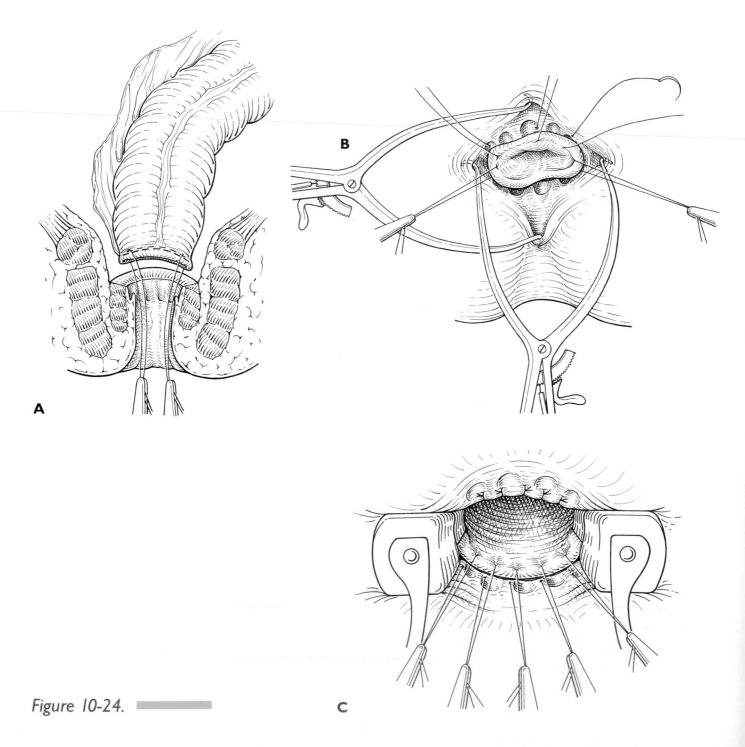

Figure 10-24.

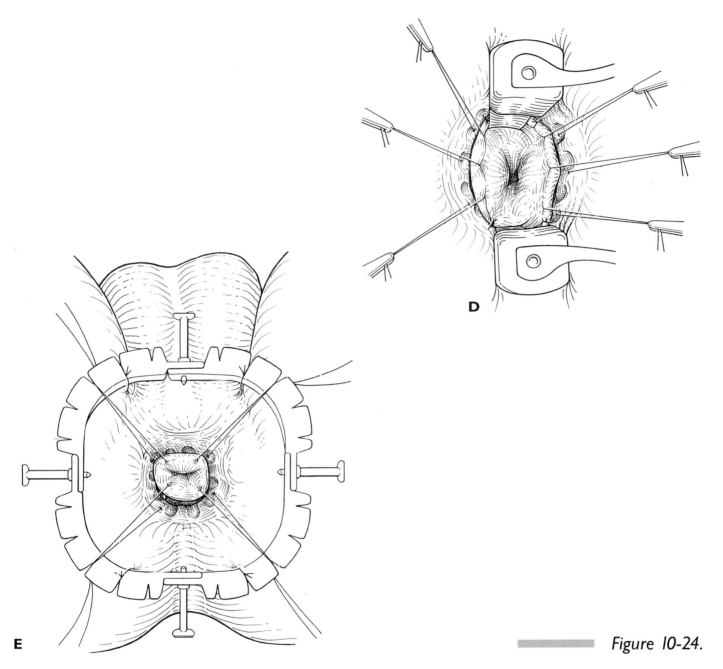

D

E

Figure 10-24.

When using a sutured technique we usually pass two narrow suction drains down into the pelvis, just deep to the intra-anal suture line, and bring the ends out through the abdomen.

Stapled End-to-Side Coloanal Anastomosis with a Colonic Pouch

Usually a 10 × 10 cm colonic pouch is created. The proposed apex of the pouch is first determined and held in a Babcock forceps. The apex of the proposed colonic pouch is then placed in the pelvis to ensure that it will reach the anal staple line without being under any tension (Fig. 10-25A). Once the surgeon is satisfied that there is no tension at the proposed end-to-side anastomosis, a series of stay sutures is used to appose the antimesenteric borders of the colon and longitudinal enterotomy approximately 2 cm long is then made in the taenia coli at the apex of the colonic "J." Hemostasis is secured and a linear staple cutter is advanced along both limbs of the colon (Fig.10-25B). We generally use a PLC 75 staple cutter, but the GIA 95 or the 100-mm 3M linear staple cutter is equally satisfactory. The staple cutter is then closed, the knife is advanced, and two rows of staples are applied to achieve a side-to-side anastomosis. If the proximal end of the colon was closed at the time of tumor excision, it is important to ensure that the linear staple cutter is advanced right to the closed proximal end of the colon. If, on the other hand, the proximal end of the colon has been left open, which is preferred by some surgeons, then it is closed using a transverse stapler once the anastomosis has been constructed.

A pursestring is now placed in the distal pouch enterotomy, having first excised the anterior segment of the colotomy adjacent to the staple line, as this has a tendency to become ischemic. A No. 30 Foley catheter is inserted after closing the pursestring around it and placing a proximal clamp over the colon to test the integrity of the pouch (Fig. 10-25C). Not only does this technique check that there is no evidence of fluid leak from the staple line, but it also removes any blood and fecal material from the colonic pouch. The inflated catheter balloon is then gently withdrawn through the pursestring, which serves to dilate the enterotomy.

The anvil of the circular stapling device is then inserted through the apical enterotomy and the pursestring is closed around the central spindle. The cartridge section of the circular stapling device is advanced through the anal canal to the line of transection. The central pin is advanced through the middle of the anal staple line, the anvil and the cartridge section are snapped together, and the staple gun is closed, fired, and withdrawn as previously described (Fig. 10-25D). The anastomosis is again checked by insufflation with air under saline, by digital assessment, and by ensuring that two complete tissue rings have been recovered from the staple gun.

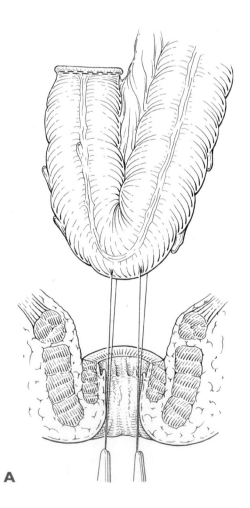

Figure 10-25. ▬▬▬   **A**

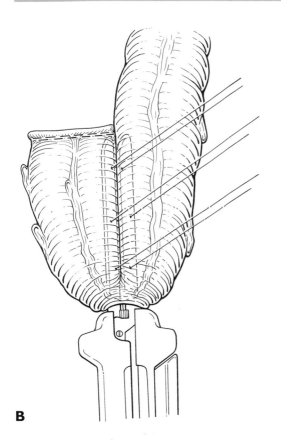

B

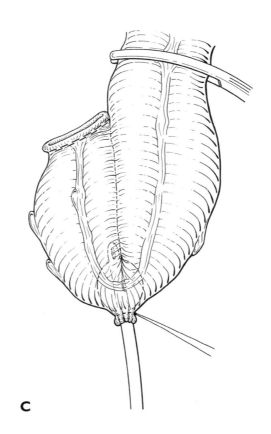

C

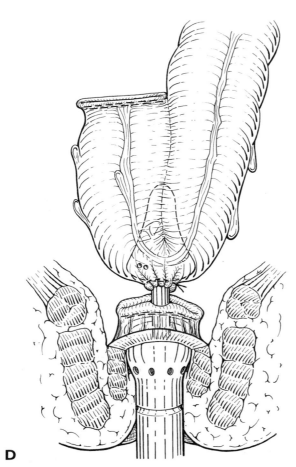

D

Figure 10-25.

Sutured End-to-Side Coloanal Anastomosis

Some surgeons prefer to suture the colonic pouch using a running extramucosal suture technique. The end of the colon is also closed by a running extramucosal suture. A sutured coloanal anastomosis may also be performed, in exactly the same manner as was described for side-to-end anastomosis, having delivered the apex of the pouch to the dentate line.

Completion of the Operation

Once the coloanal anastomosis has been completed and hemostasis secured in the pelvis, two closed suction drains are placed down into the pelvis and usually a proximal loop ileostomy is raised. We believe that the risk of dehiscence from a coloanal anastomosis is significantly greater than that of leakage from an ileoanal anastomosis because the patients are generally elderly, the blood supply to the colon is less certain, and there is fecal material in the residual colon. Consequently, in almost all patients operated on for malignant disease, we raise a proximal loop ileostomy. A trephine is made in the right rectus muscle and a disc of skin and subcutaneous tissue is removed. A cruciate incision is made over the rectus sheath, the rectus muscle is split, and the peritoneum is opened widely enough to accommodate two fingers in the abdominal wall defect easily. The distal end of the ileal loop is marked with a suture at a convenient point near the apex of the loop, and a window is created between the arcades adjacent to the mesentery of the small bowel through which a tape is threaded to serve as a retractor. The apex of the loop is withdrawn through the abdominal wall defect and the abdomen is closed as described in Chapter 1. A small transverse enterotomy is made in the distal limb of the loop adjacent to the suture, and the proximal limb of the ileostomy is everted and sutured to the skin, as described in Chapter 4 (Fig. 10-26).

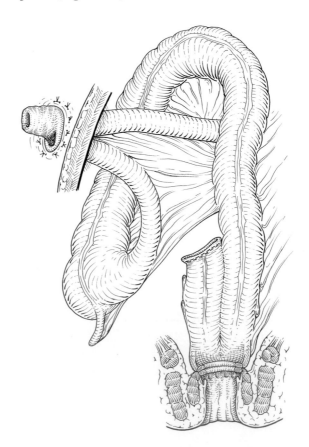

Figure 10-26.

Abdominoperineal Excision of the Rectum

Abdominoperineal excision is used for tumors of the lower third of the rectum that are bulky or that involve the pelvic floor, Denonvilliers fascia, the vagina, or the anal canal. This is often the preferred operation for the patient with a bulky rectal tumor that has not been downstaged by preoperative radiation therapy. This operation is also used where radiation therapy has failed to control cancer of the anus and anal verge. Coexisting radical lymphadenectomy may still be needed if there is residual tumor. The patient must, of course, be counseled both with respect to the need for a permanent stoma and the risk of impaired sexual function from the radical rectal excision (see Ch. 4). A stoma site must be marked preoperatively, with the patient seated as well as recumbent, and consideration given to the patient's normal attire, so that the site is optimally placed.

We use a synchronous combined approach rather than completing the pelvic dissection from above and removing the anal canal later. Synchronous combined excision of the rectum ensures that there is complete hemostasis in the perineum and pelvis, provided the patient is correctly positioned in the lithotomy position, and access from both routes is quite satisfactory.

Abdominal Dissection

Abdominoperineal excision of the rectum involves a more conservative colectomy. Although the origin of the inferior mesenteric artery is usually ligated at its origin and the sigmoid colon resected, the proximal bowel generally has a good vascular supply from the marginal artery. Hence in most cases, it is possible to deliver the end of the descending colon through the abdominal wall trephine without mobilization of the splenic flexure. In all other respects, mobilization of the sigmoid colon is exactly as described in left hemicolectomy/high anterior resection and the pelvic dissection is performed in precisely the same manner described for low anterior resection. The dissection, however, must be individualized at the level of the pelvic floor. If the tumor is situated posteriorly and involves the presacral fascia, this should be excised (taking great care not to damage the presacral veins) together with the posterior fibers of the puborectalis. The same applies for laterally placed tumors, where a wide excision of the levator ani is preferred. If the tumor is anteriorly situated, then it should be widely excised, taking the posterior wall of the vagina in female patients. We generally advise that the majority of the posterior dissection should be performed from above, but if a synchronous combined excision is performed, it is crucial that the two surgeons should work together and not against one another.

Perineal Dissection

One of the most important aspects of the perineal procedure is to secure a watertight seal around the anal canal in order to minimize contamination. We place a strong pursestring suture of Vicryl or Dexon around the perianal margin, which is tied before the operation commences. We then make a circumanal incision, the size of which is determined by the position, site, and size of the tumor (Fig. 10-27A). Once the perianal skin has been totally divided, we suture the inner margin of the divided skin to completely secure the closure of the anal canal (Fig. 10-27B). The excision, of course, involves removing the anal sphincters; hence the fat around the sphincters is divided so as to approach the ischiorectal fossa laterally and the tip of the coccyx in the midline posteriorly (Fig. 10-27C). The extent of the anterior dissection depends on the site and size of the tumor. For anterior tumors involving the posterior vaginal wall, the entire vaginal wall should be included with the perineal skin incision. In posteriorly placed tumors, the anterior dissection in female patients is along the rectovaginal septum, and in male patients the dissection lies immediately behind the prostate, unless the tumor involves prostatic tissue, in which case part of the gland may have to be excised as well. During the anterior dissection, fibers of the levator ani attached to the anorectum, vagina, or prostate will have to be divided. These fibers invariably carry branches of the internal pudendal artery and tributaries of the internal pudendal vein. These vessels must be identified and secured by diathermy while the muscle is being divided. It is often easier to split these muscle fibers in the midline using a pledget before their division. Once divided, the anterior aspect of the anorectum is free from the prostate and seminal vesicles in the male and from the vagina and cervix in the female (Fig. 10-27D). It is then possible to open the peritoneal cavity of the rectouterine or rectovesical pouch so that contact can be made with the abdominal surgeon (Fig. 10-27E).

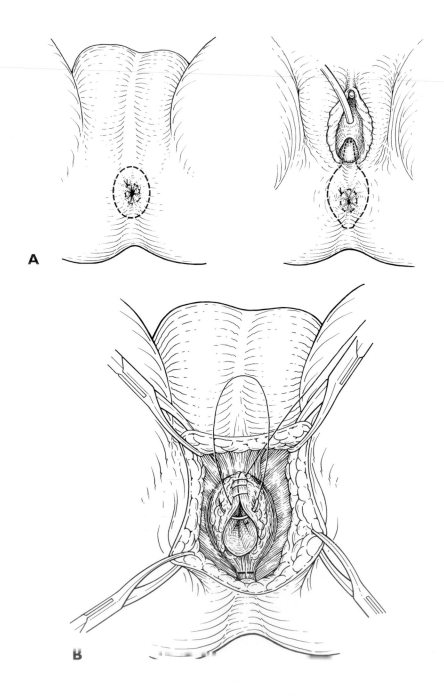

A

B

Figure 10-27.

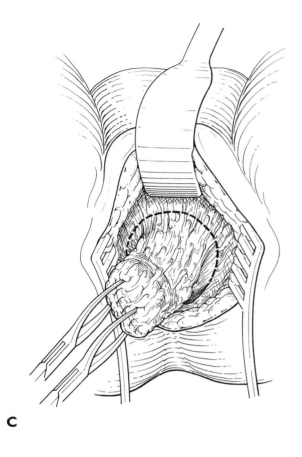

C

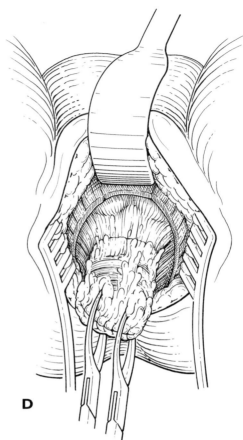

D

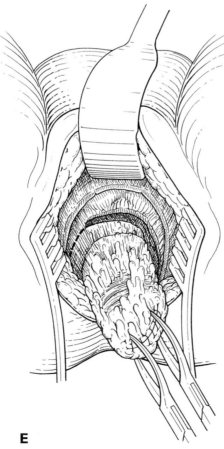

E

Figure 10-27.

We generally prefer the perineal surgeon to develop the anterior plane of excision, while the abdominal surgeon defines the posterior clearance margins. In this way there is no risk of stripping the presacral fascia, which can lead to torrential hemorrhage from presacral veins. Such damage is easily done by the perineal operation unless Waldeyer's fascia is deliberately incised. Consequently, in most cases the abdominal surgeon divides Waldeyer's fascia above the puborectalis so that the rectum and the pelvic floor muscles are taken in continuity, thereby establishing communication with the perineal surgeon from above. It is now the task of the perineal surgeon to divide the rest of the levator ani from the obturator internus. This maneuver must be done on both sides of the rectum to achieve complete rectal excision. Usually some help is needed by the abdominal surgeon. It should now be possible to remove the entire specimen once the junction between the descending colon and sigmoid has been divided, either between Zackkery Cope or Potts clamps or by using a linear staple cutter.

Having removed the specimen, meticulous hemostasis must be secured. If the posterior vaginal wall has been taken, bleeding from its cut edge is common and should be controlled using a running catgut suture (Fig. 10-27F). Provided there has been no contamination, we generally close the perineum as a primary procedure over suction drains. The suction drains are introduced into the pelvis from above and brought out through the abdominal wound. The perineal surgeon will find that it is not possible to close more than the subcutaneous fat and skin, because the levators have been completely excised. There is a substantial dead space, which should be filled if possible. Often this can be achieved by bringing the omentum down into the pelvis; if not, the omentum may be mobilized on the right gastropupleric arcade so that it can reach to the bottom of the pelvis. It is not our practice to close the pelvic peritoneum. Indeed, this is often quite impossible in radical resections for malignant disease owing to the fact that the pelvic peritoneum has been widely excised at the pelvic brim. Surgeons tempted to close the pelvic peritoneum should resist this, because if it proves difficult, a small hole will pose a much greater risk of small bowel obstruction than if the whole pelvis were left open. At this point the perineal operator closes the skin while the abdominal surgeon places drains on suction to avoid hematoma formation during abdominal wall closure (Fig. 10-27G).

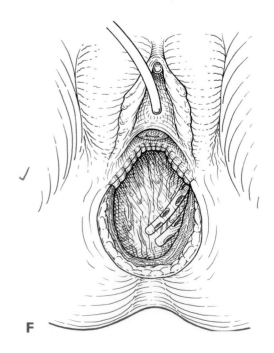

Figure 10-27.   F

A trephine for the end colostomy is made in the left rectus muscle, excising a disc of skin and subcutaneous fat, and making a cruciate incision over the rectus sheath. The rectus muscle is split, the peritoneum is opened, and the end of the colon is delivered through the abdominal wall defect, as described in Chapter 4. The abdomen is then closed as described in Chapter 1. Finally, mucocutaneous colostomy sutures complete the operation (Fig. 10-27H).

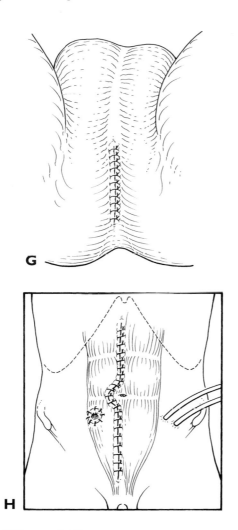

Figure 10-27.

Local Excision of Rectal Cancer

Local excision is feasible in only a highly select group of patients with rectal cancer. In our experience, less than 5 percent of all rectal cancers are amenable to local excision. Only those tumors that involve the mucosa and submucosa and that have not extended beyond the lamina propria are suitable. Furthermore, in our experience, only those tumors that are less than 12 cm in diameter are appropriate. It is important to remember that if there is any doubt whatsoever about nodal metastases, it is far wiser to embark on a radical rectal excision than to attempt complete cure by local excision but fail. This is particularly relevant now that sphincter-saving resections are feasible and are relatively easy to perform in these cases. The only exception to this philosophy is the patient in whom a radical rectal excision might be contraindicated because of coexisting disease.

These tumors must be very carefully assessed preoperatively and the precise location within the rectum determined. Intrarectal ultrasonography is particularly valuable in identifying T1 and T2 stage tumors. Information about the upper extent of the lesion is crucial because lesions with an upper margin, more than 8 cm from the anal verge, are unsuitable for local or transsphincteric procedures. Anteriorly placed lesions are best managed with the patient in the prone jackknife position; posterior lesions are best managed with the patient in the lithotomy position, although admittedly, those lesions lying just beyond the anorectal angle can prove quite difficult to remove peranally with the patient so positioned. The mobility of the tumor in the submucosal plane should also be assessed. Mobile tumors can usually be delivered into the operating field by placing six to eight sutures around the periphery of the tumor, leaving the suture tails long, and then gathering the tails together in a manner resembling the cords of a parachute, twisting them, and pulling the lesion en masse into the operating field (Fig. 10-28A & B).

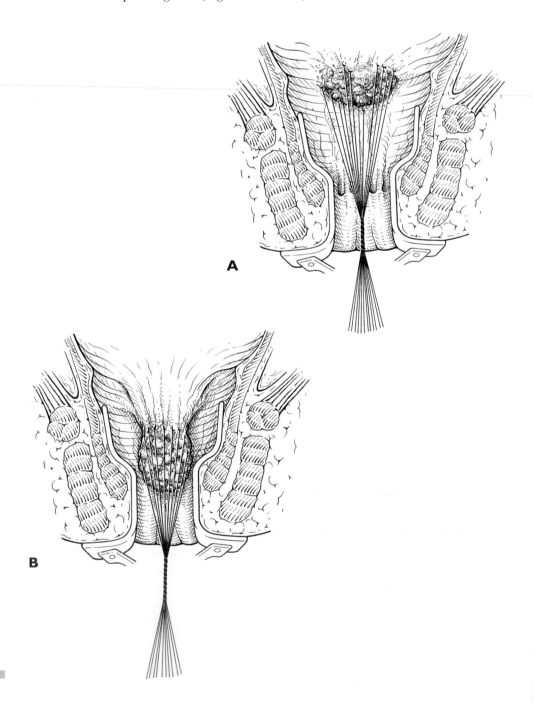

A

B

Figure 10-28.

Peranal Technique for Anteriorly Situated Lesions

The patient is placed in the prone jackknife position. An intra-anal bivalved retractor is used to display the lesion. Infiltration of the submucosa and the rectal wall around the tumor is necessary to reduce hemostasis and to develop a tissue plane of excision (Fig. 10-29A). We use a 1:300,000 epinephrine solution for this purpose. A series of sutures are placed around the periphery of the tumor, as just described. The excision should include at least 2 cm from the macroscopic edge of the tumor to ensure complete removal of tumor. The mucosa and submucosa is divided peripherally around the lesion using diathermy. All submucosal vessels must be secured during division of the mucosa and submucosa in order to maintain a dry field. If the tumor has been correctly staged, complete clearance can be achieved by excision of a disc of full-thickness rectal wall. Indeed, if rectal fat is not observed, the excision has not been sufficiently deep to achieve adequate clearance (Fig. 10-29B). It is often helpful to place a series of stay sutures beyond the resection margin to facilitate closure of the defect once the tumor has been removed. Once the lesion has been removed completely, the defect in the rectal muscle should be closed transversely using a continuous Vicryl or PDS suture, and the mucosa closed with a running chromic catgut suture (Fig. 10-29C).

for tu
lesior
anore
and f
sure s

Intra

The
demc
epine
recta
ing a
tal w

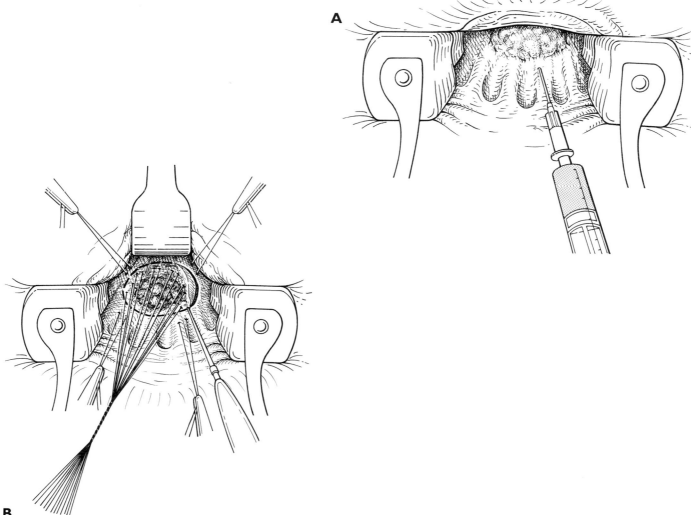

A

B

Figure 10-29.

Fig

F

Left Hemicolectomy and Hiqh Anterior Resection. The differences here are related to initiating the operation in the left pericolic gutter and the splenic flexure is mobilized routinely. A retroperitoneal approach is then made to the origin of the inferior mesenteric artery. This is identified in a way very similar to that described by Dr. Keighley in his script. For sigmoid and upper third rectal cancers, the inferior mesenteric artery is ligated flush at its origin as well the left colic artery included in the resection. The transection line of the bowel is chosen depending on the site of the tumor. For a descending colon or sigmoid colon carcinoma, the bowel will be transected at the junction of the proximal two-thirds and distal one-third of the transverse colon. For sigmoid colon cancers, the proximal line of resection is chosen at the mid-descending colon. For the upper third of rectal cancers, the line of transection is at the junction of the descending and sigmoid colons. The presacral space is then entered between the investing layer of fascia of the rectum and Waldeyer's fascia. Presacral nerves are routinely preserved and ureters are identified routinely. An occlusive tape is placed below the tumor and the distal section of bowel is washed out with 40 percent ethyl alcohol. Distal margins are a minimum of 5 cm in the fresh unfixed specimen. The technique of stapled anastomosis was mentioned earlier.

I think there is a minimal role for transecting the vasculature at the superior hemorrhoidal artery. The ligation of the inferior mesenteric artery at its origin poses no undue difficulties, but does usually enhance the ability to mobilize the left colon.

In the event that resecting of the upper third of rectum or in the case of lower anterior resection, there is deemed to be a locally extensive neoplasm, we will usually bring omentum down as a pedicle based in the left gastric epiploic vessels to quarantine the pelvis. Thus with small bowel maintained in a cephalad location, any postoperative radiation therapy deemed appropriate can be applied with less risk of small bowel injury from radiation enteritis.

For low anterior resection, this procedure involves removing the mesorectum with posterior dissection beyond the tip of the coccyx. Thus this will mean routinely the performance of an anastomosis that is either coloanal or ultralow colorectal. We use identical techniques to that of Dr. Keighley in terms of doubly ligating the inferior mesenteric vein. The principles of management of adjacent organ involvement (e.g., ureter, bladder, vagina) or apparent presacral fixation are followed according to the principles as outlined by Dr. Keighley. With fixed or tethered or poorly differentiated midrectal or low rectal cancers, preoperative chemoradiation therapy is given. In most cases rectal sonography will be used for low and midrectal cancers preoperatively. If nodal involvement is thought to be present on the basis of this, then preoperative chemoradiation therapy is also given.

Following resection and extraperitoneal anastomosis presacral sump drainage is used.

With hand-sewn coloanal anastomoses, I use effacing anal sutures of O-Dexon in lieu of a Park's retractor or Lone Star retractor. These effacement sutures have been used routinely by us for the past 10 years for coloanal, ileoanal, and most transanal procedures. The technique of resection and anastomoses are essentially as described by Dr. Keighley.

When colonic J-pouches are required, we use an 8- to 10-cm pouch, created with the use of the ILA 100-mm stapler and PI30 stapler being placed across the tip of the "J." An antimesenteric incision is made in the apex of the loop. If a stapled anastomosis is to be used, then the anvil is placed at this time and tied over a pursestring through the apex of the loop. Otherwise this area is grasped with a Babcock clamp and delivered through the open anal canal after placement of anal verge sutures.

Indications for colonic J-pouches include patients who have a narrow or contracted left colon and those with low resting and squeeze anal sphincter pressures.

With respect to abdominoperineal resection, the operation is done almost exactly as described by Dr. Keighley. The exception is that almost all the dissection is done with the electrocautery including taking the lateral ligaments widely with cautery rather than using ligatures and clamps. For anterior rectal tumors in women where invasion of the rectovaginal septum is present, a partial resection of the posterior vagina will be performed. In most cases this precludes closure of the vaginal defect. In such cases the posterolateral vaginal walls are sutured to the fat and residual levator fibers in the posterolateral portions of the perineal wound. The perineum is then sutured up to the neovaginal orifice with absorbable sutures and packing of the posterior vagina is performed. The pack is removed after 5 to 6 days. The wound is irrigated out daily thereafter with sterile saline solution.

At the Cleveland Clinic we use both these combined synchronous procedures as well as single surgeon dissection. The bias has been toward a single surgeon dissectional. The merits of the combined synchronous have been well outlined by Dr. Keighley.

Transanal resection for rectal cancer is as outlined by Dr. Keighley. I believe there is no role for transsphincteric excision of rectal cancer.

Victor W. Fazio

The Saint-Antoine group concurs with Dr. Keighley's descriptions. Insofar as the aim of this book is to describe techniques, I do not think that the Principles section is adequate. We also usually perform a midline incision, but for well-localized tumors in the cecum, ascending colon, or splenic flexure, we prefer to perform a transverse right or left subumbilicus incision in the obese patient. Although for rectal cancer we operate with the patient in the double-approach position, for colon cancer we do not. We are not sure that the frequency of leg-vein thrombosis is not increased by use of the Allen stirrups.

At the end of a rectal resection in a male patient, we routinely replace the transurethral catheter with suprapubic pelvic transcutaneous drainage, which the patient finds more comfortable. As a rule we always try to ligate the vessels before mobilizing the segment of tumor-bearing colon and to li-

(Continues)

gate the colon on both sides of the tumor provided this maneuver is easy and safe to perform.

We usually mobilize the mesocolon bilaterally from the midline to the border. This technique ensures demonstration of the position of the duodenum and right ureter on the right side and of the left ureter on the other side.

With regard to right hemicolectomy, closure of the peritoneal window is technically easier to start before the anastomosis is fashioned. Perianastomotic epiplooplasty can help to avoid any adhesions between the anastomosis and the midline incision. We have no experience with antitumor agents, but we always put a clamp just behind the tumor and wash the distal rectum before stapling.

When we have difficulty fashioning the anastomosis, especially when dealing with sepsis, we prefer to bring out both ends as ostomies rather than to protect the anastomosis with a loop ileostomy. We always try to avoid spillage during creation of anastomoses, which in our experience are mostly hand sewn, by using tapes to snare the bowel on both sides, 10 cm away from the cut ends. When the distal end is rectum, we use a transverse vascular clamp, placed at least 3 cm from the anastomosis and closed very gently. Our technique is generally to use hand-sewn running sutures, taking all layers on both sides and interrupted only at two angles, the posterior and anterior planes.

An alternative to the end-to-end sigmoidorectal anastomosis when the sigmoid is narrow and the rectum is large is to construct a side-to-end anastomosis after stapling the sigmoid end.

As far as low anterior resection is concerned, we agree that posterior dissection and retrorectal mobilization have to be performed first, although the anterior dissection can be made before the lateral one. The latter will be very easy to perform if the rectum and its mesentery have been freed anteriorly and posteriorly.

The anterior plane of dissection is in front of Denonvilliers fascia regardless of the location of the tumor.

We have never left the vagina open in such circumstances as described by Dr. Keighley. When we perform a total hysterectomy or a simple vaginal resection together with a colorectal anastomosis, we try to isolate both suture lines by interposition of a well-vascularized piece of omentum.

In our experience, it has always been possible to construct a pouch for a coloanal anastomosis. Reading the description of the stapled coloanal anastomosis reinforced our belief that to construct a hand-sewn pouch, anal anastomosis at the dentate line is much easier.

We never deliver the colon through the anus. There is no reason to dilate the anus when it is not necessary. If the hand-sewn anastomosis is built at the dentate line, after a mucosectomy of 1 cm leading to the transanal abdominal dissection field, only gentle exposure of the suture line is mandatory (using Gelpi retractors or Lone Star retractor).

If the apex of the pouch extends 2 to 3 cm beyond the symphysis pubis, it will reach the anus. This maneuver is easier and much quicker than the maneuver described by Dr. Keighley to create a pouch of sufficient length.

Two or three details are missing from Dr. Keighley's description, in my opinion. He does not mention the possibility of a transmesenteric route for the colon when the mesentery of the transverse colon threatens to crush the duodenojejunal angle, or in some cases of bringing the right colon, vascularized by the ileocecocolic vessel, through the right paracolic space. We have successfully constructed a colic pouch with the hepatic flexure in a couple of cases after using this technique to bring it down.

We think that, after any procedure involving section of the inferior mesenteric artery and vein at their origin, it is very important to fix the border of the mesocolon to preaortic fascia behind the duodenojejunal angle to avoid trapping of jejunal loops. We always mobilize the greater omentum on the left gastrocolic arcade before bringing it down to the pelvis after Miles operation and for us it is very important that well-vascularized omentum be fixed by the perineal surgeon to the site of skin closure and not simply pushed down by the abdominal surgeon, in order to avoid any dead space.

Colostomy is never transperitoneal, as it is suggested by Dr. Keighley. The left colon is brought out through a 4- to 5-cm-long subperitoneal incision. In our experience, the risk of prolapse is thus far considerably decreased using this technique.

With regard to the length of colon to be brought down to the pelvis for either low colorectal or coloanal anastomosis, we always strive to obtain enough to fill the pelvis with floppy colon.

In summary, I would like to say that the need for adequate distal margins in resection rectal cancer cannot be stressed enough. With regard to local excision, we are reluctant to perform such a procedure for tumors located in the anterior rectum.

Rolland Parc

11

Diverticular Disease
Michael R. B. Keighley

Principles

Surgical resection for diverticular disease is usually performed for complications, some of which carry a high mortality because of continuing sepsis or severe coexisting cardiorespiratory disease. The principal complications include fecal peritonitis, which still carries a mortality of approximately 40 percent; diffuse purulent peritonitis, in which the mortality is approximately 12 percent; localized pericolic abscess, with a mortality of approximately 6 percent; and an inflammatory phlegmon in the sigmoid, in which the mortality is 4 percent. Inflammatory phlegmon may or may not be complicated by a colovesical, coloenteric, colocutaneous, or colovaginal fistula. Other complications include acute or chronic obstruction, which may involve the small as well as the large bowel, and massive hemorrhage (see Ch. 15).

Most surgeons would argue that the Hartmann operation is still the safest procedure for life-threatening sepsis, particularly fecal and diffuse purulent peritonitis. Resection alone removes the perforated segment without the risk of an anastomotic breakdown. However, in a third of patients intestinal continuity is never restored after the Hartmann operation, either because of severe coexisting cardiorespiratory disease or because the patient's general condition is too poor to tolerate a second major surgical procedure in which the colostomy is taken down and a colorectal anastomosis performed. A further argument used by those who believe that the Hartmann procedure is not necessarily the optimum procedure is that restoring intestinal continuity is a difficult and a high-morbidity procedure that sometimes necessitates a covering proximal stoma anyway. Furthermore, although the Hartmann procedure should theoretically be associated with the lowest risk of subsequent sepsis, nevertheless further peritoneal contamination can occur if there is dehiscence of the oversewn rectal stump or if there is ischemia or retraction of the end colostomy. For this reason some now argue that in low-risk patients, or for localized sepsis, primary resection, on-table colonic lavage, and primary anastomosis with or without a proximal defunctioning stoma might be a more appropriate operation. We do not subscribe to this view given that the majority of patients are extremely ill, and believe that the safest life-saving procedure is a sigmoidectomy end colostomy with oversewing of the rectal stump.

In the less urgent situation of a localized pericolic abscess, there is no doubt that preoperative percutaneous drainage (Fig. 11-1) to convert an infected procedure to an elective clean operation allows an increasing proportion of patients to undergo a primary resection and anastomosis, particularly by utilizing on-table colonic lavage (Fig. 11-2) if for some reason preoperative mechanical bowel preparation is deemed undesirable or unsafe, or has been unsuccessful. We therefore propose to describe three major types of operative procedure for complicated diverticular disease: the Hartmann operation and restoration of intestinal continuity after the Hartmann operation, primary resection and anastomosis with or without on-table colonic lavage (and creation of a proximal stoma where necessary), and finally resection for colovesical fistula, the principles of which would also apply for colovaginal, colocutaneous, and coloenteric fistulas.

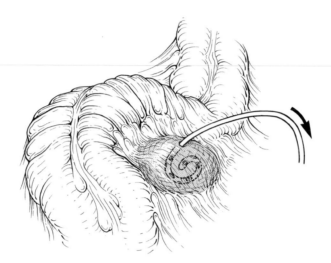

Figure 11-1. ▬▬▬▬▬▬

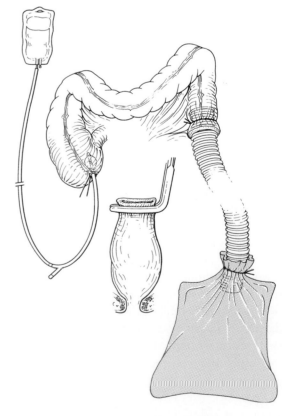

Figure 11-2. ▬▬▬▬▬▬

It goes without saying that for emergency procedures preoperative mechanical bowel preparation is impossible and dangerous. However, for elective operations (e.g., an established colovesical fistula or an inflammatory phlegmon), it is essential that fecal material be cleared from the colon and rectum by meticulous preoperative mechanical bowel preparation. In elective surgical procedures short-term antimicrobial cover would also be advised; however, for established infections more prolonged antibiotic administration with drainage and on-table peritoneal lavage is generally practiced. All patients, whether they are having an elective or an emergency procedure, are at risk of thromboembolism, hence the use of graduated compression stockings, on-table pneumatic leg bags, and subcutaneous heparin is generally advised.

Hartmann Operation

The patient is placed in the modified Lloyd-Davies position with the legs in Allen stirrups. The bladder is catheterized, and it is often a good idea to place a large Foley catheter in the rectum. In seriously ill patients it may be necessary to monitor left atrial filling pressures and an arterial line is generally advised.

A generous midline laparotomy incision is made. In perforated diverticular disease there is usually diffuse purulent or fecal peritonitis. The first consideration is the removal of all infected material from the peritoneal cavity, hence large-volume saline washouts are begun immediately. If there has been an established infective process, fibrin exudate will need to be gently wiped away from the loops of small bowel. It is likely that the omentum will be adherent over the sigmoid colon if the cause of the peritonitis is diverticular disease (Fig. 11-3). However, a careful search must be made to identify an alternative source of peritoneal contamination if no obvious perforation is immediately evident in the sigmoid. A perforation of the sigmoid colon can be assumed only if all other potential sites of perforation have been excluded and there is an inflammatory phlegmon or omentum adherent to the sigmoid.

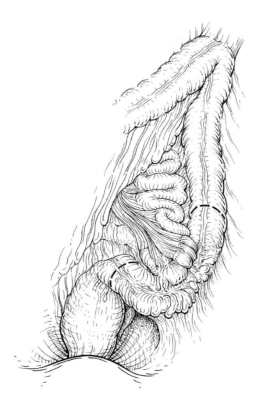

Figure 11-3.

The principle of sigmoidectomy is merely to remove the sigmoid in the quickest and safest manner while ensuring an adequate blood supply to the proximal colon for colostomy and safe closure of the rectal stump. A radical operation to remove all of the diverticular disease is not necessary; this can be done when intestinal continuity is restored.

Often the sigmoid colon is ischemic and fecal material from the perforation continues to contaminate the peritoneal cavity. In our experience, placement of a purse-string suture around the perforation is a waste of time, but the use of ties around the sigmoid above and below the perforation with delivery of any fecal material from the colon afterward minimizes contamination (Fig. 11-4). However, if there is an extensive inflammatory mass such a procedure is often not possible. Under these circumstances an antiseptic swab is placed over the hole, the segment of colon is held in the surgeon's left hand (Fig. 11-5), and the sigmoid colon is mobilized as rapidly as possible and resected between two clamps. To facilitate this, the peritoneum along the lateral border of the descending colon and the sigmoid is divided, taking care not to injure the gonadal vessels and ureter. No attempt is made to divide the peritoneum on either side of the rectum because this opens new planes that may become infected. The mesentery of the sigmoid colon is divided between clamps to the level of the proposed transection of the sigmoid colon. Transfixion sutures may be used if the mesentery is very thick (Fig. 11-6). A segmental sigmoid resection is then performed between crushing intestinal clamps and the diseased, perforated segment is removed. The risk of continued intestinal contamination is over at this point. The rectal stump is then oversewn using a running Vicryl or PDS suture. We prefer to take bites of the rectal wall from one side to the other over the clamp (Fig. 11-7). When the clamp is removed the suture is merely pulled, which inverts the rectum, and the suture is then returned to its original point to complete a two-layer closure. Today, however, we increasingly use a linear stapler, either the TA-55, RL-50, or PIA-55, depending on the size of the bowel and the surgeon's preference.

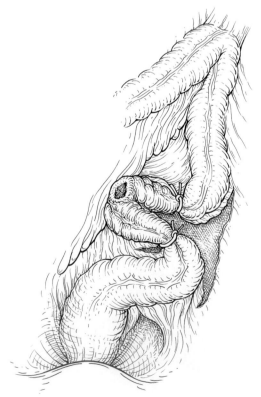

Figure 11-4.

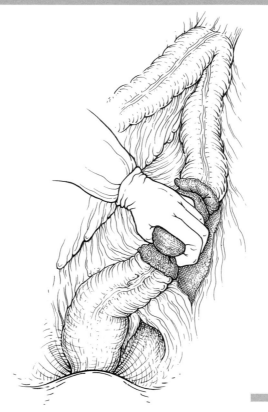

Figure 11-5.

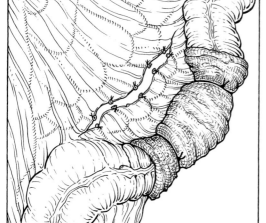

Figure 11-6.

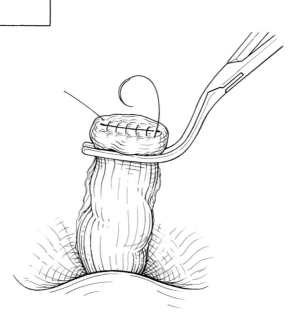

Figure 11-7.

Attention should now be directed to the proximal colon because it is essential to bring out a length of colon that is not under tension and that has an adequate blood supply. The sigmoid mesocolon may be thick and short and the abdominal wall deep, and unless sufficient attention is paid to the construction of the stoma, retraction or ischemia can occur, resulting in morbidity or death. Consequently, the entire left colon is generally mobilized and it may be necessary also to take down the splenic flexure (Fig. 11-8). Once the left colon has been adequately mobilized, a trephine is made in the left rectus muscle at the desired site, which must have been marked preoperatively. A disc of skin and fat is excised, the rectus sheath is split or divided, and the peritoneum is opened so as to allow delivery of the divided left colon (Fig. 11-9). To prevent contamination during this procedure, the bowel should be either sealed with a Potts clamp or transected with a stapler. The staple line is excised prior to mucocutaneous suturing. Further peritoneal lavage may then be performed before inserting large closed suction drains to the sites of maximum sepsis. The omentum is brought down to the site of the oversewn rectosigmoid stump and the abdomen is closed as described in Chapter 1.

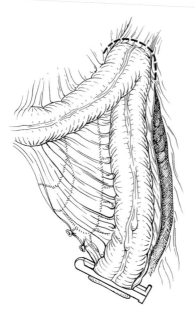

Figure 11-8.

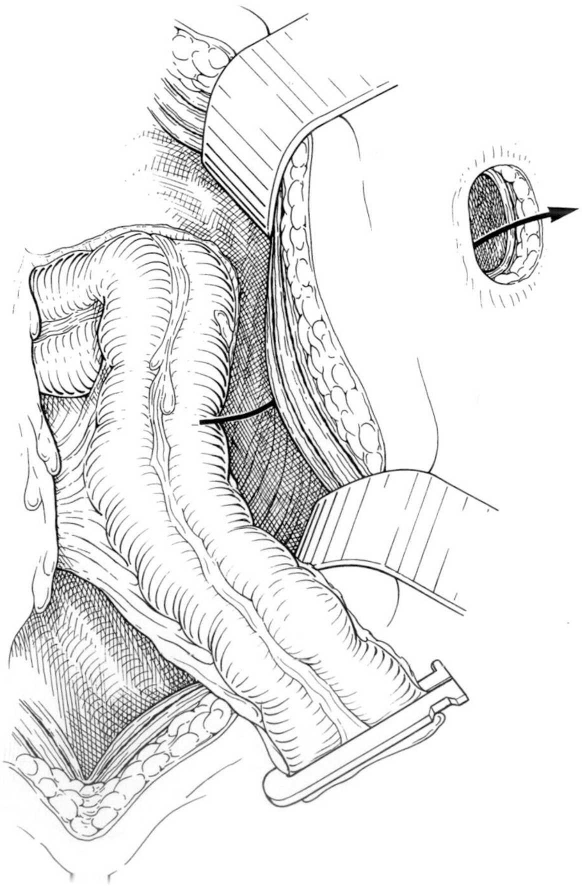

Figure 11-9.

Alternative Strategies

The sigmoid colon may be so necrotic that it is deemed unsafe to attempt to oversew the rectal stump. Under these circumstances, if the segment of colon requiring resection is short, a double-barreled colostomy may be considered as an option (Fig. 11-10A & B). This, however, is usually only feasible after mobilization of the rectum, division of the pelvic peritoneum, and retrorectal resection in order to bring the divided segment up to the abdominal wall without tension. Such a procedure increases the risk of pelvic sepsis and it is often feasible only in thin patients; it is quite impossible in grossly obese individuals or where there has been extensive fibrosis around the sigmoid colon. An alternative strategy, particularly if an extensive segment of the sigmoid colon is completely necrotic and where suture closure of the rectosigmoid is deemed unsafe, is to divide the lateral margins of the rectum, undertake a full posterior rectal mobilization, and transect the rectum below the sacral promontory (Fig. 11-11). Inevitably such a procedure opens new tissue planes, increasing the risk of pelvic abscess. However, this is far less of a risk than a necrotic rectal stump, hence staple transection at this level may be a safer option.

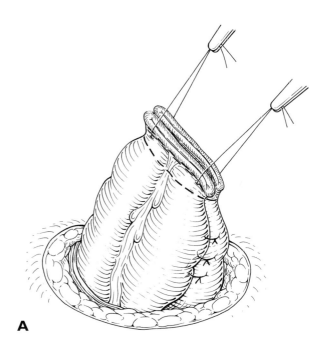

A

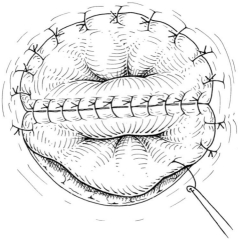

B

Figure 11-10.

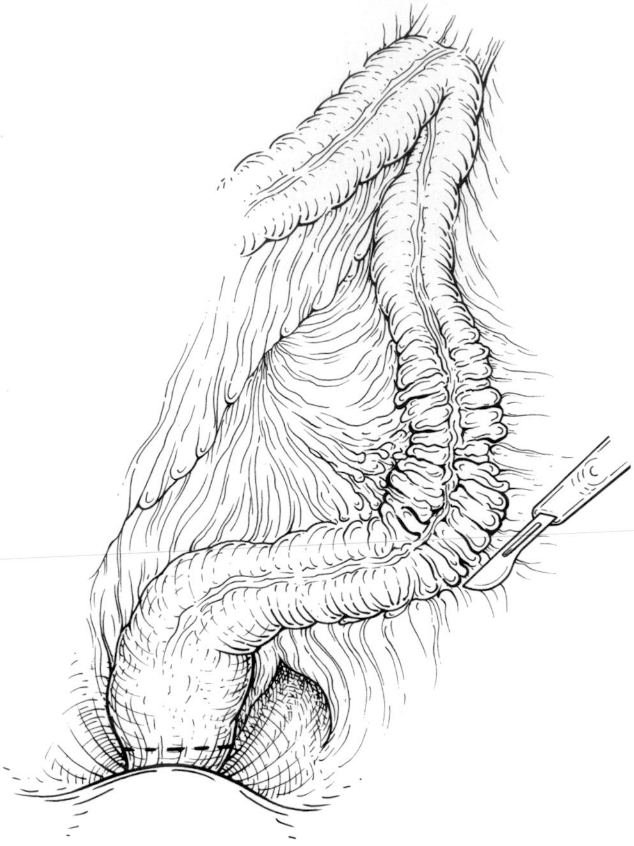

Figure 11-11.

If, as is rarely the case, the sigmoid perforation lies at the apex of the sigmoid or if the mesentery is sufficiently long after complete mobilization of the sigmoid loop, the perforated segment may be delivered to the abdominal wall as a "perforostomy" (Fig. 11-12). Such a procedure requires a large trephine in the abdominal wall and extensive division of the rectus muscle to accommodate the sigmoid. Furthermore, perforostomy is often quite impossible because of the build of the patient or because of fibrosis accompanying the inflammatory disease in the sigmoid. Nevertheless, this is an option that may have to be considered in certain circumstances.

The use of sharp dissection may be necessary if a perforation has occurred in a segment of sigmoid colon that has been the site of recurrent episodes of inflammation (Fig. 11-11). Under these circumstances, the pericolic fibrosis may be so extensive that sharp dissection may prove to be the only way in which to remove the sigmoid colon. The first stage is to mobilize loops of small intestine and omentum from the sigmoid. The lateral peritoneum is divided with a scalpel or with a cutting diathermy. Great care must be taken to keep as close to the bowel as possible and to identify the gonadal vessels and ureter above the inflammatory mass so that they can be traced down and their division avoided. Sharp dissection may also be needed between the sigmoid colon and the bladder and the sigmoid mesentery will almost certainly have to be transfixed to secure vessels in the thickened sigmoid mesentery. In the presence of such extensive fibrosis it is often quite impossible to use a linear staple cutter or linear stapler to close the distal sigmoid and the technique of suture closure, described earlier, may have to be used. Also, in these circumstances, there may be so much fibrosis in the proximal sigmoid that further mobilization may be necessary in order to deliver a healthy segment of colon to the abdominal wall for colostomy.

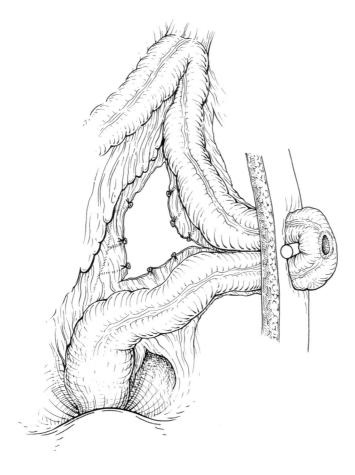

Figure 11-12.

Restoration of Intestinal Continuity

Restoring intestinal continuity after a Hartmann resection is a potentially high morbidity procedure, hence all patients should be adequately counseled about the potential risks of a further major operation. They should also have been thoroughly evaluated preoperatively to determine whether the results of restoring intestinal continuity are likely to be satisfactory. Many of these patients are elderly with impaired sphincter function. We therefore advise all patients to have anal manometry and electromyography. Some patients may have adapted so well to their colostomy that they may not wish to entertain the risks associated with restoring intestinal continuity in the hope that normal bowel function can be achieved.

A full mechanical bowel preparation is absolutely essential. The entire colon must be cleared of fecal residue; likewise, any inspissated mucus in the rectal stump should be evacuated by rectal washout. A potential stoma site should be marked on the right side of the abdomen in case a covering loop ileostomy is necessary to protect the anastomosis. The patient is placed in the modified Lloyd-Davies position with the legs in Allen stirrups so that there is adequate access to the rectal stump. Access to the rectum is absolutely crucial as the stump may be difficult to identify, particularly if it has been transected beyond the pelvic brim. Furthermore, this position allows the anastomosis to be tested underwater and enables the circular stapling gun to be utilized if this is the most appropriate method of anastomosis. The patient is catheterized. The previous midline incision is reopened. There are likely to be extensive adhesions from loops of small bowel adherent to one another and to the omentum. Loops of bowel may be adherent to the posterior aspect of the previous laparotomy incision, hence great care should be taken when opening the abdomen in order to avoid iatrogenic injury to the small bowel. The omentum is first carefully dissected from the abdominal wall and from the previous operation site. Loops of small bowel are then dissected from the pelvis and the rectal stump (Fig. 11-13A).

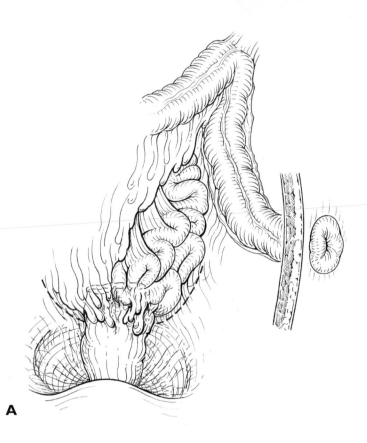

Figure 11-13.   **A**

Identification of the rectal stump may prove to be extremely difficult. Unless the rectum can be identified with confidence, there is a risk that blind dissection at the base of the pelvis may result in iatrogenic damage to the base of the bladder or even to the ureters. If the previous resection has been a limited sigmoidoscopy and the rectosigmoid junction remains in situ, identification rarely poses a problem. If, on the other hand, the rectal stump cannot be adequately visualized, an assistant should be instructed to pass a sigmoidoscope through the rectal stump. The physical presence of the instrument or its light inside the rectum should allow placement of stay sutures on the apex of the viscus. Dissection of the rectal stump should then commence posteriorly having previously identified both ureters at the pelvic brim because if there has been any previous inflammatory reaction in the pelvis the ureters can be displaced medially and may be at risk of damage. The dissection should continue posteriorly, immediately behind the superior hemorrhoidal artery.

Sometimes it is easier to enter the posterior plane laterally. Scar tissue around the front of the sacrum should be incised, if necessary, with a long-handled blade so that the thickened mesorectum can be dissected from the presacral fascia but great care must be taken not to damage the presacral veins and preferably to preserve the pelvic autonomic nerves. This plane is further developed by careful blunt dissection so that the posterior margin of the rectum can be fully delivered from the sacrum. It may be necessary to divide the superior hemorrhoidal vessel in order to achieve this but generally the plane behind the vessels is bloodless and easier to define provided the presacral fascia is intact. The sides of the rectum should then be mobilized by division of

the pelvic peritoneum, the lateral border of the mesorectum, and the lateral ligaments. Finally, the anterior pelvic peritoneum is divided to expose the anterior border of the rectum. If there is any sigmoid colon adherent to the upper rectum, this
must be resected prior to colorectal anastomosis (Fig. 11-13B).

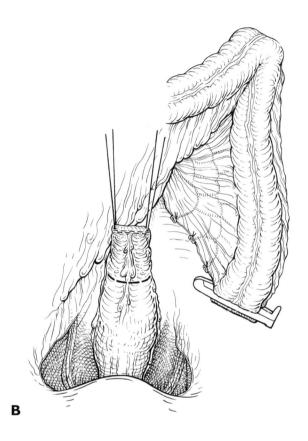

B

Figure 11-13.

The end colostomy is now taken down by dissection from the abdominal wall and
parietal peritoneum. The left colon will have to be mobilized and it may be necessary
to take down the splenic flexure in order to achieve a safe, tension-free anastomosis
between the descending colon and the upper third of the rectum. Once it is evident
that the descending colon can be brought without tension onto the rectal stump, a
colorectal anastomosis is performed.

The anastomosis may be achieved using either the circular stapling device or a single-layer hand-sutured technique (Fig. 11-14). It is safer to perform a sutured anastomosis by resecting the residual sigmoid colon adherent to the upper rectum under
direct vision than it is to perform a stapled anastomosis, because introduction of the
staple gun in a narrow, contracted defunctioned rectum may prove quite difficult and
may cause damage to the rectal ampulla. Indeed, performing a Hartmann procedure
merely by introducing the circular staple gun through the residual rectum and
advancing the pin through the transected rectal stump is a technique that is rarely
possible because of stenosis and deformity in the hypoplastic defunctioned rectum. If
a circular stapling technique is to be used, it is much safer to fully mobilize the rectum from the presacral fascia down to the pelvic floor so that a straight rectal
ampulla is available for transection with a transverse stapler and subsequent anastomosis (Fig. 11-15). This naturally involves far more rectal dissection, and a greater
risk of hematoma and sepsis in the pelvis. Consequently, we often prefer a sutured
anastomosis to establish intestinal continuity after Hartmann resection. Two closed-

suction drains are placed behind the rectum. If there has been any technical difficulty whatsoever with the colorectal anastomosis or if the mechanical bowel preparation has been less than ideal and on-table colonic lavage has not been performed, a covering loop ileostomy should be made through a trephine in the right rectus muscle (Fig. 11-16). If, on the other hand, there have been no technical difficulties and when the anastomosis is tested underwater there is no evidence of air leakage, then the abdomen may be closed as described in Chapter 1.

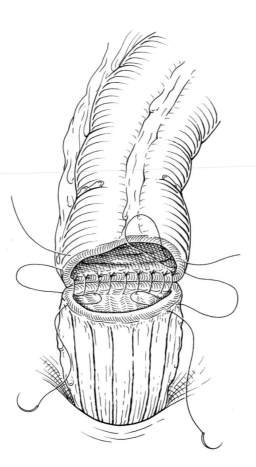

Figure 11-14.

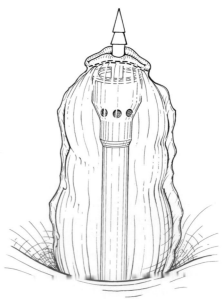

Figure 11-15.

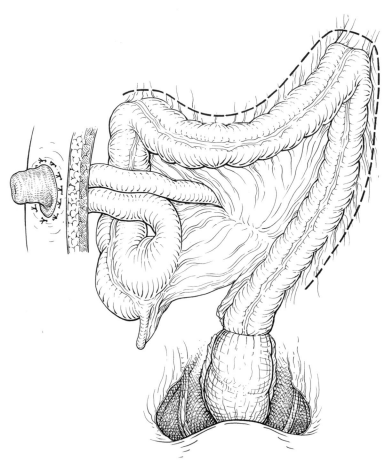

Figure 11-16.

Primary Resection and Anastomosis with or without On-Table Colonic Lavage

Primary resection and anastomosis is usually feasible in most patients with an inflammatory phlegmon in whom the operation is being performed for obstructive symptoms and in patients with a colovesical enterocolonic or colovaginal fistula provided that there is no gross sepsis around the operation site. The indications for primary resection and anastomosis have been extended in recent years to include complications of diverticular disease, particularly pericolic abscess or localized perforation. This is due in large part to improved imaging, which, by providing a method of accurate percutaneous drainage of pus, allows the conversion of an infected situation into a planned elective resection once all the local sepsis has been drained. The role of primary resection and anastomosis with on-table colonic lavage has been extended by some to include the treatment of purulent peritonitis complicating perforated diverticular disease, but we question the wisdom of such an enterprise and would still prefer to confine primary resection and anastomosis to noninfective diverticular disease.

The techniques of resection do not differ substantially from those described for Hartmann resection except that in the elective situation there may be extensive fibrosis that necessitates sharp dissection. Also, under these circumstances, it is absolutely crucial to remove all the sigmoid colon, thereby fashioning an anastomosis between the descending colon and the upper third of the rectum. Thus it is often necessary to mobilize the splenic flexure, relying on the marginal artery supplied by the middle colic artery to maintain the viability of the proximal colon. Also, it is necessary to divide the peritoneum on the lateral and anterior aspects of the rectum and to divide the mesorectum with the sigmoid mesentery so as to gain access to the upper rectum for division and anastomosis. When resection is being performed as an emergency procedure for complicated diverticular disease under circumstances in which preoperative mechanical bowel preparation has not been possible or where preoperative mechanical bowel preparation is considered ill-advised, the technique of on-table colonic lavage should always be used after resecting the diseased segment (see also Ch. 13). Once the proximal colon has been completely cleared of all fecal residue and any liquid used to perfuse the bowel has been drained from the colon, a primary anastomosis may be performed either using a hand-sutured technique or a circular stapling device (see Ch. 2).

If there is any doubt about the integrity of the anastomosis, a proximal defunctioning stoma should be raised. If the bowel has been successfully cleared of fecal residue, a proximal loop ileostomy would be preferred for decompression because it is safer to close and less likely to compromise the blood supply to the anastomosis. It is our practice to test all anastomoses by insufflation of air, as described in Chapter 2, even though a proximal stoma is considered desirable, so that any obvious defect can be closed and retested afterward. The abdomen is then closed with two soft suction drains down to the resection site, as described in Chapter 1.

Resection for Fistulas

Colovesical Fistula

Diverticular disease is one of the most common causes of colovesical fistula. It usually presents with recurrent urinary tract infection or pneumaturia in association with large bowel symptoms. The fistula may not always be demonstrated by contrast radiography or even by cystography. At operation the usual situation is that of an inflammatory phlegmon in the sigmoid colon adherent to the dome of the bladder. Almost all fistulas develop between the midsigmoid and the top of the bladder. If there is involvement of the base of the bladder, an alternative diagnosis should be considered, such as malignant colovesical fistula either from the large bowel or from the bladder. Occasionally a colovesical fistula may be associated with an enterocolic fistula, either between the cecum and the sigmoid or the transverse colon and the sigmoid, or between the small bowel and the sigmoid. There may be coexisting localized pus if the fistula occurs soon after the development of a pericolic abscess, but usually a colovesical fistula is merely a part of an inflammatory mass without a localized infective focus.

When the abdomen is opened an inflammatory mass consisting of the sigmoid colon, omentum, loops of small intestine, the dome of the bladder and, in the female, the left fallopian tube and ovary is encountered. The first stage of the operation is to dissect the omentum from the inflammatory mass; subsequently the loops of small bowel are freed from the sigmoid and bladder (Fig. 11-17). If the small bowel is perforated iatrogenically, it should be promptly repaired transversely using continuous extramucosal PDS or Maxon sutures. Similarly, if a true fistula is demonstrated between loops of bowel, the nonaffected segments (i.e., other than sigmoid colon) should merely be closed, unless there has been considerable damage to the small intestine, in which case a small resection may be preferred. The sigmoid colon is then mobilized from surrounding structures, using sharp dissection if necessary. Usually only a very small defect in a grossly thickened bladder wall is found. Resection of part of the bladder should be strongly resisted, as this would further reduce the capacity of an already compromised bladder and lead to troublesome postoperative urinary frequency. The defect in the mucosa of the bladder wall is closed with catgut followed by a second layer to approximate the detrusor. In reality, however, the bladder wall is so thickened that a mass closure of mucosa and detrusor using interrupted sutures is probably preferable. The peritoneum over the surface of the bladder is then closed as a separate layer. If a transurethral urinary catheter has not been passed prior to the start of the operation, one is then inserted into the bladder. A suprapubic catheter would cause less discomfort to the patient if bladder drainage is necessary for more than a week. However, the dome of the bladder is so thickened that the use of a suprapubic catheter may in fact be contraindicated in these circumstances.

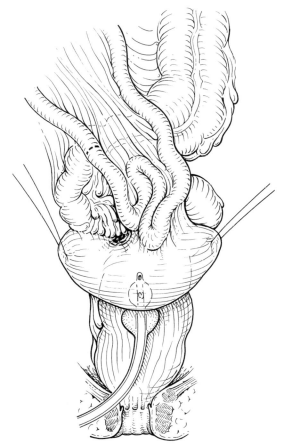

Figure 11-17.

Once the bladder defect has been dealt with and the sigmoid colon mobilized, the entire sigmoid is resected and an end-to-end anastomosis is performed between the descending colon and the upper third of the rectum (Fig. 11-18). It is rarely necessary to use a proximal stoma unless there is frank sepsis, technical difficulties in fashioning the anastomosis, or excessive bleeding at the operation site. Two closed suction drains should be placed down to the left pelvic brim after completion of the anastomosis, and the abdomen is closed as described in Chapter 1.

Other Fistulas

Occasionally diverticular disease may be complicated by a colocutaneous or colovaginal fistula. In the case of a colocutaneous fistula the sigmoid colon is resected and an anastomosis is fashioned, provided there is no gross intraperitoneal sepsis. The fistulous tract through the abdominal wall usually develops through an old wound. This tract is then cleared of any infective material and is either left open to granulate or is drained.

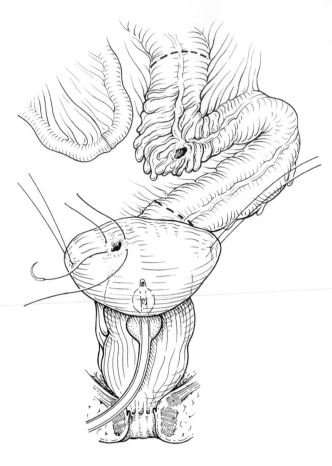

Figure 11-18.

A vaginal fistula complicating diverticular disease may be due to a leak from an existing anastomosis, such as from a sigmoid anastomosis to the posterior fornix, or to a complex coloenteric fistula tracking to the top of the vagina caused by diverticular disease (Fig. 11-19). Irrespective of the etiology, the vagina merely acts as a drain, hence the defect in it can be ignored. Because there is no vaginal disease, once the cause of the fistula has been resected, a primary anastomosis is performed as in the case of a long-standing postoperative fistula (Fig. 11-20). If it is an early postoperative fistula, a proximal loop stoma alone may suffice (Fig. 11-21).

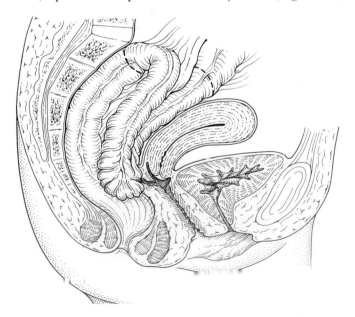

Figure 11-19.

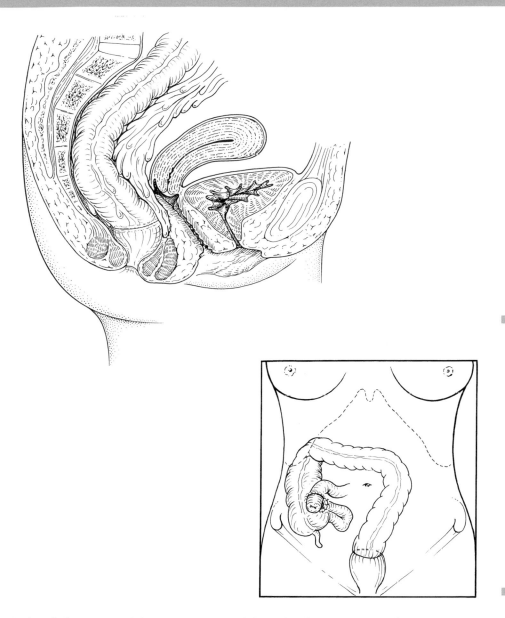

Figure 11-20.

Figure 11-21.

A detailed account of the management of these fistulas is given in Chapter 17.

Editorial Commentaries

I agree entirely with Professor Keighley's statement that the Hartmann procedure is undoubtedly the safest operation to perform in the seriously ill patient suffering from purulent or fecal peritonitis after perforation of sigmoid diverticular disease. The disturbing fact remains, however, that in at least a third of these patients, intestinal continuity will never be reestablished. In those in whom continuity is reestablished, morbidity following the second operation is often as high as that following the first. Anything to eliminate the difficult closure stage would be welcome. We tend to resect the diseased segment and if there is no peritonitis and no gereralized puru-

(Continues)

lent or fecal peritonitis, perform an anastomosis and construct a loop ileostomy. If the fecal load is large, an on-table bowel preparation is used. If the fecal load is minor, no preparation is performed. This is an excellent approach in the patient who is not septic. If the patient is septic, the diseased segment is resected and a sigmoid colostomy constructed. If a mucous fistula can be performed, that, too, is done. If a mucous fistula cannot be performed because of anatomic constraints, which is usually the case, then a Hartmann procedure is performed as high on the rectum as possible and the presacral space is not entered. I perform staple closure almost exclusively, and leave long Prolene sutures at either side of the stapled-over Hartmann closure.

I agree that before surgery to reestablish intestinal continuity, the patient should be counseled that the result may be poor, particularly if the patient is older. I do not staple the colorectostomy, as the rectal and proximal bowel tissues are not completely normal. I tend not to staple any tissues that are abnormal (i.e., edematous, granular, inflamed fibrotic, or dilated).

My final comment relates to the treatment of the bladder after resection of a sigmoidovesical fistula, which is the most common type of fistula seen in patients with diverticular disease. Often the bladder is so densely woody with fibrosis, edema, and acute and chronic reaction to the fistula that nothing can be done to close the fistula. Because the fistula is usually tiny, resecting the fistula and leaving a suction drain between the bladder and rectum for 5 to 8 days after the procedure is an approach with which I have had excellent results.

John H. Pemberton

We subscribe to Dr. Keighley's view that the Hartmann procedure is the best operation in the management of emergencies such as fecal or diffused peritonitis. Primary anastomosis has no place in the treatment of these conditions, even with a proximal diverting stoma. Resection and primary anastomosis can be undertaken in the case of localized pericolic abscess provided the abscess is at a good distance from the anastomotic site. We agree that, if possible, preoperative percutaneous drainage of such an abscess should be done.

Regarding the Hartmann procedure, we agree that it is not necessary to remove all of the diverticular disease during the first stage of the operation. The sigmoid colon is transected at the level of or just proximal to the rectosigmoid junction, which will be resected during the second stage of the operation when intestinal continuity is restored. The distal colon is closed with staples reinforced with a running Vicryl suture. The angles of the rectal stump can be sutured to the posterior parietal peritoneum to prevent its slipping down.

In the case of diffuse peritonitis, we always drain the pelvis and place a Mikulicz pack in the pouch of Douglas covering the rectal stump. This minimizes the consequences of dehiscence of the rectal stump and prevents the loops of small bowel loops from slipping down in the pelvic cavity. Restora-

(Continues)

tion of intestinal continuity is technically easier because of the tenacity of the postoperative adherences in the pelvic space.

The sigmoid colon is divided a few centimeters proximal to the perforation. The left colon is generally mobilized, but we try to avoid taking down the splenic flexure at this stage, as peritonitis and distension of the colon make this maneuver dangerous and open new tissue planes to the risk of infection.

If the distal segment of the colon is viable and sufficiently long, it can be brought up to the abdominal wall either in a double-barreled colostomy or in the inferior extremity of the midline incision. This option is selected only if two conditions are present: perforation is distant from the rectosigmoid junction, and the distal colon has a good aspect and is long enough to avoid any retrorectal or lateral mobilization of the rectum.

With regard to closure of the Hartmann procedure, the delay between the two stages is never less than 3 months and is usually 4 months. Contrast radiography of the defunctioned rectum is performed a few days prior to the operation to visualize any possible blind fistulas.

We do not routinely perform manometry or electromyography. Many elderly patients have impaired anal sphincter function; the most important factor for us is their preoperative clinical status.

Dr. Keighley's description of Hartmann closure is perfect. He is right to insist on the importance of resection of the rectosigmoid junction. The anastomosis must be at the upper third of the rectum. For us, the splenic flexure is always taken down if not done previously.

Just a few comments on primary resection and anastomosis: Again, the splenic flexure is always taken down, often at the first stage of the procedure. Hand-sewn anastomoses are not tested with air insufflation and intraperitoneal colorectal anastomoses are not routinely drained.

We agree with Dr. Keighley's treatment of colovesical fistulas and follow the same principles for these conditions. We try if possible to interpose omentum between the colorectal anastomosis and the site of the fistula, particularly in colovaginal fistulas.

In summary, there are no great differences between Dr. Keighley's principles and ours, except for the drainage of the pelvic cavity in the case of purulent or fecal peritonitis.

Rolland Parc

12

Inflammatory Bowel Disease

Proctocolectomy, Brooke Ileostomy, and Continent Ileostomy

John H. Pemberton

Proctocolectomy

Total proctocolectomy involves excision of the cecum, the entire colon, the rectum, and the anus. The abdominal and perineal components of the dissection are performed simultaneously.

The more detailed technical aspects of abdominal colectomy are illustrated in discussions on right hemicolectomy and anterior resection. In brief, the bowel to be resected is mobilized along the right gutter, the hepatic flexure, the gastrocolic ligament, the left gutter, the splenic flexure, and the pelvic attachments, in that order. It is important that proctectomy proceed along anatomic cleavage planes. It is unnecessary to mobilize the rectum using an intrarectal mesenteric technique; the presacral nerves do not traverse the mesorectum and are, in fact, quite distinct from it. Finally, if the rectum has been mobilized sufficiently from above (transabdominally), the surgeon should have no difficulty in completing the dissection from below.

Mobilizing the Right Colon

The distal ileum, cecum, and ascending colon are freed from their lateral peritoneal attachments by lifting the bowel and sweeping the attachments posteriorly (Fig. 12-1). Next, the gastrocolic ligament is severed in the avascular plane at about the midtransverse colon. The gastrocolic and phrenocolic ligaments are sequentially taken, thus freeing the transverse colon and the hepatic flexure (Fig. 12-2). Taking precautions not to injure the duodenum, the surgeon wipes it posterolaterally, away from the field of dissection. Moreover, great care is taken not to avulse a mesenteric vein at this point; if

the bleeding point retracts under the pancreas, the operation then becomes more difficult. After entering the lesser sac, the gastrocolic omentum is transected as far to the
left as possible; in this way, the splenic flexure is advanced upon from the left.

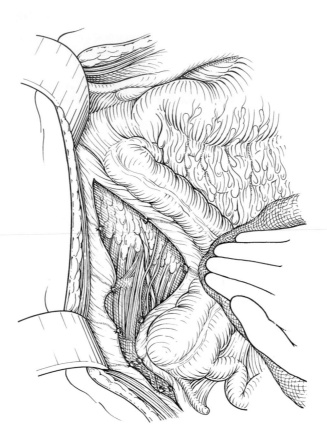

Figure 12-1.

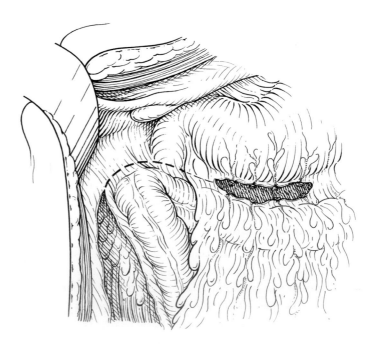

Figure 12-2.

Transecting the splenocolic ligament is facilitated by approaching the flexure from the left gutter, freeing the descending colon laterally and posteriorly allowing precise visualization of the splenocolic ligament (Fig. 12-3). In this way, the splenic flexure is approached from the left and right. Excessive caudal traction on the ligament is avoided. Because the splenocolic ligament is avascular, it may be divided without clamps.

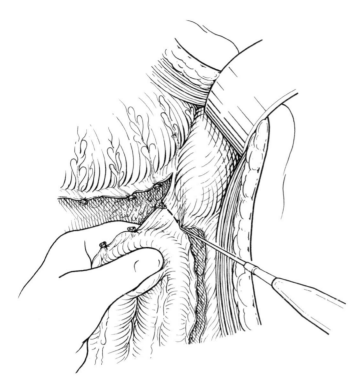

Figure 12-3.

The sigmoid colon is then mobilized from its lateral, peritoneal attachments. The mesentery is then transected and ligated (Fig. 12-4). Maintaining position on the patient's left, the surgeon retracts the colon and sigmoid medially and mobilizes both (Fig. 12-5) along Toldt's line. The vascular mesentery is then clamped, transected, and ligated.

Mobilizing the Proximal Rectum

Scissors are used to incise the posterior peritoneum. Thereafter, blunt dissection along natural cleavage planes allows quick, safe, and easy mobilization of the rectum from the hollow of the sacrum without injury to the presacral veins. Anterocephalad traction on the rectum is the key (Fig. 12-5).

The surgeon exerts cephaloanterior traction on the distal sigmoid and proximal rectum. The base of the mesosigmoid is incised with scissors and "air dissection" is used to develop the natural plane posterior to the sigmoid and rectum, yet anterior to the presacral venous plexus (Fig. 12-5). As appropriate, traction is applied on the junction of rectum and sigmoid, and the base of the mesosigmoid is likewise retracted. Having delineated and opened the natural cleavage plane, scissors are used to push areolar tissue out of the way (Fig. 12-5).

As the bowel is pulled more medially (away from the operator), Toldt's "white line" is incised and the lateral peritoneal attachments are swept off the sigmoid and rectum to visualize the left ureter (Fig. 12-6). This maneuver effectively frees the sigmoid and upper rectum laterally.

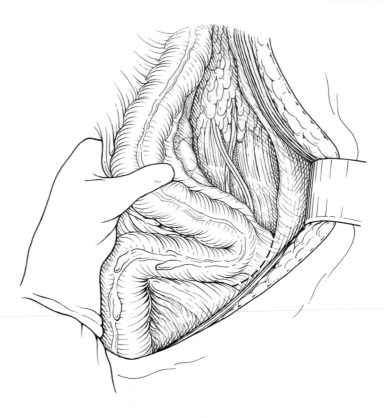

Figure 12-4.

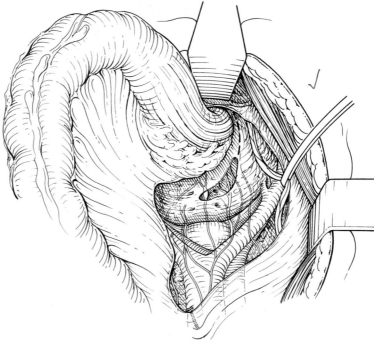

Figure 12-5.

Mobilizing the Distal Rectum

With the left hand pulling the rectosigmoid anterocephalad, the surgeon slides the right hand over the presacral veins, finger-dissecting all the way to the levator ani. Waldeyer's fascia is incised with the scissors to prevent tearing either the mesorectum or the presacral veins There are no nerves traversing this plane. The lateral midrectal attachments are loosened. The rectovesical (or rectovaginal) peritoneum of the cul-de-sac and underlying vesicosigmoid attachments are then incised with scissors and the plane between the seminal vesicles and prostate (or rectum and vagina) is developed.

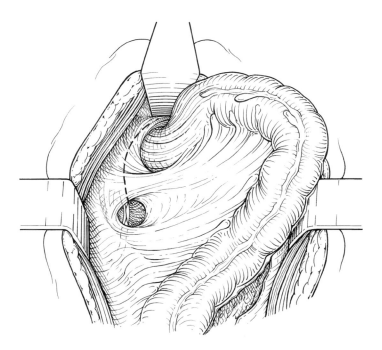

Figure 12-6.

Next, the lateral ligaments, which have been loosened, are developed by finger dissection and ligated (Fig. 12-7). The rectum is now free circumferentially. The last
structure to sever is the anococcygeal ligament (Fig. 12-8).

At this point, the entire rectum from the level of the levators has been circumferentially freed and mobilized from the hollow of the sacrum, out of the pelvis. Packs
are placed in the hollow of the sacrum posterior to the rectum to tamponade any ooz-
ing. Finally, the superior hemorrhoid and left colic arteries (Fig. 12-9) are divided,
with care taken to spare the presacral nerves located at the base of the pedicle. The
distal ileal mesentery is next ligated and the terminal ileum transected with the GIA
stapler (Fig. 12-10).

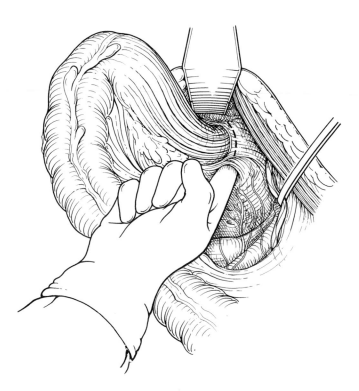

Figure 12-7.

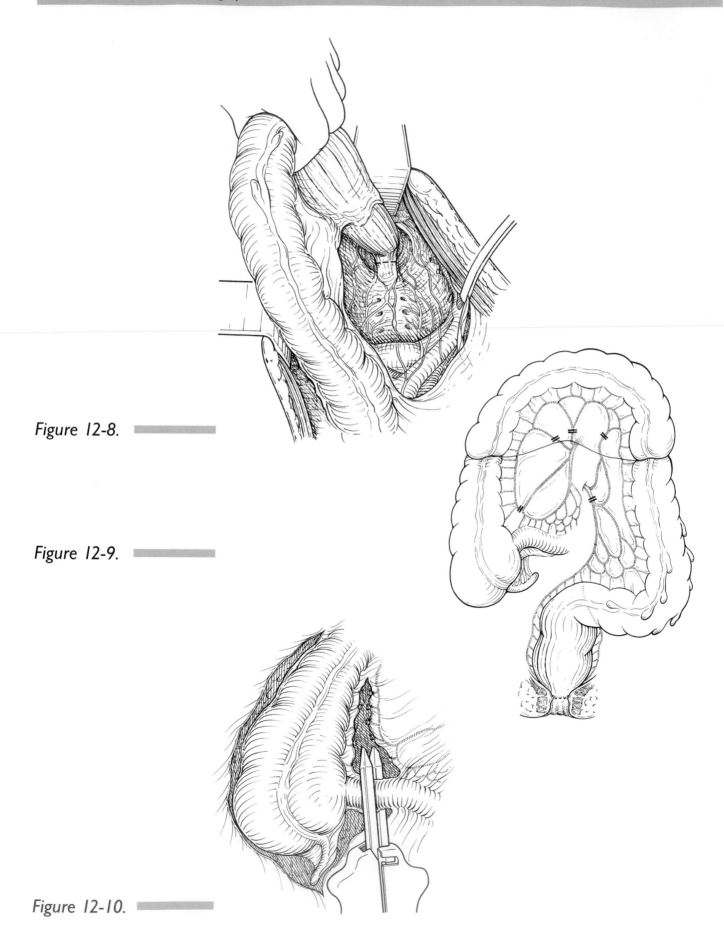

Figure 12-8.

Figure 12-9.

Figure 12-10.

Proctectomy

The distal rectum and anus are freed from their three attachments; the anococcygeal ligament, the levator ani, and the inferior hemorrhoidal vascular pedicles.

An elliptical incision is made about the anus (Fig. 12-11). Kocher clamps are placed so as to coapt the incised skin margins, obliterating the anal lumen (Fig. 12-12). Kraske and Murphy (rake) retractors are inserted as shown in Figure 12-12 beneath the wound edges. An intersphincteric dissection is then performed as described in Chapter 1.

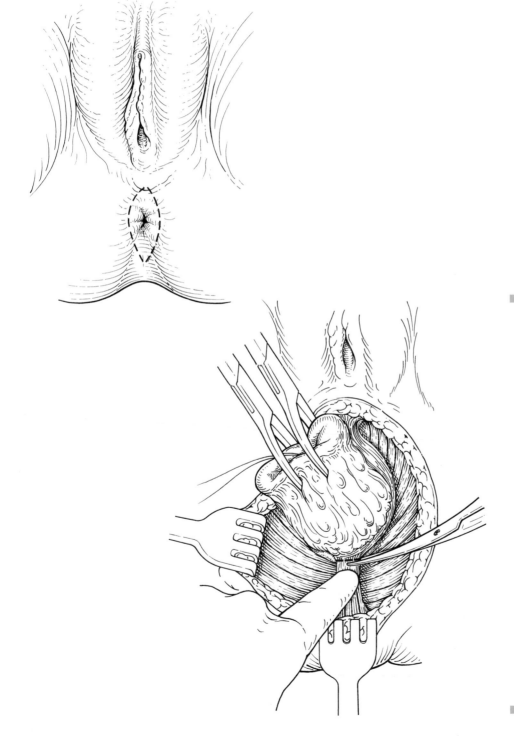

Figure 12-11.

Figure 12-12.

Using cautery, the incision is deepened until the coccyx is palpated in the posterior midline; scissors are used to open the incision onto the laparotomy pads placed previously in the dissected presacral space (Fig. 12-13). The anorectal specimen has now been freed posteriorly.

The forefinger is placed into the presacral space and the levator muscle on the left is hooked and pulled outward toward the surgeon. The levator is then incised from the 6-o'clock and the 3-o'clock positions using cautery. The finger is reinserted and the levator muscle on the patient's right is incised the same way from the 6-o'clock and the 9-o'clock positions (Fig. 12-14).

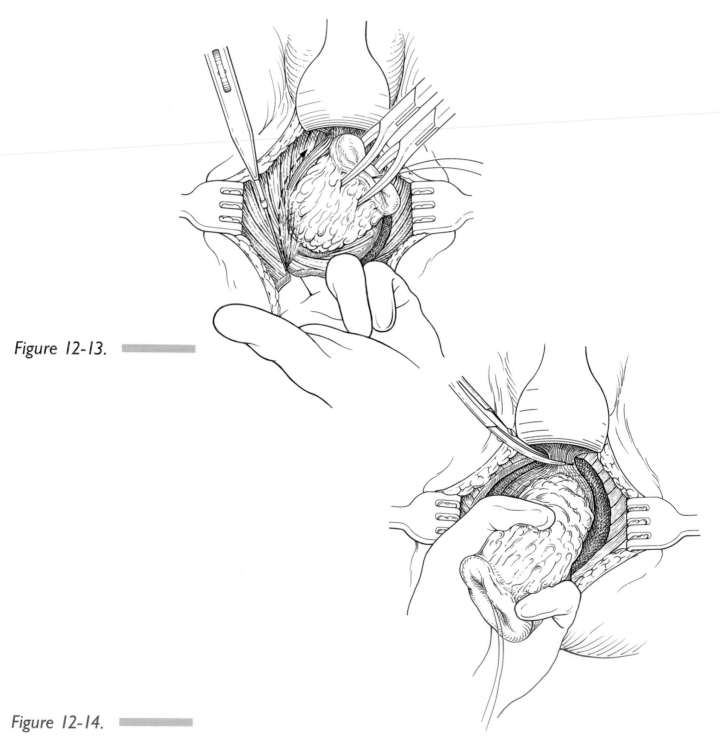

Figure 12-13.

Figure 12-14.

Reaching into the presacral space, the surgeon extracts the entire colonic specimen (Fig. 12-15). The anterior attachments are transected with the cautery. In women, the surgeon's left index finger palpates within the vagina to avoid opening into it. In men, the surgeon strives to stay away from the prostate, its adjacent plexus of veins, and the membranous urethra. The urethra can be located in both men and women by palpating the Foley catheter within it.

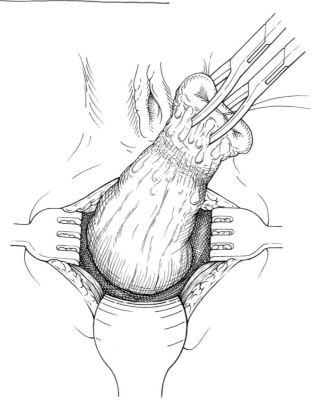

Figure 12-15.

Perineal Closure

Working from the deeper to the more superficial plane, the levator ani muscles are reapproximated and the perineal wound is closed. Two round closed suction drains are first inserted as shown in Figure 12-16. The more superficial portions of the wound are closed with interrupted Vicryl sutures.

Conventional Brooke Ileostomy

Through an appropriately placed incision over the premarked stomal site, a circular defect 2 cm in diameter is dissected through the skin, subcutaneous tissue, and fascia (with the inferior epigastric vessels ligated as necessary). The distal ileum is pulled through the right abdominal wall defect (Fig. 12-17). The seromuscular portion of ileum is then anchored to the subcuticular tissue with interrupted 2-0 chromic catgut sutures. When doubled back upon itself, the stoma should protrude some 3 to 5 cm anterior to the skin margin. The stoma is finally established by suturing the distal ileum (all layers) to the skin (Fig. 12-18).

Continent Ileostomy

The continent ileostomy is made up of four distinct parts: (1) the reservoir itself, (2) the nipple valve, (3) the conduit of ileum extending from the reservoir through the abdominal wall, and (4) the stoma.

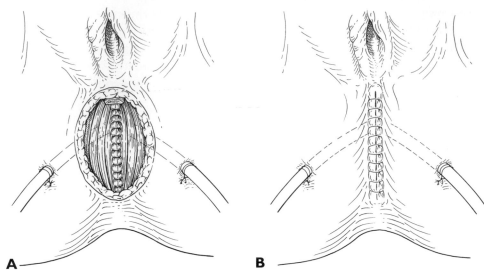

Figure 12-16.   A   B

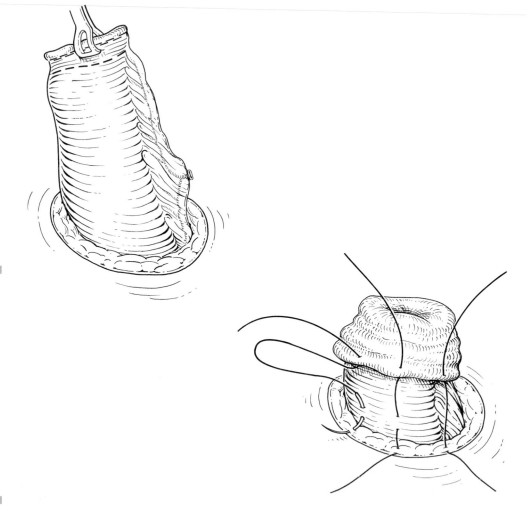

Figure 12-17.

Figure 12-18.

The distal 45 cm of ileum is marked off for use as the pouch, and the nipple and conduit to the ileostomy (Fig. 12-19). A 15-cm length of ileum proximal to the cut end of the terminal ileum is marked off; this portion will serve as the nipple and conduit. An Allis clamp is then placed another 15 cm proximal (30 cm proximal to the end of the ileum). The surgeon stands on the patient's right side (all illustrations are from that vantage point).

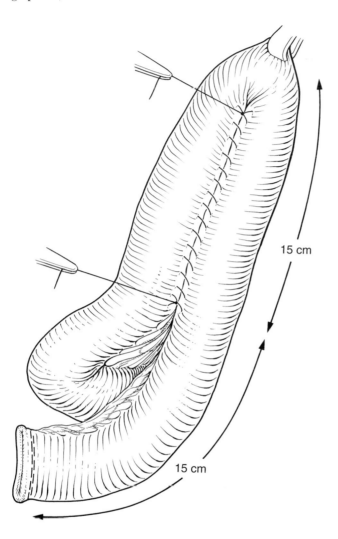

15 cm

15 cm

Figure 12-19.

Anterior Suturing

At the apex marked by the Allis clamp (Fig. 12-19), the surgeon approximates the seromusculature with running 2-0 absorbable suture. For the pouch, "inner" and "outer" layers are approximated with a layer of absorbable suture material, so that with time the pouch can increase in size, thus decreasing the frequency with which the patient must evacuate the internal reservoir. At the 15-cm point, as marked from the transected end of the ileum to demarcate the conduit, the suture is tied.

Opening the Ileum

Using cautery and beginning at the antimesenteric aspect of the bowel, the surgeon opens the ileum as shown (Fig. 12-20A). Opening the proximal limb of the loop 2 to 3 cm beyond the distal loop separates the afferent (inflow) tract from the efferent (outflow) limb. Next, the "posterior" mucosa and submucosa bilaterally are reapproximated with another 2-0 absorbable suture (Fig. 12-20B). When this row has been completed, hemostasis has been achieved.

The two opposed limbs of ileum have now been sutured together in two separate layers. The pouch is then approximated to the inflow tract as shown in Figure 12-20C.

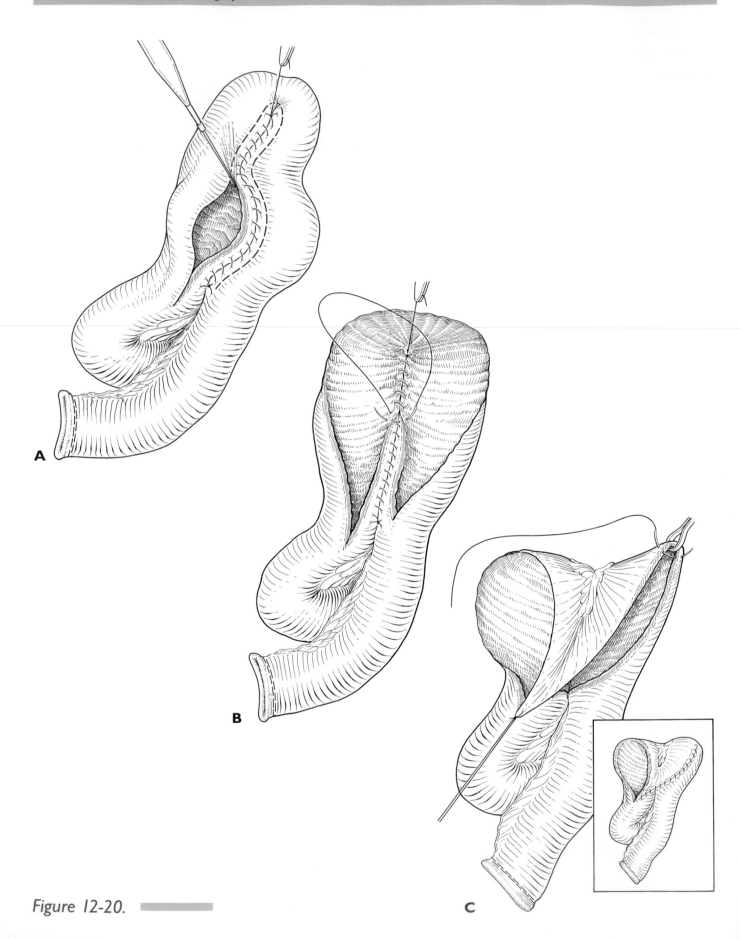

Figure 12-20.

A

B

C

Efferent Side Closure

With a 2-0 absorbable suture, the surgeon closes the efferent portion of the pouch in two layers as shown in Figure 12-20C. The Allis clamp assists in approximating both sides of the efferent limb of the pouch equally.

Constructing the Nipple

The afferent aspect of the pouch remains open to construct the nipple. The surgeon inserts the index finger into the efferent limb of ileum (Fig. 12-21). Russian forceps are used next to invaginate 6 to 7 cm of ileum into the pouch (Fig. 12-22). Slight cauterization of the ileal serosa will facilitate the formation of adhesions. ✓

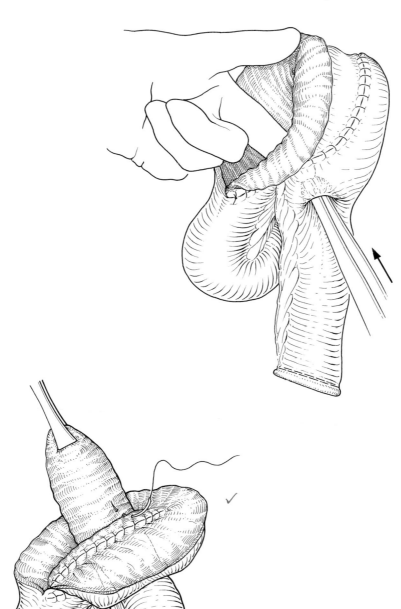

Figure 12-21.

Figure 12-22.

Then, to permanently affix the intussuscepted ileum, sutures and three staple lines are constructed using either the TA instrument (without the pin) or an S-GIA stapler (without a knife) (Fig. 12-23). To prevent dislodging of the nipple, sutures are placed at the junction of the pouch and the efferent limb of ileum, where the ileum emerges from the pouch on both sides of the mesentery (Fig. 12-24). The opening on the afferent side of the pouch is now closed in two layers.

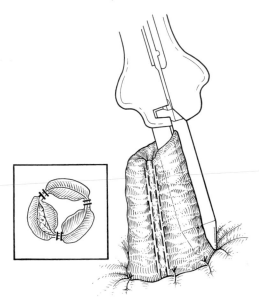

Figure 12-23. ▬▬▬▬

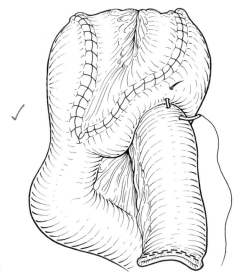

Figure 12-24. ▬▬▬▬

Testing the Integrity of the Pouch and Continence of the Nipple

The integrity of the pouch and the continence of the nipple is tested by clamping the afferent limb of ileum and then injecting into the pouch through the efferent limb about 150 to 200 ml of air using a large (60-cc) Medina catheter-tipped syringe. When the pouch is inflated, the surgeon removes the pouch tube. If the nipple is competent, the pouch remains inflated until the Medina tube is reinserted, which then promptly evacuates the air.

At the premarked site, a two fingers-width stoma opening is made; 2-0 silk sutures are used next to affix the lateral aspect of the pouch and the base of the nipple to the internal abdominal wall (Fig. 12-25A). These anchoring sutures should *not* be placed through the full thickness of the pouch, or fistulae may develop.

The ileum is then delivered through the stomal opening (Fig. 12-25B), suturing the distal ileum (all layers of the distal end of the conduit) *flush* to the skin and subcuticular tissue (Fig. 12-26).

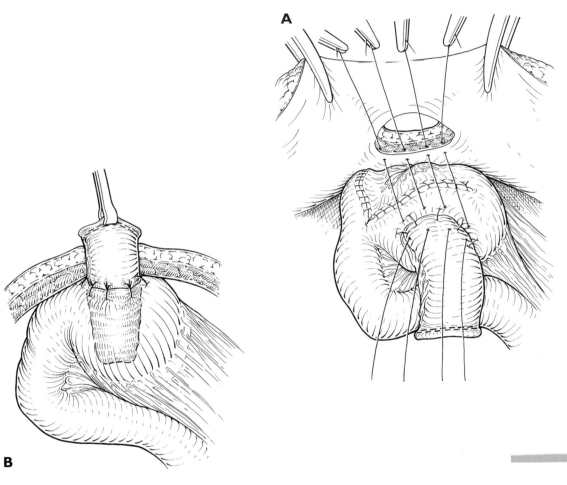

Figure 12-25.

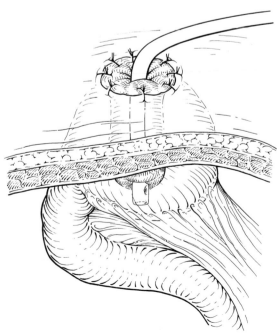

Figure 12-26.

The pouch, nipple, conduit, and stoma have now been completed. A tube is inserted into the pouch to keep it decompressed for 1 month as it heals (Fig. 12-26). The position of the tube is marked and the tube secured in position by suturing it to the skin. Marking the tube facilitates the patient's learning to intubate the pouch.

Reperitonealizing the Pelvic Floor

After proctectomy and Brooke ileostomy or continent ileostomy, the pelvic floor is reperitonealized with a running 3-0 chromic catgut suture, taking care not to gather the ureters into the closure.

Editorial Commentaries

Proctocolectomy and Ileostomy. In inflammatory bowel disease we invariably preserve the omentum, provided it does not shred into numerous finger-like processes, in which case adhesion formation afterward is probably increased. We take a good deal of time and care in dissecting the omentum from the transverse mesocolon in the avascular plane forming the roof of the greater omentum. We also entirely concur with Dr. Pemberton that a close rectal dissection is not necessary. The whole of the mesorectum is removed because it provides a bloodless plane posteriorly and posterolaterally. The presacral nerves can be easily identified and, in our experience, are in greatest danger of damage as they cross the pelvic rim. They should be carefully identified at this point and dissected from the mesorectum and traced as they diverge laterally to the base of the bladder. In our experience, autonomic nerve damage should also be prevented by close anterior dissection of the lower aspect of the rectum. By hugging the lateral fibers of the rectum, Denonvilliers fascia is not opened and the seminal vesicles and prostate are not really exposed since they are protected by the fascia. This maneuver not only protects the nerves but overcomes troublesome bleeding from the prostatic venous plexus. We tend to bring out our perineal drains through the abdominal incision. They are placed below the levator plate and are then brought out in the flank so as to avoid drains on the perineum. Only suction drains are used in our clinical practice.

Kock Reservoir Ileostomy. We fashion a Kock reservoir ileostomy in very much the same manner as described by Dr. Pemberton. However, we tend to use a single continuous extramucosal suture; it takes less time and is hemostatic, and it does not compromise the lumen of the pouch. We only suture the back row of the pouch in the first instance, leaving the whole of the front of the pouch open for construction of the nipple valve. We use three procedures that we believe help overcome the problems of desusception of the nipple valve; they are as follows:

1. Defatting of the ileal mesentery that is to be intussuscepted as the valve.
2. Use of a fascial collar to stabilize the valve.

3. Use of a linear staple technique. Our method of stapling involves using either the GIA or PLC without a blade. We take great care not to incorporate the ileal mesentery in the staple line.

Only when the nipple valve has been constructed do we close the anterior aspect of the pouch with a single layer extramucosal continuous suture. When using stapling procedures for nipple valve construction we tend only to decompress the pouch for between 7 and 10 days. We, of course, use a low stoma site just above the symphysis pubis through the rectus muscle.

Michael R. B. Keighley

Proctocolectomy and Ileostomy. In inflammatory bowel disease and familial adenomatous polyposis, we usually resect the omentum, thus dividing the gastrocolic ligament. We have found that this may decrease the rate of postoperative bowel obstruction.

Close rectal dissection is not necessary for the upper rectum. The sympathetic nerves can be identified in front of the aorta and then dissected and spared as they diverge laterally. For the mid- and lower rectum, in the absence of rectal cancer, the dissection is conducted close to the rectal wall to prevent sacral and autonomic nerve damage.

To avoid the inconvenience of perineal drainage, we use suction drains exteriorized through the lower quadrant of the abdominal wall.

Continent Ileostomy. We fashion a Kock reservoir ileostomy with the modifications described by W. O. Barnett. The end of the ileum is closed; a 10-cm segment of the distal ileum is preserved to serve as a collar and a stapled J pouch with 14-cm limbs is constructed using the GIA 90 stapler. The proximal portion of the intestine is transected 14 cm above the pouch, and the serosa and underlying fat removed from both sides of the mesentery supplying this segment. An isoperistaltic valve measuring 5 cm in length is fashioned by intussuscepting the segment of intestine into the pouch by the anterior defect corresponding to the introduction of the GIA. Three rows of SGIA staples (without a knife) are applied along the entire length of the valve in quadrants other than the mesenteric area. The proximal intestine is hand-sewn to the anterior defect of the mesentery at the base of the valve and sewn around the base of the valve to form a collar similar to that used in Nissen fundoplication. Resorbable sutures (4-0 polyglycolic acid) are placed between the musculoperitoneal layer of the abdominal wall and the intestinal collar. A catheter is placed in the pouch to test for valve competence and for postoperative decompression. The stoma, sited above the symphysis pubis through the rectus muscle, is sewn to the skin.

Rolland Parc

With respect to the proximal colectomy component of the proctocolectomy, in my practice, there is no difference from the way in which Dr. Pemberton does the proximal colectomy component of the proctocolectomy procedure. In terms of mobilizing the proximal rectum, my technique of

(Continues)

proctectomy is outlined in the final part of this chapter, Crohn's Disease. There is a departure from, but also agreement with, the opinions expressed by Dr. Pemberton. My first comment is in the form of an agreement: There is no doubt that the caution advocated by many surgeons in the past who operate "closely against" the rectum was based on a well-meaning but erroneous belief that this practice would ensure the preservation of sexual nerve function. Indeed, it has been amply demonstrated that dissecting in the plane immediately anterior to Waldeyer's fascia, but extraneous to the rectal mesentery, will allow for a bloodless dissection that is both rapid and free of the risk of injury to the nervi erigentes as well as the risk of blood transfusion. On this, we are in total concordance with Dr. Pemberton's views. However, I depart from his viewpoint on blunt dissection. There is, in fact, no role for blunt dissection during the course of a proctectomy. To quote a British author, surgeons "rejoice in the pneumatic squelch" that accompanies placing a hand in the presacral space and levering the rectum forward. In fact, this may cause injury and one would prefer to do the dissection under direct vision using lighted retractors. The rest of the dissection is very similar to that described by Dr. Pemberton; indeed, it is reflected in an earlier chapter of mine.

Similarly, my discussion of the conventional Brooke ileostomy is the same as that described by Dr. Pemberton, except that we do not use seromuscular sutures.

With respect to construction of the continent ileostomy, there are some points of distinction here. First, we use three 12- to 15-cm long loops of small intestine to make an S-shaped pouch. This has been standard practice since 1975, when the author observed Dr. Charles Ripstein performing continent ileostomies this way. The nipple valve is made such that it is 6 cm in length; therefore, a 12-cm segment is dedicated to its construction distal to the 35 to 45 cm dedicated to the S pouch itself. Distal to this is an additional 7 to 8 cm that is used for the exit conduit that will traverse the abdominal wall aperture. The three limbs are brought together in the conventional fashion using a running 2-0 absorbable suture. An S-shaped incision is made to open up the dimensions of the pouch. The posterior layers are then reinforced with a continuous 2-0 absorbable suture. Intussusception of the nipple valve is done using a Babcock clamp placed halfway along the length dedicated to the valve. The valve is then fixed in position. A variety of techniques have evolved over the years. Our preference is to use the TA 55 instrument without the pin for the part of the valve on either side of the mesentery. Thus, the two rows of TA 55 staples actually straddle the mesentery of the valve. The S-GIA or equivalent may be used, but one has concerns about the trauma that the very tip of this instrument may produce. The sequel to this may very well be a high fistula into the valve itself.

The major change that we have made in the past 5 years has been the stapling of the valve to the wall of the pouch itself. This is done via a 1-cm enterotomy made on the side of the pouch at the junction of the mesenteric margin and vasa recti supplying that part of the pouch. The antimesenteric tip of the valve is then brought to that enterotomy, the TA 55 is placed through the enterotomy into the valve, and the valve is stapled to the wall of the pouch. This helps secure the valve and has been a significant factor in reducing the risk of dessusception of the valve. The other advantage of the three-loop pouch is that it separates the afferent from the efferent limb. In the event of a complication, such as dessusception of the valve or difficulty in intubation, or a valve fistula, it is technically not excessively difficult to resect the valve, rotate the pouch, and use the previous afferent limb to fashion the neovalve.

The tube is left in position for 3 weeks. Prior to discharge, the patient is instructed on how to intubate the pouch.

Victor W. Fazio

Ileal Pouch-Anal Anastomosis

John H. Pemberton

Among the various alternatives to Brooke ileostomy for chronic ulcerative colitis or familial adenomatous polyposis (FAP), ileal pouch-anal anastomosis (IPAA) is today deemed the procedure of choice in suitable patients. Thousands of such operations have been performed to date. Naturally, IPAA itself has undergone innumerable modifications and some rethinking of its goal. Essentially, there are two views. One is that the goal of IPAA is to eradicate disease, *and the possibility of further disease.* If patients have some problem with fecal control, that is the tradeoff for cure. To these proponents, complete mucosal excision is mandatory. The other view is that the goal is to give the patient as good a chance as possible to be continent. A small cuff of anal canal mucosa (the transition zone) will remain. If patients have some irritation and bleeding from the retained anal canal mucosa, that is the tradeoff for continence. Randomized trials have been and are being done to see if one operation is superior functionally.

At this juncture, it seems reasonable to take the following moderate (diplomatic) stance. For young (<30 years) patients with chronic ulcerative colitis who have excellent continence mechanisms (and who have up to six decades more to live), it seems reasonable to excise the mucosa completely. In older patients with less secure continence mechanisms (and who may have a shorter life span ahead) mucosal preservation is an attractive choice. For FAP patients, all of the mucosa should be excised.

Principles

I will describe my approach to complete mucosa resection first, and then the newer double-stapled technique (which is, quite truthfully, slick indeed).

Length of Rectal Muscular Cuff

A rectal muscular cuff of 3 to 5 cm seems to be satisfactory. Longer cuffs were made initially, but the dissections were tedious. Moreover, the long cuff sometimes obstructed outflow from the pouch to the anal canal. The short cuffs decrease operating time, bleeding, and contamination, and allow full expansion of the neorectum. In addition, the likelihood of leaving islands of mucosa is minimized. Preserving a 3- to 5-cm rectal cuff ensures adequate protection of the anal sphincter.

Type of Ileal Pouch

The J-shaped ileal pouch is the preferred design. This pouch, made from the terminal 30 cm of ileum, is easy to construct, provides an adequate reservoir, and empties readily.

Other pouch designs are also satisfactory, but much more tedious to construct. Initially, functional results, such as completeness of emptying, were better with the J pouch than with the S pouch, but it was discovered that this was due largely to a long efferent limb and a long (10- to 15-cm) rectal cuff that was sometimes left in place. As the rectal muscular cuff *and* efferent limb have been shortened, results of the S pouch have become more similar to those of the J pouch.

The S and the W pouches provide larger reservoirs, which should theoretically lower the stool frequency. However, the degree of improvement in reservoir function has not been dramatic using these more complex pouch designs. Moreover, these pouches are not as easy to construct with staples and so require longer operative times. In the Mayo series, the J pouch has been the predominant pouch configuration. We have found the functional results to be excellent.

Use of Ileostomy

Although most surgeons use a temporary diverting ileostomy constructed proximal to the pouch and the ileoanal anastomosis, some authors have reported good results in patients in whom no diverting stoma was used. It is important to emphasize that patients who do not have a diverting loop ileostomy and who undergo a one-stage procedure should have absolutely no tension on the ileal anal anastomosis, should not be on steroids, should have a complication-free operation, and be in good general health. Patients should be counseled preoperatively about the relative risk of a one-stage procedure as opposed to the two-stage operation. Usually, the postoperative course is somewhat more difficult for the patient, in that they must recover from the operation and from their antecedent disease while at the same time they must adjust to an ileal reservoir, which functions almost immediately.

In general, the IPAA should be covered by a diverting stoma in nearly all situations; only in highly selected patients (double-stapled; FAP patients) should a single-stage procedure be contemplated. It is easier and far more successful to treat complications associated with the diverting stoma than the complications of pelvic sepsis.

Operative Technique

The operation is usually performed in two stages. In the first stage, the cecum, colon, and proximal rectum are removed and the distal rectal and proximal anal canal epithelium resected endoanally. A J-shaped pouch is made from the terminal ileum. The pouch is then anastomosed to the anal canal at the dentate line. The anastomosis is protected by a diverting loop ileostomy. At the second stage, performed 2 months later, the ileostomy is closed. By contrast, in Europe, stage one sometimes means abdominal colectomy, whereas stage two involves constructing the pouch, and stage three is closure of the ileostomy.

With the patient in the Lloyd-Davies position and using the Allen stirrups, abdominal colectomy is performed in the standard manner, with the following exceptions. With regard to the blood supply to the terminal portion of the ileum, a number of options exist. In most of my patients having a J pouch, the ileocolic artery must be ligated to obtain adequate length for the ileoanal anastomosis. Thus, I choose this option most often. The blood supply is thus ligated as shown in Figure 12-27. The ileum is transected with a stapling device just proximal to the cecum. If necessary, the mesoappendix is divided separately. The retroperitoneal attachments of the terminal ileal mesentery are divided to the level of the duodenum, thus providing complete ileal mobility (Fig. 12-28). Before proceeding with the pelvic dissection, the sigmoid colon is divided. The abdominal colon is submitted for histologic examination while the operation proceeds. The diagnosis of chronic ulcerative colitis in patients with inflammatory bowel disease must be confirmed before the ileal pouch or anal anastomosis is constructed.

Proctectomy

The proctectomy must be performed without injuring the nervi erigentes. This can be accomplished by staying within the correct fascial planes. A close rectal dissection

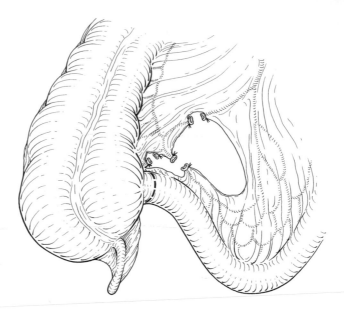

Figure 12-27. ▬▬▬▬

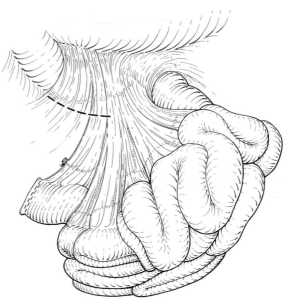

Figure 12-28. ▬▬▬▬

is not necessary; by retracting the rectum out of the pelvis the distinct fascia propria becomes conspicuous. The nerves do not run in the rectal mesentery. This plane is developed sharply down into the pelvis as far as exposure permits (Fig. 12-29). Waldeyer's fascia is incised with the scissors to prevent avulsion of the mesorectum on one side and of the pelvic venous plexus on the other. It is important to keep in mind that the rectum makes a right angle turn anteriorly at the level of S3.

Throughout the pelvic dissection, firm traction on the rectum is essential. The anterior peritoneal reflection is incised. The dissection is carried down to the level of the coccyx posteriorly and circumferentially about the rectum as far distally as possible (i.e., the seminal vesicles or alternatively, most of the vagina, should be visualized). Care is taken not to violate Denonvilliers fascia anteriorly. This is best done by blunt dissection between the rectum and vagina or prostate (Fig. 12-30). The lateral attachments of the rectum are divided sharply and ligated close to the rectum. A laparotomy pad is placed deep in the pelvis abutting the levators. This pad provides a landmark above which the endorectal mucosectomy need not be extended.

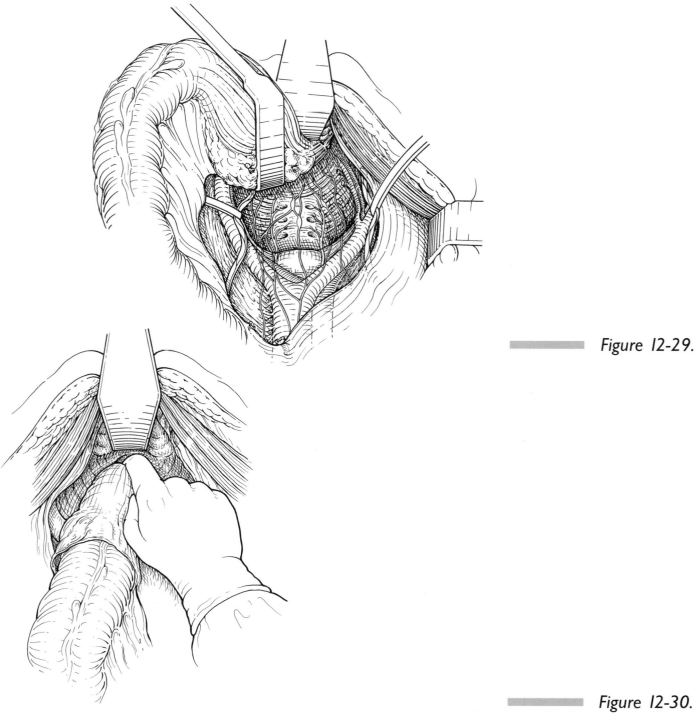

Figure 12-29.

Figure 12-30.

Constructing the J Pouch

The mobility of the terminal ileum is checked. Adequate length is available if a point on the antimesenteric aspect of ileum approximately 12 to 15 cm from the stapled end can be easily pulled beyond the skin overlying the symphysis pubis. If this cannot be done, tension is placed on the loop of bowel and the area of tethering identified. Often the ileocolic vessels foreshorten the ileal mesentery. Under these circumstances, they are isolated with vascular clamps. If vascular pulsations remain visible along the terminal ileum, and the pouch remains viable, the vessels on tension are divided and ligated. Occasionally, secondary branches of the superior mesenteric vessels cause the tethering. These can be sacrificed if the ileocolic vessels are preserved (Fig. 12-31).

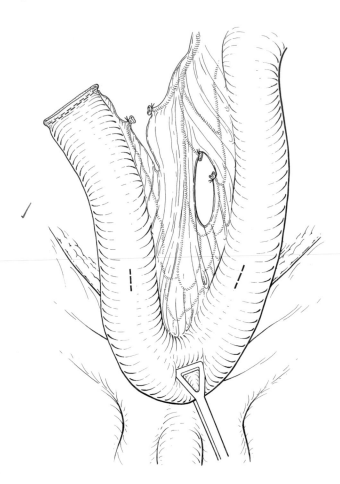

Figure 12-31.

Small enterotomies are then made 5 cm proximal to the apex, along the antimesenteric border of both limbs of the loop (Fig. 12-31). The GIA stapling device is first passed toward the pubis and fired (Fig. 12-32A). Care is taken that no mesentery is included in the jaws of the stapler. A septum of tissue remains at the apex of the pouch where the stapler blades did not reach; this septum is divided with the stapler. The long 90- to 100-mm linear stapler is then passed cephalad through the same enterotomies and fired (Fig. 12-32B).

The resulting enterotomy is closed longitudinally with two layers of sutures. There is sometimes an "ear" of terminal ileum not included in the long staple line. This portion of ileum can elongate over time and twist, causing a blowout of the pouch. This complication is avoided by merely securing the end of the ileum to the inflow tract using permanent sutures.

The apex of the pouch is inverted through its own mesentery, exposing the posterior staple line. This is a critical step because the continuity of the overlapping staple lines posteriorly must be confirmed or the pouch will leak. Sometimes interrupted sutures are required to reinforce gaps where the GIA stapling device was not properly placed (Fig. 12-33). The pouch is passed back through its mesentery.

The Lone Star retractor is positioned about the anus, exposing the dentate line (Fig. 12-34). This device effaces but *does not* dilate the anal canal.

The bulge produced by the laparotomy pad mentioned above should be easily palpable and clearly visible within several centimeters of the dentate line posteriorly.

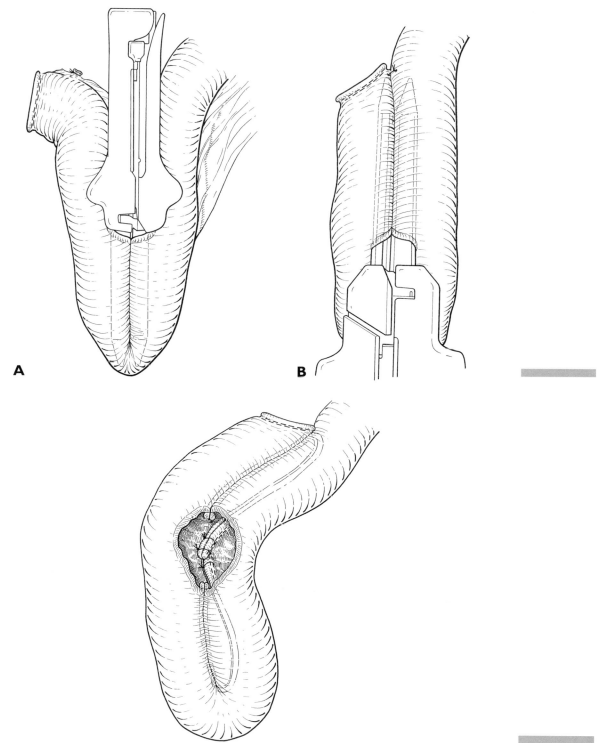

A   **B**

Figure 12-32.

Figure 12-33.

The endorectal mucosal dissection is then begun posteriorly. Submucosal injection of saline with epinephrine is used to aid the dissection. The mucosa is incised along the dentate line. The layer of loose connective tissue just below the mucosa is entered. This is followed with blunt and sharp dissection circumferentially until the level of the laparotomy pad is reached posteriorly. I prefer to perform this dissection with the scissors. Often pushing the cut end of the anal canal mucosa cephalad aids in visualizing the correct submucosal plane (Fig. 12-35). The length of dissection ranges from 3 to 5 cm and determines the length of the rectal cuff. The muscular wall

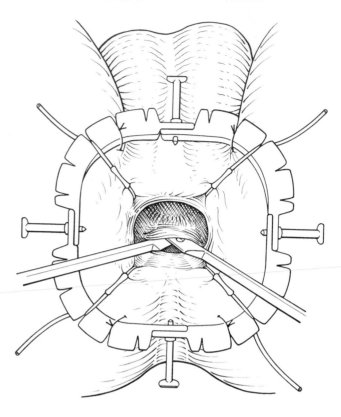

Figure 12-34.

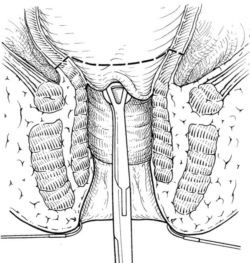

Figure 12-35.

of the rectum is transected over the laparotomy pad entering the presacral space. The laparotomy pad is removed from above. A finger is passed into the presacral space and used to guide the remaining dissection. The muscular wall is divided laterally on both sides, leaving the rectum attached anteriorly. A finger then hooks the rectum and draws it out through the anal canal. Traction is applied dorsally to the remaining rectal segment, better exposing the remaining anterior attachments. This expedites the dissection, especially in men, and decreases the likelihood of injury to the prostate. Before cutting the remaining attachments, the perineal wound should be inspected for hemostasis. Traction on the rectum everts the wound, providing good exposure; bleeding sites that can be easily cauterized at this point may be lost into the pelvis once the rectum is removed. The remaining attachments are transected and the rectum is submitted for histologic examination.

Ileal Pouch-Anal Anastomosis

The perineum and the pouch are now ready for the IPAA. A long Allis clamp passed through the muscular cuff from below is used to grasp the apex of the pouch and to deliver it through the perineal wound. The mesentery must be carefully inspected to ensure no twisting has occurred. It is quite common that the mesentery is on no small degree of tension. Once the pouch sits within the rectal cuff with its apex extending beyond the sphincters, a second Allis clamp grabs the pouch below, dorsal to the first. Four sutures of 2-0 absorbable material are used to circumferentially anchor the seromuscular layer of pouch to the puborectal muscle (Fig. 12-36). These sutures are placed about 2 cm proximal to the apex of the pouch. The wall of the ileum between the two Allis clamps is then incised transversely for a distance of approximately 1 cm. The one-layer anastomosis is made using a 2-0 absorbable suture on a UR needle.

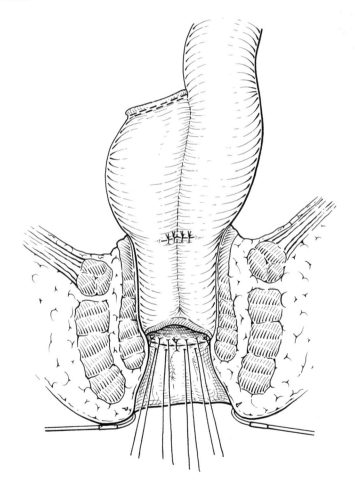

Figure 12-36.

Exposure during the anastomosis can be best maintained by sewing the dorsal half of the suture line first. Sutures are placed in the 3 and 9 o'clock positions. These initial stitches include a generous full-thickness bite of ileum, muscle at the level of the internal sphincter, and anoderm. The dorsal Allis clamp is removed, allowing placement of a dorsal suture similar to the first two. Additional stitches incorporating the ileum, sphincters, and anoderm are then placed. After completing the posterior half of the anastomosis, an anterior suture is placed at 12 o'clock and the anastomosis completed.

The suture line is checked most easily by the surgeon's finger. An index finger should easily pass through the anastomosis.

Closure

Prior to closing the midline incision, an ileostomy site is constructed. A 2-cm-diameter disc of skin and subcutaneous fat is excised from the preoperatively marked site, exposing the rectus sheath. A cruciate incision is made in the lateral one-third of the anterior rectus sheath. The fibers of the rectus abdominal muscle are separated with a curved clamp. The posterior rectus sheath is incised in a similar manner. Two fingers should pass easily through the defect.

The terminal ileum is identified as it enters the pouch. A loop of ileum approximately 20 to 25 cm proximal to the pouch, which easily reaches the level of the skin, is chosen for the ileostomy. A Penrose drain is passed through the mesentery of the ileum at the chosen point and used to withdraw the ileum through the stoma site. The loop should extend approximately 6 cm outside the level of the skin so that an adequate nipple can be constructed. There is no reason to use a supporting ileostomy "rod" except in the heaviest of patients.

The abdomen is liberally irrigated with warmed saline. The pelvis is drained with two large round catheter drains. These are introduced into the abdomen through separate stab wounds in the left lower quadrant. Both are positioned posterior to the pouch, deep within the pelvis. The midline incision is closed.

Maturing the Ileostomy

A scalpel opens the ileum at the level of the skin on the downstream side (distal limb) of the ileal loop. The incision extends 270 to 300 degrees around the circumference of the bowel, leaving only the mesenteric border intact. The distal edge of the bowel is secured to the dermis with several sutures of 3-0 chromic catgut. Four sutures are then placed in the 2-, 4-, 8-, and 10-o'clock positions of the proximal ileal edge. These sutures include the full thickness of the ileum, the ileal serosa at skin level, and dermis. These sutures are not tied until all four are positioned. As they are tied, the proximal ileum intussuscepts, forming a nipple of everted ileum. Simple sutures, including the full thickness of bowel wall and dermis, are placed between the previous stitches.

A sterile dressing is placed over the abdominal incision and a stoma pouch over the loop ileostomy. A perineal dressing is likewise placed.

Double-Stapled Ileoanal Anastomosis

The anastomosis between the pouch and the anorectal junction may be constructed using a double-staple technique. The technique is readily performed and there is invariably much less tension on the anastomosis than when peformed by hand. The obvious reason is the anus must be averted to suture the IPAA while it is pushed upwards to staple: this difference of 3–4 cm facilitates IPAA in obese and very tall patients.

The distal rectum is transected as close to the levator ani muscles as possible by pulling upward on the rectum and pushing the perineum superiorly. A 35-mm staple gun can be used because the anal canal, and not the thick and wide rectal muscular wall, is being stapled. It is extremely important that the linear staple line be no more than 3 to 4 cm above the dentate line. Liberal use of the index finger and regloving ensures proper placement of the cross-staple line. After firing the circular stapler, the resulting anastomosis will be within 2 cm of the dentate line. If the rectum and not the upper anal canal is transected, a long cuff of anal canal mucosa (anal transition zone) and *rectum* will be present, which is unacceptable. Alternatively, if the linear staple line is too low, the circular stapler will transect the internal sphincter and a portion of the external sphincter at the level of the puborectal muscle. Alternatively, a purse-string suture may be placed in the rectal cuff from below. This seemingly defeats one aim of stapling, that is, double stapling does not dilate the anal sphincter. Placing a pursestring suture by hand will dilate the canal.

The double-stapled approach facilitates constructing the pouch differently. An enterotomy is made at the apex of the soon-to-be-constructed pouch. Then, a 90- or 100-mm stapler is introduced and *one* firing is performed. A pouch with limbs of up to 15 to 17 cm can be constructed in this way without difficulty. The anvil (diameter 28 to 31 mm) is then inserted into the enterotomy in the apex of the pouch and secured with a 2-0 polypropylene pursestring suture. The stapling gun is placed into the anal canal, and the trocar is advanced through the linear staple line. The trocar is removed and the anvil connected to the stapler. The stapler is then fired in the usual fashion, and the tissue "doughnuts" are examined for complete integrity. The level of the anastomosis may range from the dentate line to 2 cm above the dentate line (See Fig. 10-15).

In some centers the ileal pouch is not diverted if it has been constructed in this way; reports are actually quite encouraging. I divert the pouch still, preferring to deal with the possible complications of stomal closure, rather than overwhelming pelvic sepsis.

Using an S Pouch

Although I do not use this pouch design, for reasons stated previously, illustration of the technique is shown (Fig. 12-37). I do not believe the outflow tract will reach any further into the pelvis than the apex of the J pouch. For that reason, and given the problem with even very short outflow tracts elongating, if a complex pouch design seems necessary, the W pouch is a better alternative (Fig. 12-38). It is larger and has no outflow tract like S pouches. However, W pouches *are* big and may be too big for the pelvis of some patients.

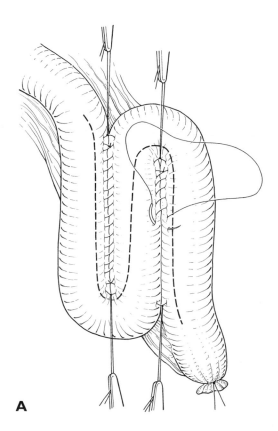
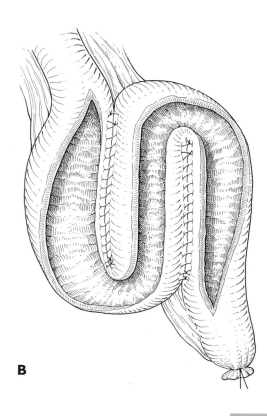

A   B

Figure 12-37.

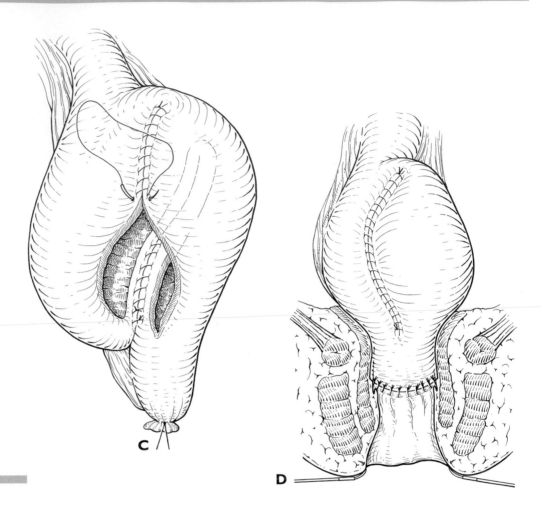

Figure 12-37.

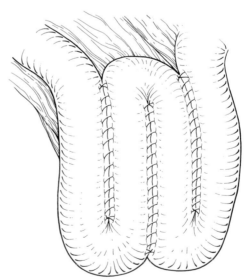

Figure 12-38.

Closing the Ileostomy

About 2 months after ileoanal anastomosis, the patient returns for closure of the stoma. I mobilize the stoma into the peritoneal cavity, resect it, and perform an end-to-end ileo-ileostomy. Others prefer to "unfold" the mucosa and close without resecting. I had two patients in whom leaks from punctured enterotomies occurred in the extraperitoneal portions of the proximal limb of the stoma after such a closure.

Editorial Commentaries

Level of Anastomosis. In our own randomized trial, stapled ileoanal anastomosis 1.5 cm above the dentate line (at the top of the anal columns) was associated with significantly better clinical results than stapled ileoanal anastomosis at the dentate line. The incidence of bleeding was comparable, there was significantly less soiling when the anastomosis was performed at the top of the anal columns, and the quality of continence was significantly better at the high level of anal anastomosis. Nevertheless, we would agree with Dr. Pemberton that anal mucosectomy is probably indicated if there is a coexisting carcinoma, particularly associated with dysplasia, and that a mucosectomy and sutured ileoanal anastomosis is probably the preferred operation for patients with FAP.

Sutured Ileoanal Anastomosis. We avoid leaving any retained rectal stump because in our experience the presence of a rectal cuff has been associated with an increased incidence of pelvic sepsis. If a mucosectomy is performed, it is extremely short, rarely measuring more than 1 to 1.5 cm in length. The technique that we use for sutured ileoanal anastomosis is that of interrupted 2-0 Vicryl sutures on a 25-mm round-bodied needle. We have performed the anastomosis with the intra-anal speculum, Gelpi retractors, and the Lone Star retractor. Of these three, we find the Gelpi retractors provide the best access for sutured ileoanal anastomosis. We do not think that two Gelpi retractors placed 90 degrees to one another causes excessive anal retraction or perineal damage.

Pouch Design. Like Dr. Pemberton, we prefer the J pouch. However, we make a slightly larger pouch using two 20-cm lengths. Also, we always make the pouch through an apical enterotomy using a linear staple cutter. We excise the anterior lip that is left at the apical enterotomy because it tends to become ischemic. Occasionally an S pouch is used if it is impossible to bring the apex of a J pouch down to the dentate line. In a previous randomized trial, we found no advantage of W pouches over J pouches.

Covering Ileostomy. We generally only omit a covering ileostomy in a patient who has already had a colectomy and is therefore off steroid medication, where two complete rings of tissue are recovered from the circular staple instrument using the double-staple technique, where there have been no technical difficulties with pouch construction or pouch-anus anastomosis, where there is no evidence of coexisting sepsis, and where intraoperative testing of the pouch and ileoanal anastomosis reveals no evidence of leakage. We totally agree with Dr. Pemberton that complications at the ileoanal anastomosis, which might occur from not using a covering stoma, are much more serious than potential stoma-related complications when a protecting ileostomy is used. Nevertheless, in our experience, over 70 percent of patients who have

(Continues)

had a previous subtotal colectomy can safely have a pouch constructed without a covering ileostomy.

Previous Subtotal Colectomy. By and large we prefer two-stage restorative proctocolectomy; stage one involves subtotal colectomy, end ileostomy, and oversewing of the rectal stump. Such a policy ensures that there is no evidence of Crohn's disease in the resected specimen; it also allows the patient to become familiar with an end ileostomy; it allows the patient to be weaned off steroid medication before pouch construction is undertaken and in 70 percent of cases subsequent pouch formation can be performed without a covering ileostomy.

Vascular Mobilization to Achieve a Tension-Free Ileoanal Anastomosis. It is sometimes necessary to divide vessels in the small bowel mesentery. If it is possible to avoid this, the risk of subsequent ileoanal stenosis, and pouchitis, might, however, be minimized. Either a critical vessel in the small bowel mesentery or the main trunk of the superior mesenteric artery may need to be divided, provided, of course, that there are adequate arcades peripherally to maintain viability of the small bowel. We nearly always mobilize the origin of the superior mesenteric artery under the pancreas and completely mobilize the duodenum and the duodenojejunal flexure.

Closure of Loop Ileostomy. We now favor stapled closure of loop ileostomy (see Ch. 4).

Michael R. B. Keighley

We agree with the general principles and goals of IPAA described by Dr. Pemberton. Nevertheless, some technical details are quite different in the procedure we employ.

Indications for a Two-Stage Procedure. The goal of surgery in these cases is to save the patient's life during a severe attack and to preserve the possibility of a sphincter-preserving procedure in the future. Subtotal colectomy with ileostomy and sigmoid mucous fistula is the rule in our clinic for fulminant colitis. It is also advisable in elective cases when the patient is on a long-standing course of corticosteroids and/or azathioprine because of their poor tissue healing.

Positioning the Patient. The patient is placed in the modified lithotomy position. The rectal lumen is washed with several hundred milliliters of povidone-iodine solution to reduce the risk of pelvic contamination. During positioning great care must be taken to protect nerves from pressure, and mobilization of the legs must be possible during the procedure.

Colectomy. In ulcerative colitis the greater omentum is often inflamed and adherent to the colon (a possible site of sealed perforations), and we prefer to divide the gastrocolic ligament en bloc and to remove all the omentum. Mobilization of the colon is limited to avoid a large area of deperitonealization in the paracolic gutters, where hemorrhage and fluid collection may result in abscess formation.

Proctectomy. At this stage, the technique we employ is quite different from Dr. Pemberton's. The lower sigmoid is not divided, and colectomy and proctectomy are performed en bloc. The dissection of the rectosigmoid is conducted as close as possible to the bowel wall to preserve parasympathetic and hypogastric nerves. A real intramesenteric dissection of the rectum is realized. The lower limits of the dissection are the tip of the coccyx posteriorly, the lower third of the vagina or midlevel of the prostate anteriorly, and the upper limit of the levators laterally. The rectum is closed at this level with the TA 55 stapler and then transected between the stapler and a clamp to avoid pelvic contamination. The entire specimen is delivered through the abdomen. The retained rectal stump is short, measuring 2 cm. As a consequence the mucosectomy is also very short, the upper limit of the mucosectomy being delimited by the staple line.

Construction of the J Pouch. The J pouch is our preferred technique also. The ileum is mobilized to allow the pouch to reach the anus. The mesentery is severed from the posterior parietal peritoneum up to the third part of the duodenum, and the left side of the superior mesenteric vein is denuded. These maneuvers allow the reservoir to reach the anus without excessive tension. We use the same criteria to ligate the tethering vessels. Two ileal limbs, both 18 cm in length, are held side by side with the antimesenteric edge anterior. A small enterotomy is performed on each limb on the antimesenteric side and at the midlevel of the limb, and the GIA 90 stapler is introduced. The pouch is created by two applications of staples. Like Dr. Pemberton, we often obtain an "ear" of terminal ileum that was not included in the staple line. In such cases another application of the stapler corrects this fault and provides a larger reservoir, 18 cm in length.

Mucosectomy. The anus is gently dilated and the anal canal exposed with two Gelpi retractors positioned at right angles. Now, we use the Lone Star retractor, which provides the best exposure, in our opinion. The mucosectomy starts a few millimeters above the dentate line to preserve discrimination and is conducted circumferentially up to the staple line. At this level the rectal muscle is transected, and the specimen (mucosa and staple line) removed and sent to the pathologist.

Ileal Pouch-Anal Anastomosis. Our technique at this time is the same; anastomosis is made using a 4-0 absorbable suture. A Penrose drain is inserted in the pouch through the anastomosis to evacuate blood and intestinal fluid.

Ileostomy. As a rule we protect the IPAA with a diverting loop ileostomy. We fully agree with Dr. Pemberton that it is preferable to deal with the com-

(Continues)

plications of stomal closure than pelvic sepsis. However, we sometimes do not divert IPAA in very select cases: in patients with FAP in good health, if the procedure was performed without any difficulty or complications, and if there is no tension on the mesentery and anastomosis.

Double-Stapled Ileoanal Anastomosis. We have no experience with this technique. We have only two questions: (1) Why is the rectum transected as close to the levator ani as possible with a TA stapler with this technique and not with the hand-sewn technique, and (2) Is it safe to perform the anastomosis within 2 cm of the dentate line?

Rolland Parc

My first comment is about the level of anastomosis. In the 1,300 patients undergoing ileoanal anastomosis at the Cleveland Clinic up until August 1994, almost 1,000 have had a stapled anastomosis. These have generally been 1.5 cm above the dentate line, and, like Dr. Keighley, we have observed singular improvement in function as well as lessened morbidity with the stapled technique as compared to the hand-sewn anastomosis following mucosectomy. Patients experience a lessened need to wear pads and lower rates of soiling as well as nocturnal soiling. In addition, there were lessened rates of anastomotic complications. Mucosectomy and hand-sewn anastomosis is then reserved for patients with coincident colorectal cancer or rectal dysplasia.

Lessons learned from proctocolectomy and the pelvic pouch include the lack of need for a rectal muscular cuff, that a temporary ileostomy is not always necessary but is a wise precaution, that the procedure should never be performed in patients who are toxic or malnourished, and that Crohn's disease is a contraindication to the procedure. The shape and dimensions of the pelvic pouch appear to play little role in functional outcome; however, we use an S pouch when difficulty in reaching the anus is likely or is present.

Victor W. Fazio

Crohn's Disease

Victor W. Fazio

Principles

The following description of operative techniques, with the exception of surgery for fulminant colitis, assumes that local and systemic circumstances will allow bowel anastomosis to be done safely. The principal indications for operation are obstruction, abscess, and fistula. Occasionally perforation, bleeding, or malignancy will also call for resection.

In most elective circumstances, mechanical bowel preparation is given, although among patients with some degree of bowel obstruction, tolerance is variable. Intravenous antibiotic cover is begun just prior to the abdominal incision. Where the possibility of stoma construction exists, preoperative siting is carried out with the patient in the supine and sitting positions.

Occasionally, intraoperative tube decompression of the proximal dilated small bowel will be required. When necessary, this may be done expeditiously by passage of a sterile nasogastric tube through the line of proposed resection of the proximal small bowel. The tube is coaxed through the linen tape that has been applied to occlude the bowel segment. By intermittently occluding the tube suction, decompression is achieved without enteric spillage.

Incision

A midline incision is used, thus sparing both lower quadrants of the abdomen for possible future stoma sites. We prefer an initial 15-cm incision, centered on the umbilicus. In many cases, this provides adequate exposure and can always be extended. Wound drapes and a self-retaining (Balfour) retractor with a bladder blade are used. At laparotomy the abdominal contents are checked; particular attention is paid to assessment of the entire small bowel, colon, and gallbladder.

Operative Recognition of Crohn's Disease

Although overt phlegmonous disease, especially in the terminal ileum, is usually obvious, as are local complications such as perforation or fistulas, there may be other features present that are more subtle. Chronically obstructed, but otherwise normal, small bowel may be edematous or thickened, simulating Crohn's disease. Palpation of the mesenteric margin is a useful index of assessment. A mesenteric margin thickened compared to proximal and clearly normal bowel is often an indicator of underlying Crohn's disease and is frequently due to a linear mesenteric ulcer on the luminal (mucosal) surface. Although enlargement of the lymph nodes commonly occurs along the length of the ileocolic vessels in Crohn's disease, the enlarged paraileal nodes, especially the most proximal node at the suspected proximal margin of disease, will help provide a guide to the extent of disease. Fat wrapping, the encroachment of fat onto the serosal surface of the bowel, is a feature of Crohn's disease. It usually indicates that there is mucosal ulceration. In a more subtle form, this may be manifested by the absence of scalloping between the vasa recti branches of the marginal vessel. Alternatively, small deposits of fat may be seen along attenuated hyperemic vessels on the serosal surface. These probably indicate that this segment of bowel is affected by Crohn's disease. However, unless this segment is strictured or harbors overt ulceration, in the interest of bowel conservation, resection of this extra segment may not be appropriate.

Assessment of colonic involvement in Crohn's disease may also be difficult. Serositis may not necessarily denote Crohn's disease in that segment. Furthermore, noninflamed serosa does not exclude frank mucosal ulceration. In certain cases, especially if preoperative colonoscopy has not been used, intraoperative endoscopy may be advised to avoid the risk of leaving behind frank ulcerated colonic disease.

Margins of Resection

There is no compelling evidence that radical (i.e., greater than 15-cm margins) resection lessens the rate of recurrent Crohn's disease. Accordingly, we use margins of 5 cm in most cases. This implies that the resected specimen has been opened on a side table in the operating room in order to ensure that overt ulceration or cobblestoning is not present at the lines of resection. Exceptions to this include patients with the short-bowel syndrome and those undergoing strictureplasty procedures; however, in no circumstances are anastomoses made to strictured bowel ends.

Small Bowel Resection

Techniques of Resection

The basic principles of resection include obtaining adequate exposure and illumination, and "quarantining" the abdominal cavity with packs so as to minimize contamination if there is any risk of fecal spillage. When the bowel is divided and the anastomosis is fashioned, care is taken to place these packs appropriately and to use bowel occluders, such as linen tapes, above and below the evacuated diseased segment (Fig. 12-39).

The special resectional problems posed by Crohn's disease include grossly thickened mesentery and lymph node enlargement, possible fixation or tethering of the bowel

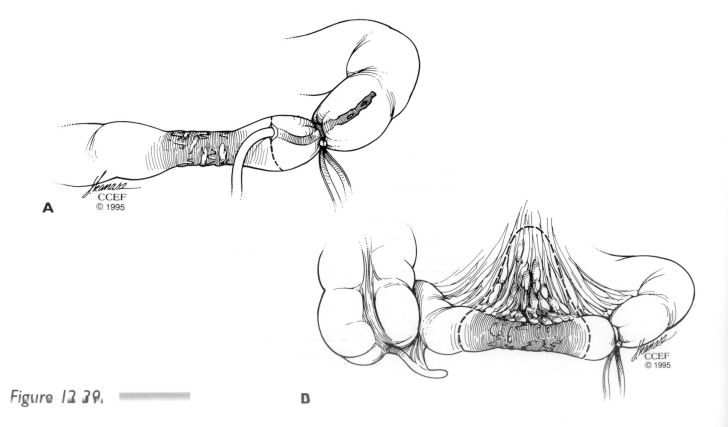

Figure 12-39.   A   D

loops to the retroperitoneum, and adherence to adjacent bowel loops or intra-abdominal organs. There is no evidence that resection of enlarged lymph nodes will influence recurrence rates (although some nodes will harbor enteric bacteria and, in a few cases, frank suppuration is present), thus we do not attempt a radical lymphadenectomy. In many cases, the majority of the enlarged lymph nodes can be safely encompassed by the resection. This is appropriate and even desirable provided no "normal" bowel requires resection (because of ischemia) other than what was originally planned.

The ordinary techniques of vessel identification and mobilization prior to selective clamping are usually impossible to use for the mesenteric vessels in Crohn's disease. A much safer technique, one designed to prevent retraction of the proximally clamped vessel and thus the production of a hematoma advancing toward the origin of the superior mesenteric vessels, is to use a series of Kocher clamps in an overlapping fashion, with suture ligation of the pedicles (Fig. 12-40). A Kocher clamp is placed on the side of the mesentery that will remain after the resection. A curved Kelly clamp is placed on the specimen side at a distance sufficient to allow mesenteric division, leaving a cuff of mesentery. We divide the tissues closer to the specimen (Kelly clamp) side than the in situ side. Note the tied marginal vessel (Fig. 12-40A). To avoid a chordee effect, that is, the in-curving of the divided bowel end, the mesenteric division is begun by placing a fine curved forceps through the mesentery at the bowel wall level. The jaws of the clamp are spread. Cautery is used between the vasa recti up to the marginal vessel. This is individually ligated and divided. From this point, the overlapping technique is used (Fig. 12-40B). A series of overlapping Kocher and Kelly clamps are placed, dividing the mesentery and then adding additional clamps as necessary. A No. 1 chromic catgut suture (on a CTX needle) is placed beneath the tip of the Kocher clamp (Fig. 12-40C). The needle is passed beneath the next overlapping Kocher clamp to ensure that it encompasses all the vessels in the clamped mesentery. Thus when the suture is tied down, hemostasis is assured. For a very bulky pedicle (e.g., that of the ileocolic vessels), the peritoneum on the proximal side of the clamp can be incised or scarified. The tying of this vessel pedicle is then done by seating the catgut along this line, which will prevent suture slippage (Fig. 12-40D). The enteric contents are milked proximally and the bowel is occluded with a linen tape. The bowel is then transected with sharp scissors or electrocautery (Fig. 12-40E), after completing division of the mesentery.

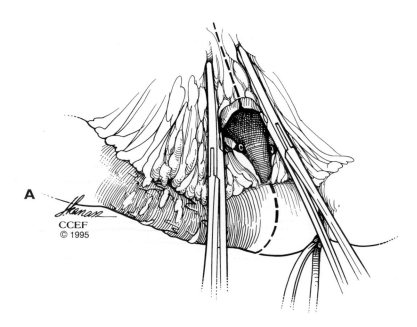

A

CCEF
© 1995

Figure 12-40.

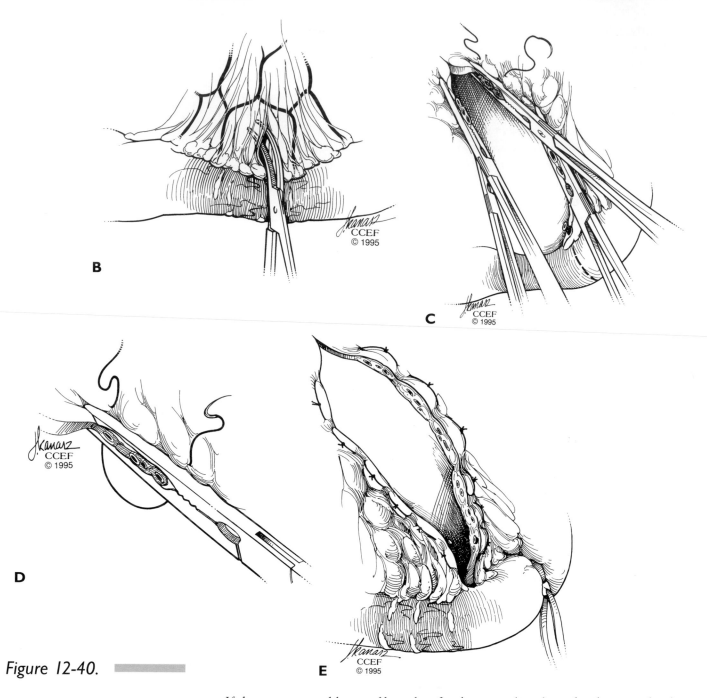

Figure 12-40.

If there are matted loops of bowel or fistulas extending from the ileum to the duodenum, colon, stomach, bladder, or fallopian tubes, these are detached or separated. The ileal Crohn's disease is the primary segment and will need resection. The secondarily involved organ (such as the transverse or sigmoid colon, or loops of proximal small intestine) may be safely treated by wedge or sleeve resection and repair. In the case of bladder or uterine/tubal involvement, simple suture repair is adequate. Intra-abdominal or retroperitoneal abscesses are drained and the omentum is used to protect the small bowel, especially the anastomosis, from the residual abscess cavity.

Anastomotic Techniques

Our preference is for stapled anastomotic techniques because they are speedier and are particularly appropriate for bowel ends of disparate caliber. An exception to this,

for which we prefer a hand-sewn end-to-end anastomosis, is the uncommon situation
where a short segment of preserved terminal ileum remains. Where feasible, following ileal resection for Crohn's disease, we preserve the ileocecal valve, as this seems to reduce postoperative bowel dysfunction. Although usually the ileal Crohn's disease extends right up to the ileocecal valve, necessitating ileocecal resection, occasionally the prevalve ileum can be preserved. Provided one can retain 5 to 7 cm or more of normal distal ileum, an ileoileal anastomosis is constructed using an end-to-end hand-sewn technique. Hand-sewn and stapled methods are illustrated in Figures 12-41 and 12-42.

Hand-Sewn Technique. A full-thickness bite of the bowel edge is taken using 3-0 Vicryl, starting on the mesenteric side of the midline. To assure an inverting anastomosis, a mattress suture is used (Fig. 12-41A); a detail of the posterior aspect is seen in Figure 12-41B. Mattress sutures are continued posteriorly until the bowel edge is free of the mesenteric fat (Fig. 12-41C). As the posterior mattress sutures are tied beyond the mesenteric margin, the serosa of the bowel becomes clear of the mesenteric fat. 3-0 Vicryl is then placed in a seromuscular fashion for the anterior layer of the anastomosis—excluding mucosa (Fig. 12-41D). The mesenteric defect is then closed with 0-0 chromic catgut, carefully avoiding injury to the mesenteric vessel. This complication, which could lead to a hematoma or ischemia of the bowel edge, is minimized by suturing opposing, previously ligated, mesenteric pedicles (Fig. 12-41E).

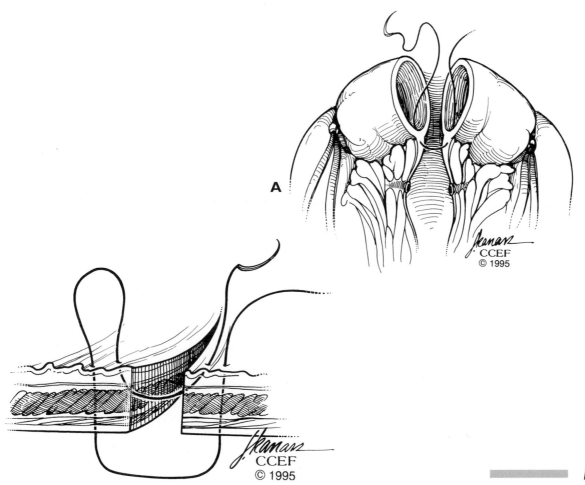

Figure 12-41.

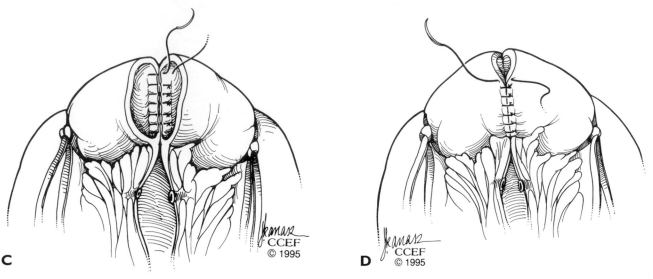

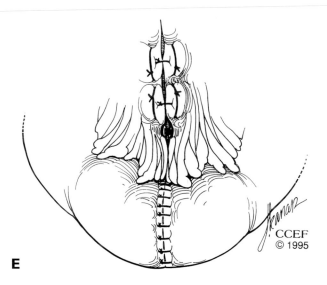

Figure 12-41. ▬▬▬ **E**

Ileo-Ascending Colon Stapled Anastomosis. With open, hand-sewn anastomoses, the luminal aspect of the bowel is visible and can therefore be assessed for evidence of overt or significant Crohn's disease and the need for revision of resection limits. When stapling techniques are used, examination of the bowel can only be done after the lines of resection have been chosen and the resected specimen examined. In a few cases, further resection may be required prior to stapled anastomosis. Frozen sections of the margins are not used. Although there is still some controversy about using stapled anastomosis in patients with Crohn's disease, there is little evidence of adverse outcomes with this technique; certainly operative contamination by enteric contents is minimized.

Unless there is sparing of the distal 5 to 7 cm of terminal ileum, allowing the formation of an ileoileal anastomosis and preservation of the ileocecal valve, the ileocecal resection includes both the terminal ileum and the lower pole of the cecum, which may or may not have some cecal Crohn's disease. The mesentery is divided and ligated as described above. We generally aim for a 5- to 7-cm margin distal to the ileocecal valve (Fig. 12-42A). In many cases, especially if the abdominal incision is small, the right colon is mobilized to facilitate the anastomosis.

The bowel segment is again "quarantined" with occluding tapes to minimize contamination. A linear staple cutter such as the GIA 60 (Autosuture, U.S. Surgical Co., Norwalk, CT) or PLC-75 (Ethicon Inc., Livingston, NJ) is used to divide and staple the bowel ends (Fig. 12-42B). The margins of the open resected specimen are checked before proceeding with the anastomosis. ✓

An enterotomy is made into the proximal colon and distal ileum 2 cm from the stapled bowel ends to allow the anvil and the cartridge of the stapler access to the lumen (Fig. 12-42C). Care is taken to displace the mesenteric margins as far as possible from the proposed staple line. The enterotomies are then closed with continuous 3-0 Vicryl reinforced by interrupted 3-0 Vicryl (Fig. 12-42D & E).

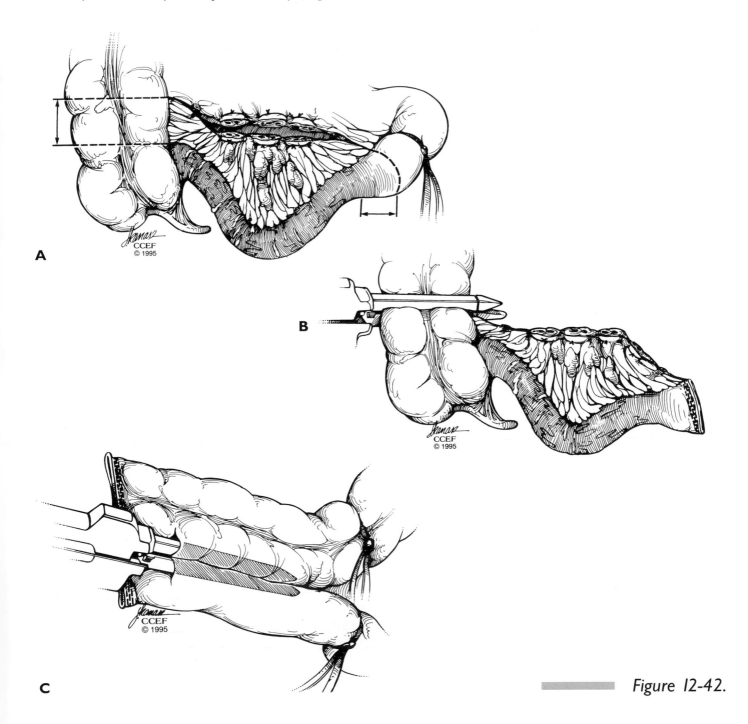

A

B

C

Figure 12-42.

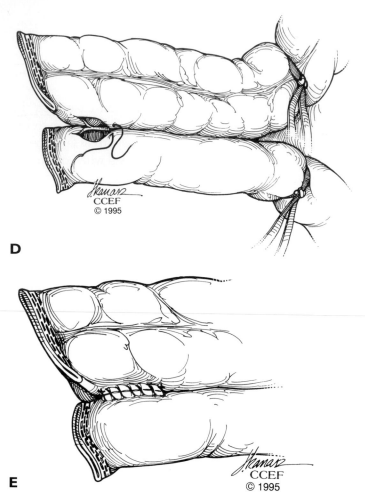

D

E

Figure 12-42.

Strictureplasty

Resection is still the most common surgical procedure in the treatment of Crohn's disease. However, a small proportion of patients with small bowel Crohn's disease may exhibit multiple or extensive proximal strictured segments (skip lesions). Management of these strictures may involve chronic anti-inflammatory medication, hospital admission, and courses of hyperalimentation, including home parenteral nutrition in some cases, or surgical procedures such as multiple resection and internal bypass. Patients having resection are vulnerable to the development of the short bowel syndrome. Likewise, risk groups also include those with recurrent disease and an already foreshortened small intestine. An alternative to resection for such patients is that of strictureplasty, a procedure in which the diseased segment is left in situ but is widened surgically by a procedure similar to a Heineke-Mikulicz pyloroplasty for short segments up to 8 to 10 cm, or a Finney strictureplasty for segments 10 to 25 cm in length. These procedures alleviate obstructive symptoms in almost all cases with acceptably low (6 to 7 percent) rates of suture line or septic complications.

The contraindications to strictureplasty include peri-intestinal sepsis (fistula at the stricture site, paraintestinal abscess, stricture perforation), phlegmonous inflammation, long segments (e.g., 25-cm stricture), stricture in close proximity to a proposed resection, multiple strictures in a short segment of bowel, malignancy or suspected malignancy, and colonic strictures.

Short Strictureplasty (<8 cm)

The bowel above and below the proposed strictureplasty site is isolated between tapes. Using cutting cautery, the seromuscular layer is incised down to the submucosal level. The incision is made 3 cm proximal and distal to the stricture, to reach supple, nonconstricted bowel (Fig. 12-43A).

An enterotomy is made over the nonstrictured bowel end and angled forceps are used to spread the enterotomy. The exposed submucosa and mucosa of the anterior wall of the stricture are then divided using coagulating current, as this layer is quite vascular (Fig. 12-43B). The enterotomy is then completed. A fibromuscular mound or thickened bowel wall is usually seen on the posterior (mesenteric) wall of the stricture. Seromuscular sutures of 3-0 Vicryl are placed opposite one another at the approximate midpoint of the defect. The mucosa is biopsied with sterile colonoscopy forceps (Fig. 12-43C). Using lateral traction, the longitudinal enterotomy is converted to a transverse defect (Fig. 12-43D). A one-layer extramucosal closure is used to complete the strictureplasty (Fig. 12-43E). A metal clip is applied to allow subsequent radiographic identification when/if follow-up contrast studies are performed (Fig. 12-43F).

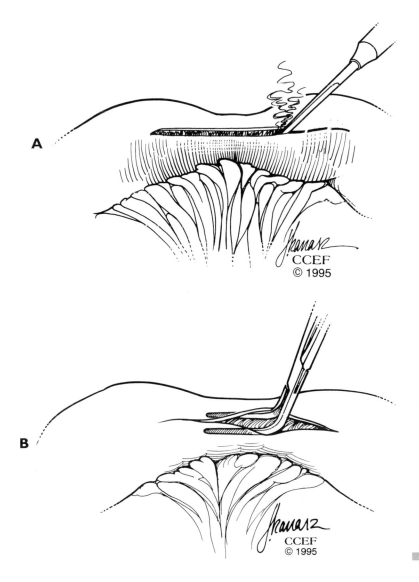

A

CCEF
© 1995

B

CCEF
© 1995

Figure 12-43.

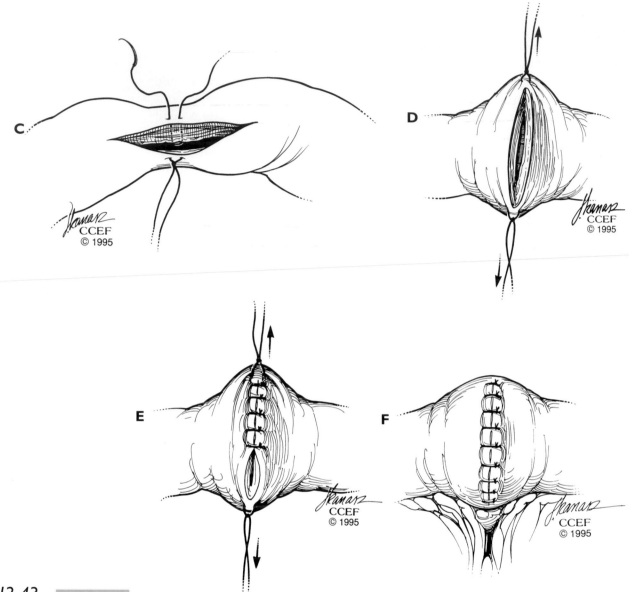

Figure 12-43.

Long (Finney) Strictureplasty (10 to 25 cm)

An enterotomy similar to that previously described for short strictureplasty is used. In these cases, the enterotomy is made anterolaterally, not directly anteriorly (Fig. 12-44A & B). Thus when the bowel is aligned side-to-side, tension in both the anterior and posterior suture lines is minimized. Some strictures may have some small "dilated" segments within the stricture, like a mini chain of lakes. Where possible, it is useful to align a tightly strictured segment against a relatively "normal-caliber" segment.

A continuous 2-0 Vicryl suture joins the medial (posterior) edges of the defect. Sutures are placed through all coats of the bowel edge. This layer is reinforced with interrupted 2-0 or 3-0 Vicryl to further approximate any nonopposed mucosa where possible (Fig. 12-44C). The anterior layer is then closed with interrupted 2-0 Vicryl in one layer using seromuscular sutures (Fig. 12-44D). A metal clip is placed on the mesentery to facilitate future radiographic identification.

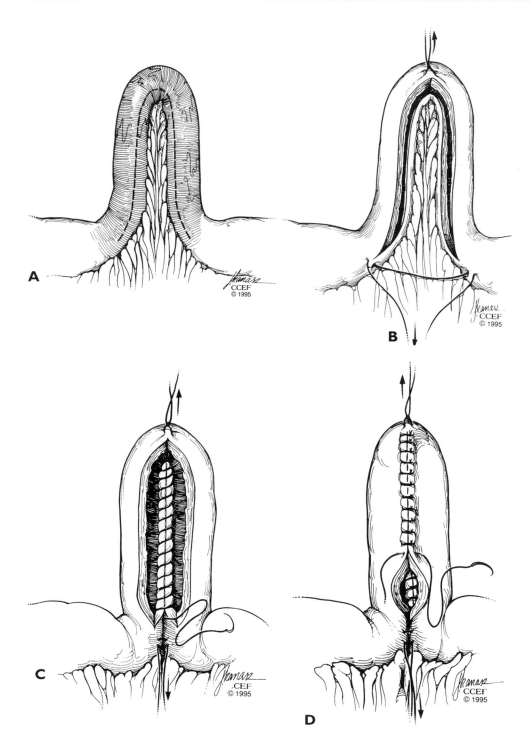

Figure 12-44.

Segmental Colectomy

The principles of resection and anastomosis are similar to those described for small bowel Crohn's disease. The most common areas of segmental colonic involvement are the sigmoid and transverse colon. Presently, strictureplasty is not recommended ✓ for isolated colonic strictures, except at stenosed ileocolic or ileorectal anastomoses, and resection is advised. Recurrence rates are very high following anastomosis of large bowel ends, but compared to total colectomy and ileorectal anastomosis, segmental restorative resection results in less diarrhea. ✓

Figure 12-45A illustrates the lines of resection, leaving 5 to 10 cm of clearance beyond overt disease. The patient may require on-table colonoscopy if the colon has not been fully assessed preoperatively. This will ensure identification of other involved areas of diseased colon in need of removal. Thus, positioning the patient in the Trendelenburg position with the legs placed in Lloyd-Davies stirrups is advisable. This is the preferred position for patients requiring sigmoid resection for segmental Crohn's disease. The presence of aphthous ulcers or scattered punctate mucosal ulcers, although indicative of Crohn's disease, does not warrant extending the colectomy to include these areas.

For delivery of the splenic flexure, the omentum is raised upward onto the chest wall. The left colon is mobilized along the white line in the lateral gutter, retracting the descending colon upward and medially. This exposes Gerota's fascia over the kidney (Fig. 12-45B).

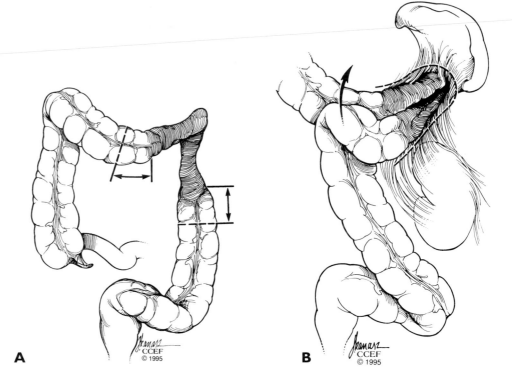

Figure 12-45.   **A**   **B**

Combined traction on both the transverse and descending colon in a downward and medial fashion allows the lateral peritoneal incision to be extended about 1 to 2 cm lateral to the splenic flexure of the colon. This procedure involves a combination of both cutting and coagulating electrocautery.

Mobilization of the transverse colon is facilitated by one of two methods. If the omental attachment is not too thickened and fused to the mesocolon or bowel, cautery dissection will separate the omentum from the colon and mesocolon, allowing entry into the lesser sac. This will aid in the complete delivery of the splenic flexure. If the omentum is inextricably fused to the colon, then partial omentectomy is necessary, with en bloc resection of the attached distal transverse colon.

The hepatic flexure may need to be mobilized if deemed necessary for a tension-free midtransverse colon to middescending colon anastomosis, as in the case illustrated.

The lines of resection for segmental excision are defined (Fig. 12-45C). The proximal and distal colon segments are occluded with tapes. For resection of the splenic flexure, the marginal vessels, left branch of the midcolic vessels, and ascending branch of the left colic vessels are ligated and divided.

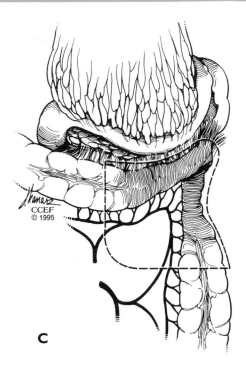

C

Figure 12-45.

Segmental Resection of the Sigmoid Colon for Crohn's Colitis

In older patients, Crohn's disease of the sigmoid colon is commonly mistaken for diverticulitis; however, many patients with Crohn's disease have perianal disease. In Crohn's disease, examination of the opened specimen will show an ulcerated mucosal surface, whereas in diverticular disease the surface is almost always normal. The resection lines are shown in Figure 12-45D, with high ligation of the inferior mesenteric artery (to enable added mobilization of the proximal colon, if needed), transection/ligation of the left colic and marginal vessels, and colon division approximately 5 cm above and below the diseased segment. Mobilization of the sigmoid is performed in a lateral to medial direction, incising the peritoneum of the left colic gutter while identifying and preserving the left ureter. The alternative approach is that of conservative resection with division/ligation of the sigmoid vessels instead of high ligation, which is appropriate if anastomotic tension is not a consideration.

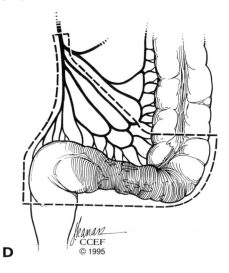

D

Figure 12-45.

Anastomosis may be performed using the ILS-29 or CEEA 31 circular stapler. This is a rapid, safe, and an eminently satisfactory method when the anastomosis is within the range of the transanally placed stapler (i.e., <20 cm from the anal verge). The modified stapler with detachable anvil/shaft complex is illustrated in Figure 12-45E. A pursestring suture is placed in the cut ends of the bowel using 0-0 or 2-0 Prolene. Minute bites of the cut end of bowel are taken with the Prolene suture at 7-mm intervals. This will minimize extrusion of bowel around the shaft once the pursestring has been tied. Upon union of the anvil and shaft of the cartridge, the two are approximated into the firing range and the anastomosis is completed (Fig. 12-45F).

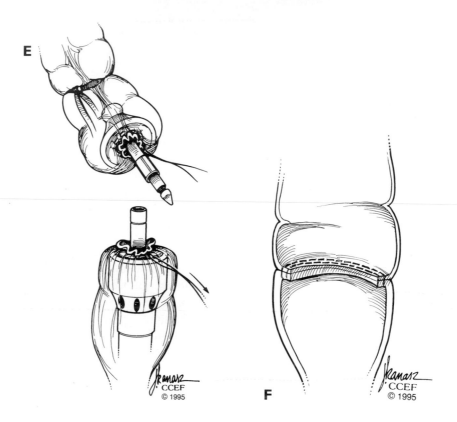

Figure 12-45.

The tissue rings are checked following instrument withdrawal and the integrity of the anastomosis assured with air insufflation or povidone-iodine transanal injection.

Subtotal Colectomy and Ileostomy for Fulminant Colitis

This procedure is usually performed in an urgent or emergency situation. Commonly, the underlying diagnosis is uncertain; in western countries, ulcerative colitis and Crohn's disease are the usual causes. The principles of the operation include the following:

1. Preoperative siting of the ileostomy.
2. Rectal assessment by proctoscopy.
3. Adequate exposure using a midline incision.
4. Assessment of the peritoneal cavity and colon for existing perforation, which if present must be controlled immediately.
5. Avoidance of fecal contamination through inadvertent colotomy.
6. Mobilization of the abdominal colon.
7. Conservative (usually) vascular pedicle ligation for subtotal colectomy.
8. Assessment of the small bowel for Crohn's disease.

9. Transection of small bowel with preservation of as much length of normal bowel as possible.
10. "Conservative" resection margin of the distal sigmoid where possible, leaving enough so that the distal segment can reach the anterior abdominal wall without tension.
11. Extraperitonealization of the distal segment.

For patients with toxic dilatation of the colon, the gas- and stool-filled segment may make splenic flexure mobilization difficult. Stool cannot be evacuated, but dilatation by gas can be reduced by aspiration with a large-bore (No. 14) needle placed through the tenia. On needle removal, a 3-0 Vicryl suture will help seal the puncture site.

For patients who have associated major colonic hemorrhage, opinion is divided as to the need for completion proctectomy. Our own view is that this is rarely necessary, even when there is evidence of colonic hemorrhage. Intraoperative proctoscopy may help quantify the amount of hemorrhage from the rectal stump. Should bleeding be deemed significant, we would prefer to perform an extended proctectomy with stapling of the distal rectum at the anorectal ring. This will still allow for later ileoanal anastomosis if the diagnosis proves to be ulcerative colitis. Should completion proctectomy ever be required, this can be done fairly easily by the perineal route described above.

Preoperative Siting of the Ileostomy

With the patient in the sitting position, and later in the supine position, a standard-sized faceplate is applied to the lower right quadrant so that the following criteria are met (Fig. 12-46A).

1. The skin over the center of the plate is visible to the patient.
2. The site is at the summit of the infraumbilical fat mound.
3. The plate fits within the area defined by the lateral border of the rectus abdominis muscle, a horizontal line drawn at the level of the umbilicus, and the midline.
4. There is no encroachment on the iliac crest, the planned incision, the groin, or any creases or scars.

An indelible mark, made by pricking the skin site after placement of a drop of india ink, facilitates intraoperative identification.

Lines of Resection

In Figure 12-46B, the dotted lines indicate the limits of bowel resection and conservative vascular pedicle ligation for subtotal colectomy. The ileum may be transected with a linear staple cutter or between bowel clamps. Distally, the colon is often too thickened. I prefer to use a proximal bowel clamp, such as a Kocher clamp, and a distal linear stapler (e.g., PI55 or TA 55 [US Surgical]). Longer transverse staplers are available if the bowel is very wide.

We prefer to preserve the omentum, although some surgeons will routinely remove it along with the colon.

Mobilization of the Colon

Mobilization of the colon may be performed in several ways. A convenient starting point is a cautery incision of the peritoneum lateral to the cecum with extension in a

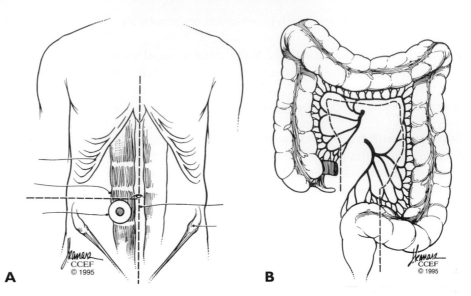

Figure 12-46.   **A**   **B**

cephalad direction to the hepatic flexure. A V-shaped exposure of the retroperitoneum results when the peritoneum of the left leaf of the small bowel mesentery is incised upward toward the duodenojejunal flexure (Fig. 12-46C). The cecum and terminal ileum are retracted upward and to the patient's left, exposing the right ureter and gonadal vessels. By retracting on the hepatic flexure downward and medially, cautery may be used to incise the retroperitoneal attachments as well as any adhesions to the gallbladder (Fig. 12-46D). Some of these unnamed vessels in the peritoneum may require ligature.

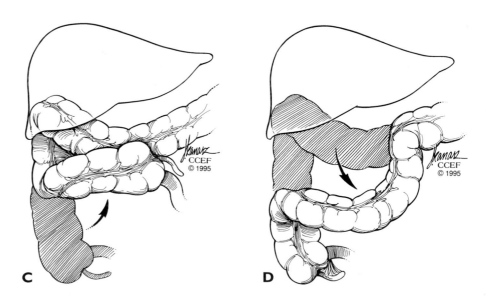

Figure 12-46.   **C**   **D**

The mobilization of the splenic flexure, omentum, and left colon with the sigmoid colon and entry into the lesser sac were discussed in the segment on segmental resection of the splenic flexure.

Management of the Distal Rectosigmoid

Because it is so easy, the surgeon is tempted to extend the distal line of resection into the rectum—perhaps even to the peritoneal reflection anteriorly. This is often done in the erroneous belief that the more inflamed bowel that is removed, the better the outcome. However, there is a strong likelihood that further surgery will be required, such as proctectomy or ileorectal anastomosis for Crohn's disease or ileal pouch-anal anastomosis in the case of ulcerative colitis. In any of these situations, the operation is made much more difficult and there is perhaps a greater risk of complications if the rectal stump is foreshortened or receded.

The three main alternatives for stump management are as follows:

1. Suture reinforcement of the stapled end of the rectosigmoid and exclusion from the peritoneal cavity.
2. Construction of a mucous fistula.
3. Exteriorization of the stump outside the abdominal wall.

Exteriorization is used when the colon wall is particularly fragile and any attempt at suturing or stapling leads to the sutures cutting out. This is a problem particularly in toxic megacolon. In this case, the distal segment is withdrawn 5 to 10 cm beyond the skin level, the end is left open, and a 2-inch-wide gauze roll is wrapped around the end of the colon. This maintains exteriorization. The construction of a mucous fistula is *not* generally employed because if the bowel end is too fragile, sutures will simply cut through; if the bowel end is not too fragile, stapling will suffice and negate the disadvantages of a second discharging stoma.

The extraperitonealization method involves stapling the cut end of the colon and reinforcement of this closure with 2-0 Vicryl (Fig. 12-46E). The appendices epiploicae of the bowel, about 3 cm from the cut end, is then sutured to the peritoneum of the anterior wound, circumferentially around the stump. This ensures its extraperitoneal location. In the event of a stump perforation, there will be no resultant peritonitis and the end of the bowel will ultimately form a small mucous fistula. The fascia and muscle superficial to the end of the stump is closed with widely spaced interrupted 0-0 Prolene.

The management of the fragile distal rectosigmoid stump should involve no suturing of the bowel at all. The stump is exteriorized for 5 to 10 cm beyond the skin, and a 2-inch-wide gauze roll is wrapped snugly around the base and stapled to itself. The fascia is closed with nonabsorbable Prolene and the skin is approximated with staples (Fig. 12-46F). One week later, the stump is amputated at skin level and a mucous fistula is created.

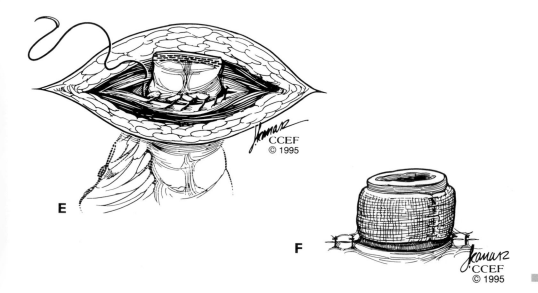

E

F

Figure 12-46.

Ileostomy Construction

Kocher clamps are applied to the skin and fascia opposite the marked ileostomy site and medial traction is applied. A 3-cm-diameter disc of skin is excised. The surgeon's left index and middle fingers support a gauze pack that is pushed anteriorly from within the abdomen over the site of the future internal ileostomy aperture. The left thumb stabilizes and retracts on the Kocher clamps. Using cutting cautery, a vertical incision is made in the fat of the ileostomy aperture, exposing the anterior rectus sheath. This is incised vertically for 3 cm. The rectus muscle is separated with a medium Kelly clamp. Three or four short, right-angled retractors will retract the separated fibers of the rectus as the Kelly clamp is withdrawn. The inferior epigastric artery and vein are retracted to one side, if seen at this time. With further upward traction of the surgeon's left hand, the cutting cautery is used to make a vertical incision in the posterior fascia and peritoneum onto the gauze pad. A "snug" two-finger aperture is thus created and hemostasis is checked. This technique is illustrated in Chapter 4.

The end of the ileum is brought through the aperture for 3 to 4 cm. A series of eight sutures of 3-0 chromic catgut are placed, but not yet tied, between the cut end of the ileum and the subcuticular layer of skin (Fig. 12-46G). This is in contradistinction to full-thickness skin, so as to avoid implants of mucosa in the needle tracts. The handle of a pair of tissue forceps helps displace the ileum for easier suture placement when all eight sutures are placed (Fig. 12-46H). The ileostomy is then matured by tying the sutures (Fig. 12-46I).

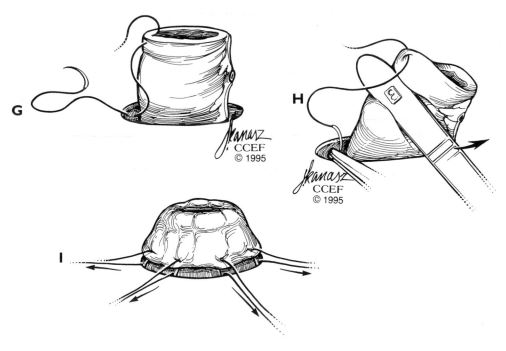

Figure 12-46.

The mesenteric defect is closed by placing 0-0 chromic sutures between the cut edge of the mesentery and the anterior peritoneum about 3 cm to the right of the main wound. This is carried upward (cephalad) and sutured to the falciform ligament to complete the partitioning of the abdomen (Fig. 12-46J). In elective or semielective cases, the end of the ileum is left occluded and the stoma is matured after the abdomen has been closed. A postoperative skin barrier and transparent pouch appliance is applied to assess more easily viability of the stoma in the postoperative period.

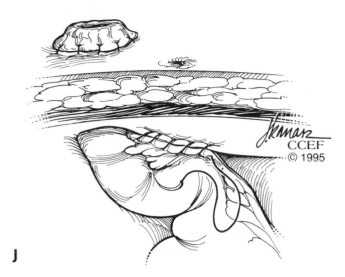

J

Figure 12-46.

Subtotal Colectomy and Ileorectal Anastomosis

The operation involves total abdominal colectomy, taking as much as possible of the resection close to the ileocecal valve. The distal line of resection is usually at or above the rectosigmoid junction at the sacral promontory. For Crohn's disease, one will also favor colonic preservation where feasible. For example, if the distal sigmoid colon, or all of the sigmoid for that matter, is spared of ulceration and the rectum is uninvolved and compliant (i.e., distends well on air insufflation), then an ileosigmoid anastomosis is desirable. If the lower half of the rectum is free of overt Crohn's disease, but the upper one-half to one-third has frank active disease, one option is that of colectomy, resection of the proximal half of the rectum, and ileo-midrectal anastomosis. One may add a small (10 cm) J pouch for augmenting the neorectal reservoir function. ✓

The operation is contraindicated if there is extensive small bowel disease, if there is active perianal suppuration or fistulas, if the anal sphincter function is poor, or if rectal compliance is low. We usually add to this list of contraindications the presence of Crohn's disease in the rectum; however, mild or modest involvement may be acceptable to some surgeons, provided the patient is aware of the probable long-term outcome.

The conduct of the abdominal colectomy has already been described (Figs. 12-45B–D and 12-46C & D). Both ureters are identified and preserved. If the lumen of the small bowel is adequate (i.e., will accept an ILP-29 or EEA31), then we prefer to use a circular stapled ileorectal anastomosis. This is similar to the colorectal anastomosis (Fig. 12-45E & F) (see Ch. 2). Otherwise, a hand-sewn one-layer 3-0 Vicryl anastomosis is used.

For the sutured ileorectal anastomosis, it is useful to place stay sutures of 3-0 catgut at the cut edge of the bowel ends. Two of these will be on the posterolateral edge and two on the anterolateral edges. The vertical mattress technique of sutured anastomosis is used as described for small bowel anastomosis.

If the proximal small bowel caliber is significantly smaller than that of the rectum, then a linear midline incision, or Cheatle slit, on the antimesenteric aspect of the bowel is made. This can be tailored to suit the caliber of the small bowel and rectum. Cutting cautery is very effective for fashioning the Cheatle slit. The antimesenteric defect of the anastomosis is closed with interrupted 3-0 Vicryl using seromucosal sutures.

Where the situation permits (i.e., a wide-caliber small bowel and a relatively short rectosigmoid stump), a circular stapled anastomosis is used. The tissue rings from the staple gun and anastomotic integrity are checked. The posterior edge of the small bowel mesentery is then sutured to the posterior retroperitoneum and the defect between the mesorectum and mesentery adjacent to the anastomosis is closed.

Protectomy and Proctocolectomy

The indications for these two procedures are almost always elective. Proctocolectomy is used for the following indications.

1. Poor response to medical therapy (i.e., continued activity of the disease with failure to thrive, continued fatigue, diarrhea, malnutrition and weight loss, anal incontinence).
2. Side effects of medication (e.g., Cushing's disease).
3. Certain extraintestinal manifestations of the disease.
4. Extensive perianal disease associated with rectal disease.
5. Colonic hemorrhage.
6. Colonic and rectal strictures that preclude adequate surveillance or there is significant concern regarding malignancy.
7. Carcinoma of the colon or rectum.

With respect to proctectomy, the most common indication is that of completion proctectomy following subtotal colectomy for toxic colitis, toxic megacolon, or accompanying colectomy for Crohn's disease associated with severe malnutrition or other illnesses. There is a place for proctectomy with preservation of the proximal colon in patients who have had previous small bowel resection and the colon is free of overt Crohn's disease. There are certain centers where proctectomy is used with creation of colostomy in patients with rectal disease and colon sparing even when no previous small bowel resection has been performed.

The principles of proctectomy and related issues for benign disease include:

1. The preparing and positioning of the patient using the modified Trendelenburg lithotomy position. These principles have been previously outlined for proctectomy for other diseases in previous chapters.
2. The combined synchronous versus single surgeon approach. My preference is to use the single surgeon approach.
3. The management of either the mucous fistula or the buried stump in the abdominal wall. These are the two most common presentations to the surgeon embarking on a completion proctectomy. A less common variety encountered is the buried intra-abdominal or pelvic stump. In this latter instance, ureteric catheters are recommended. Small bowel loops have to be carefully detached from these buried stumps. The mucous fistula, if present, has to be mobilized and closed before proceeding with the rest of the operation.
4. Identification of the ureters. This is required practice for proctectomy especially in a patient who represents a reoperative pelvic procedure.
5. Ligation and division of the superior rectal vessels. In most patients, this proceeds without undue difficulty. In the case of the patient who has had residual pelvic sepsis, the identification of these vessels is best obtained by entering the presacral space between the investing layer of fascia of the rectum and Waldeyer's fascia in the midrectal portion itself. Thus, dissection can be carried out in a cephalad direction to adequately identify these vessels. Thus, the presacral nerves will be preserved.

6. Preserve presacral nerves. These nerves are commonly reflected anteriorly with close attachment to the superior rectal vessels. The surgeon is well advised to carefully look for these nerves especially in the male patient in whom retrograde ejaculation may be a consequence of injury.

7. Mesorectal incisions. Dissection of the pelvis is carried out using cautery dissection and while the upper portion of the rectum is mobilized in the traditional "bloodless" plane, the lower third is kept in close proximity to the rectum itself. ✓

8. Dissection in the "bloodless" plane between Waldeyer's and investing layer of fascia in the rectum. This is done in the upper two-thirds of the rectal dissection and by keeping in this plane, and not straying into the Waldeyer's fascia posteriorly, a nerve-sparing operation can be achieved without undue difficulty and without risking excessive blood loss. At the point where the lateral ligaments are encountered, the posterior dissection is carried down to the coccyx exactly in the midline without straying laterally. From this point on, the dissection is kept flush on the rectal wall itself, staying on the rectal side of the fascia of Denonvilliers.

9. Keep the dissection "anterior" in the caudad extent of the presacral mobilization.

10. Unite the mesorectal incisions anteriorly just cephalad to the cul-de-sac. This prevents excessive or too deep dissection anteriorly to the vagina or the seminal vesicles.

11. Use of cautery with tissues under traction and countertraction, especially the lateral pelvic attachments of the rectum. This technique precludes the need for excessive ligation and tying the vessels. This also allows for rapid and safe dissection close to the rectal wall.

12. Anterior rectal dissection *behind* the fascia of Denonvilliers. Thus, the vesicles are avoided and careful identification of the vagina is possible.

13. Transection of the anorectum versus perineal mobilization and delivery of the large bowel. In patients who have extensive perianal sepsis it is preferable to transect the anorectum at this point. Thus, the perineal dissection can be confined to intersphincteric dissection of the sphincters.

    In most patients without significant perianal sepsis, a tape is tied around the proximal end of the rectum, a metal ring attached to this, and this ring placed in the presacral space so that it is readily deliverable from the perineal aspect.

    For the perineal approach, the perineum is reprepared as well as placement of povidone-iodine in the vagina.

14. Oversewing the anus versus leaving it open during dissection. My preference is to leave this area open during dissection. Mobilization of the anus starts with a circumferential incision immediately below the dentate line; large Allis clamps are placed on the end of the anus and this permits the next procedure.

15. The use of adrenalin. This is placed intersphincterically to minimize bleeding during the course of the procedure.

16. The technique of resection can be endoanal versus mucosectomy versus conventional wide abdominoperineal resection. The principle here is to preserve as much "ordinary" perianal skin as possible. Wider skin excision is carried out when there are redundant excessive tags or if external orifices of fistulas-in-ano are in close proximity. Our approach is to use the endoanal proctectomy with intersphincteric dissection.

17. Management of perianal rectovaginal fistula tracts and openings. This is done by excising such fistula tracts. If this can be achieved with minimal contamination, the perineal closure is effected as usual. If the perianal fistulas are extensive,

wide, or septic and preclude the safe closure of the perineum, the skin is left partly open. It is critical, however, to close the levator complex from both below and intra-abdominally to exclude the possibility of a perineal infection ascending to become a presacral sinus. Rectovaginal fistula defects upon removal of the rectum are managed by coring out the tract and simple closure of the internal sphincter using absorbable suture material.

Upon intersphincteric dissection, the presacral space is breached posteriorly. At this point, the end of the rectum is identified by the previously placed metal ring. The rectum is delivered through the perineum and anteriorly angulated on the vagina or the prostate.

18. Irrigation of the presacral space is carried out from above and careful hemostasis is applied to the posterior prostate and vagina.

19. Closure of levators and layered closure of the external sphincters. This is reinforced as well with a transabdominal closure of the supralevator fascia. The perineal wound is closed with absorbable suture material.

20. Sump drainage of the presacral space. This is done to eradicate exudate that gravitates into the pelvis postproctectomy.

With respect to the issue of the role of perineal proctectomy, there is very little place for this. However, in some patients requiring proctectomy, the operation can be rendered much faster with less blood loss and less trauma to the patient by transecting the rectum at the anorectal ring using a stapler and delivering the specimen out transabdominally. In such cases the surgeon may omit the removal of the anorectum itself. The patient may, however, develop evidence of sepsis later, usually as the result of delayed leakage from the end of the stapled-over stump. In such cases perineal proctectomy is required at a later date. This is relatively easy to achieve.

Perhaps the best case that can be made for abdominal proctectomy leaving an anorectal stump in situ, is in the patient who has extensive perianal fistulas where a completion proctectomy would likely lead to an unhealed perineal wound. The rationale is that by allowing the fistulous tracts to become quiescent, the subsequent perineal proctectomy can be done with minimizing the possibility of a later unhealed perineal wound. Notwithstanding the "logic" of this approach, it is not uncommon for these fistulous tracts to continue to be active, causing disability and pain. There is also a small but definite risk of malignancy supervening in fistulous tracts that have not been excised.

Management of Perineal Sinus

The patient having proctectomy for inflammatory bowel disease, particularly Crohn's disease, is vulnerable to development of a persistent perineal sinus. This may result from the perineal wound never healing or may appear after apparent healing, sometimes even years after the surgery has been performed. Persistent perineal sinus can be classified into those that extend above the levator muscles into the presacral space and to those where the extent of the sinuses is below the level of the levators. Within the same categories, there are also variations including those with secondary fistulous tract openings into the posterior vagina and even extension of the presacral sinus to the anterior abdominal wall. In addition to this, there may be associated cavities and side extensions resulting from these complications following proctectomy.

In general, the assessment of the persistent perineal sinus includes assessment of the extent and level of the sinus by clinical examination including probing as well as by radiologic means. Frequently, a perineal sinogram is helpful in outlining the various communications and extent and direction of the sinus tracts. In rare circumstances, communication with structures such as seminal vesicles has been shown. Additionally, however, it is important to exclude the possibility of an enteroperineal wound fistula. This can be done by a combination of sinogram from below as well as by a small bowel series. Clearly any local attempts to correct the sinus are doomed to failure if indeed there is a communication with the small intestine.

Thus, there is a spectrum of procedures available for patients with a perineal nonhealed wound or persistent perineal sinus depending on the extent and severity of such sinuses.

In the first instance, curettage and cautery with silver nitrate is used for two separate sets of circumstances. The first is that of the patient who has the small persistent sinus occurring shortly after surgery; the second is in the patient who has a somewhat larger sinus extending up to the levators but it is not clear if there is a supralevator component. In all such patients curettage will help excise debris, lint, hair balls, and foreign matter that may have gravitated into this region by virtue of the suction effect of the buttocks. This curettage will allow for further wound contracture, which will help close some of this defect. Cautery with silver nitrate is used in the form of gauze soaked in silver nitrate 2 percent. These are left in situ for 24 hours before removal. The reason curettage has a poor reputation is that recurrences are the rule rather than the exception and hence further curettage for recurrence is abandoned. Thus, when using this program, it is important to stress to the patient that this is indeed a *program* and that it will require treatments approximately every 2 to 3 months for 2 years or more. This can usually be done in the ambulatory surgery setting after the first treatment is given, under a general anesthetic. This latter will help confirm the dimensions and direction of the sinus tracts. Thus, even for large sinuses, curettage is a very safe, minimally traumatic, and frequently beneficial procedure for the patient to immediately decrease drainage and pain, and can buy some time before embarking on larger procedures. In my practice, almost all patients who have an initial presentation with the complication under discussion will have curettage as a first-time procedure.

The second procedure for this condition is that of excision and primary closure. This is appropriate for recurrent persistent perineal sinus or persistent perineal sinus that has failed to respond adequately to curettage, yet where the dimensions of the sinus are accessible from a perineal approach. This is not appropriate for patients who have a presacral sinus extension. In essence, the entire septic tract is excised, which requires a careful dissection around the probe that is placed in this until the granulation tissue lying in the tract has been excised entirely, using irrigation with antibiotic solution throughout the procedure and meticulous hemostasis. Primary closure can then be effected and is usually successful.

The third procedure is that of excision of the perineal sinus with split-thickness skin grafting. This procedure, popularized by Turnbull and Anderson in the mid 1960s, was used for patients with persistent nonhealed perineal wound or persistent perineal sinus. This was even used for some patients with presacral sinus extensions. The principle of the surgery was to excise widely the perineal wound, taking the proximal line of dissection up to the presacral space. The perineal sinus in this location was thought to be something akin to an empyema cavity. Anteriorly there is a rigid boundary, namely, the posterior vagina; posteriorly the rigid boundary is the sacrum; and laterally there is a fairly rigid boundary, the circumferential layers of the puborectalis and external sphincters. By excising these tissues in a cone-shaped fashion, there would be left at the end of this a small cephalad extension of the sinus tract. A split-thickness skin graft, taken by one's plastic surgery colleagues, could then be layered into the cone-shaped defect left and packed off. A small catheter could be placed inside the packing up to the very tip of the sinus extension to allow for any drainage that may occur cephalad to the graft. The grafts here usually took quite well leaving either complete coverage or a minor sinus at the apex of the cone. This, however, was frequently asymptomatic or at most required a small piece of gauze or cotton ball to keep the patient asymptomatic. Such a graft could be placed directly on the posterior vagina in certain circumstances.

The fourth procedure is abdominoperineal excision of the perineal wound. This is a rather large operation and requires excision of the complete presacral sinus extension as well as the infralevator part of the perineal wound. This requires a conventional abdominoperineal approach and in most ways is at least as vigorous an operation as that of abdominoperineal resection of the rectum. Ureteric stents are required. The operation depends for its success upon excising all infected scar tissue (or inadvertently retained rectal mucosa) allowing for collapse of the residual cavity and filling in the dead space by either available omentum or small intestinal loops. This has become this author's preferred procedure for the extremely problematic persistent perineal sinus.

Option number 5 is the myocutaneous flaps of which the two most commonly used are the gracilis muscle and the rectus abdominus muscle. I have used both techniques. The difficulty with these approaches, especially the gracilis, is that it suffers from the liability of the split-thickness skin graft. In neither case can there be 100 percent certainty that the graft is occupying the entire volume of the perineal sinus extension. The concern is that a small dead space will appear cephalad to the gracilis, which will gradually get infected, form an abscess, and after a delayed period of time, cause tracking of sepsis along with the gracilis emerging at the midthigh level as a very complex fistula sinus. In addition, trigger points of pain are not infrequent following such an operation. The failure rate is high. The operation, graciloplasty, is formidable and has some significant cosmetic deformity.

The rectum abdominis flap, of course, makes much more sense in that it occupies entirely the presacral sinus and can even allow for perineal reconstruction by leaving attached a diamond of skin and subcutaneous fat overlying the belly of the rectus muscle as it is reflected off its anterior costal attachment. The muscle is reflected in a presacral fashion down to the perineum based on the inferior epigastric artery. These flaps are of greater use following primary reconstruction for advanced malignancy surgery especially recurrent malignancies.

Editorial Commentaries

The Birmingham group entirely concurs with Dr. Fazio's description of his strategy for small bowel resection and strictureplasty, particularly with the view that the mesentery in Crohn's disease should be transfixed. Indeed, the mesentery is sometimes so thickened in Crohn's disease that it is often helpful to divide the peritoneal covering of the mesentery so that less tissue is enclosed in the Kocher clamps. We also find that pinching the mesentery allows dispersal of fat from the mesenteric vessels—a technique that also reduces the bulk of tissue in the clamps. This pinching maneuver is also helpful in our experience when separating a segment of involved Crohn's disease from uninvolved but adherent gut.

We entirely agree with Dr. Fazio that frozen sections really do not assist in defining the most appropriate resection margins.

We increasingly use stapling techniques for ileo-ascending colon anastomosis but prefer the technique of dividing the mesentery, placing enterotomies in the resected segment of bowel, and performing a side-to-side anastomosis with a linear staple cutter (PLC-75), followed by resection of the two enterotomies and the specimen to close the two bowel ends.

We rarely find that it is possible to preserve the ileocecal valve but agree that its retention is desirable.

We agree with the author that absorbable suture material should be used for ties and for transfixation in Crohn's disease. We tend to perform a peripheral vascular division, keeping close to the bowel, rather than a policy of high ligation.

The word "quarantining" is rarely used in this context in the British Isles but it is a good expression and serves to remind surgeons that every effort must be made to avoid spillage, or the consequence of spillage, during operations in Crohn's disease. The concept of using tapes to snare the bowel is an attractive one and is certainly to be preferred to the use of noncrushing clamps, which often slip off, particularly in involved segments of Crohn's disease.

We confine strictureplasty to short segments only, longer segments are resected and proximal skip lesions may be incorporated into the stapled side-to-side anastomosis.

We agree that there is a place for segmental colectomy and that ileosigmoid anastomosis should be used if the rectum and sigmoid are spared.

Our experience of conservative proctocolectomy with retention of the anal stump has been disappointing in Crohn's disease. There is a high incidence of persistent perineal sepsis and in most patients the anus must be removed.

Persistent perineal sinus is easily managed by the technique of local perineal excision as described by Dr. Fazio if it is short. If there is a presacral cavity abdominoperineal excision is the only technique that in our experience cures the problem. We fill the defect with the rectus abdominis myocutaneous flap based on the inferior epigastric vessels.

Michael R. B. Keighley

I always use a midline incision in patients with Crohn's disease in whom I have no idea what course the operation might take. Any incision other than midline interferes with potential stoma sites.

I agree entirely with Dr. Fazio that external assessment of the colon is particularly difficult with regard to whether a particular area harbors Crohn's disease. Intraoperative colonoscopy is therefore an invaluable tool in determining the extent and the involvement of Crohn's disease in the colon.

Mayo became involved in a controversy regarding margins for Crohn's disease. I think it is accepted by nearly everyone that margins need to be grossly free of disease before anastomosis. I personally strive to achieve

(Continues)

microscopically free margins, but not too hard; if the microscopic margin is involved, I will resect another 2 to 3 cm and check again. If the margins are still involved, I resect no further, but perform an anastomosis. We have shown some benefit to microscopically free margins, but I will not sacrifice macroscopically normal bowel to achieve microscopically free margins. The guiding principle must always be that Crohn's disease is panintestinal and that the operation being performed at the moment is to remove only the current manifestation of the disease.

I also agree that radical lymphadenectomy is not indicated in the patient with Crohn's disease. Dr. Fazio presents an interesting and very important technical point, "suture ligation of the mesentery." The mesentery is often extremely thick and it is easy to have a vessel retract and cause unmitigated havoc in the mesentery. Slowly going across with small bites and suture ligating each pedicle is an excellent idea and one that I happen to practice.

Likewise, I agree that wedge or segmental resections are all that is indicated in bowel that is secondarily involved. With regard to enterovesical fistulas caused by Crohn's disease, I often find that after pinching the bowel off the bladder, the bladder is quite indurated and accepts sutures poorly. I will then lay a suction drain in the cul-de-sac of Douglas and not suture the bladder at all. The drains are nearly always dry from the beginning and can be pulled within 2 to 3 days. With regard to saving the ileocecal valve, I rarely can do this in patients with distal ileal disease.

Strictureplasty is efficacious, safe, and should be used when patients have shortened bowel and in whom resection will shorten it dangerously further. I have not performed strictureplasties on particularly long segments of bowel, but rather will resect these. The rationale has been that the strictureplastied bowel will function; whether this is true or not is unknown. I agree entirely with Dr. Fazio's principles of abdominal colectomy and Brooke ileostomy. I tend to exteriorize the distal sigmoid colon as a mucous fistula nearly invariably.

John H. Pemberton

Concerning the determination of the extent of small bowel that needs to be resected, we agree with Dr. Fazio that fat wrapping, a thickened mesenteric margin, and the absence of scalloping are good indicators; we do not obtain frozen resection margins but instead examine the resected specimen on a side table. Intraoperative endoscopy may also be useful, because the extent of mucosal lesions is sometimes greater than that of serosal lesions. We also look for infracolonic stenosis by passing a balloon catheter through the lumen via an incision in a section of bowel to be resected. If the inflated balloon cannot be pulled through, an additional "resection," consisting of a strictureplasty, is performed.

We also perform mesenteric resection close to the bowel wall and do not hesitate to leave behind enlarged lymph nodes, as described by Dr. Fazio.

Involvement of a second organ is managed by wedge or sleeve resection and repair, and we also use omentum to protect the anastomosis from the residual abscess cavity.

For anastomosis, we use a single-layer, full-thickness, end-to-end closure using a 4-0 resorbable continuous polyglycolic suture. The technique is quicker and easier to perform, allows the visualization of the luminal aspect of the bowel, and facilitates further endoscopic surveillance of an ileocolic, ileorectal, or colocolic anastomosis compared to a side-to-end anastomosis, where the stump can make endoscopy more difficult.

Our technique of short or long strictureplasty is similar to the one described by Dr. Fazio, and we respect the same indications and contraindications.

As far as large bowel resection is concerned, we perform a segmental resection if at least one-third of the colon can be preserved; otherwise, an ileorectal or ileosigmoid anastomosis is considered.

When performing subtotal colectomy and ileostomy for fulminant colitis, a mucous fistula is placed in the left iliac fossa; sometimes placement of the fistula in the lower part of the midline incision is our preferred option. Further treatment of the rectal remnant by lavage is easy via the sigmoidostomy, the risk of peritonitis or perirectal abscess is avoided, the sigmoid is easily recognized and dissected during the second operation, and every kind of re-establishment of intestinal continuity is possible, including ileosigmoid anastomosis.

Rolland Parc

13

Large Bowel Obstruction

Michael R. B. Keighley

Principles

There is still very little consensus on the optimum management of large bowel obstruction. This is hardly surprising given that the causes are protean and the condition of the patient when first admitted to the hospital extremely variable. The common causes of obstruction are malignancy, diverticular disease, Crohn's stricture, ischemic stricture, postoperative stenosis, and endometriosis. Other causes are mechanical, such as intussusception and volvulus of the large bowel. It is important to differentiate complete from incomplete obstruction, because many patients with incomplete obstruction can be resuscitated and sometimes decompressed, thereby avoiding emergency surgery. Complete obstruction requires urgent surgical intervention, the most common cause being large bowel malignancy. Even though the physical signs and radiographs seem to provide incontrovertible evidence of mechanical large bowel obstruction, the surgeon should always consider the possibility of pseudo-obstruction, and in our view patients should never be submitted to laparotomy for large bowel obstruction unless the mechanical cause and site have been identified by water-soluble contrast radiography.

Many patients admitted to the hospital with acute large bowel obstruction are gravely ill, with gross abdominal distension, cardiorespiratory embarrassment, dehydration, and gross malnutrition. There is always a risk that in some of these patients with a competent ileocecal valve the mechanical obstruction may have caused cecal ischemia with perforation and septicemia. By contrast, others may be only slightly distended with a history of altered bowel habit. If a patient in the latter group is generally fit with no coexisting cardiopulmonary disease, radical resection and primary anastomosis may be entirely appropriate. Consequently, it is necessary to describe a spectrum of options, the choice of which will depend on the site of obstruction, the competence of the ileocecal valve, the secondary effects of obstruction, the duration of the obstruction, patient risk factors, and the extent of disease. Hence the surgical management of an obstructed colon in a patient with advanced liver metastases might be very different from that caused by a constriction in the sigmoid colon resulting in cecal perforation in a patient with eminently curable disease.

It is essential to resuscitate these patients on admission to the hospital with intravenous fluids, to commence antimicrobial therapy, and to institute antiembolism prophylaxis. The patient must be thoroughly investigated by plain radiography, sigmoidoscopy, and water-soluble contrast radiography. If there is any suggestion of impending perforation or established peritonitis, laparotomy is, of course, mandatory. On the other hand, if there is no such evidence and yet the patient is grossly distended, some would argue that the construction of a proximal stoma as a blind procedure to decompress the patient causes minimal morbidity and facilitates a safe and complete cancer resection 10 to 14 days later. In describing the various options available we will commence with more conventional methods of management before considering newer alternatives.

Right-Sided Obstruction

It must be stressed that the management of right-sided colonic obstruction differs considerably from that of left-sided obstruction. Most patients with a right-sided obstructive lesion can be safely treated by primary resection and anastomosis because the distal colon is empty and a dilated proximal portion can easily be sacrificed without morbidity (Fig. 13-1A). Indeed, there is rarely any disparity between the diameters of the bowel ends, thus facilitating primary anastomosis (Fig. 13-1B). If, on the other hand, there are any risk factors that would mitigate against a safe primary anastomosis, the two bowel ends may be delivered to the abdominal wall as a double-barreled stoma (Fig. 13-1C), or an end ileostomy and mucous fistula may be raised to facilitate a secondary anastomosis at another stage (Fig. 13-1D).

Left-Sided Obstruction

The main controversy relates to left-sided colonic obstruction. Here the traditional method of management was by a three-stage procedure involving (1) the creation of a proximal stoma usually well away from the obstructing lesion, such as in the mid-transverse colon (Fig. 13-2A), (2) subsequent resection of the obstructing lesion with a primary anastomosis protected by the original stoma (Fig. 13-2B), and (3) eventual closure of the original stoma (Fig. 13-2C). This method of management, although safe, involves three anesthetics and there is potential morbidity in each stage; indeed, some patients are never fit enough to undergo either the second or third stage of the treatment, some patients refuse to have further treatment, and some are lost to follow-up and can never be offered definitive resection. Furthermore, three-stage management is expensive and the whole process takes the best part of a year to restore a patient to normal health. By this time, if the underlying cause was malignancy, the patient may have developed advanced disease. Hence alternative options are constantly being explored as a means of minimizing the duration of therapy, expediting the primary resection, and at the same time ensuring standards of safety carrying a low morbidity and mortality.

Three-Stage Resection

Classically, a laparotomy incision is made and the site of the obstruction is determined. This also allows the surgeon to examine the right colon to determine whether there is any evidence of cecal necrosis in patients with a competent ileocecal valve. Under these circumstances, a more radical procedure is probably advised, such as a cecostomy. If there is a localized area of potential perforation but no actual leakage, a subtotal colectomy and ileorectal or ileocolonic anastomosis may be performed (Fig. 13-3). Alternatively, resection, ileostomy, and a mucous fistula may be performed if the obstruction is in the proximal left colon. However, for most patients

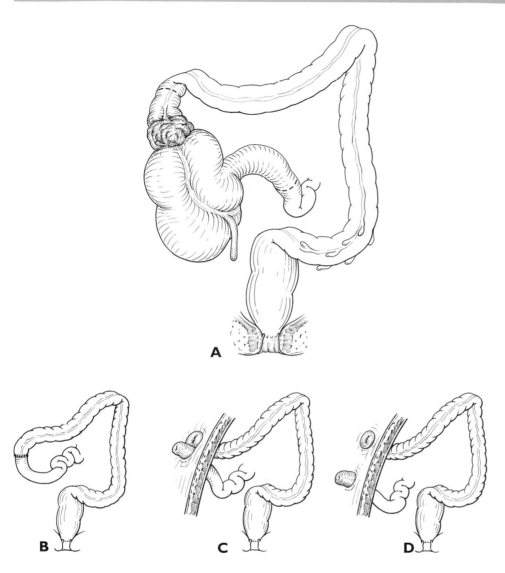

A

B   C   D

Figure 13-1.

there is merely some dilatation of the proximal colon, hence the preliminary procedure is the placement of a transverse colostomy, preferably as close to the obstructing lesion as possible. In most patients, the stoma is placed in the left side of the transverse colon through a wide trephine in the rectus muscle.

Stage 1: Loop Transverse Colostomy

The construction of a loop transverse colostomy in patients with obstruction can be quite difficult. The site may not have been marked beforehand and in any case will, to some extent, depend on the mobility of the transverse colon. Where possible, the stoma should be sited in the left upper quadrant. The omentum is dissected from the transverse colon at the site selected for decompression. A window is identified in the middle colic arcades, having dissected the omentum from the transverse mesocolon. A tape placed through this window will facilitate delivery of the bowel to the skin surface (Fig. 13-4). A trephine is constructed through the left rectus muscle. It is usually necessary to divide a part of the rectus muscle to accommodate the dilated bowel so that it is not under tension and thus prevent it from becoming ischemic (Fig. 13-5A & B). The bowel is then opened longitudinally along one of the taenia coli and the stoma is matured using direct mucocutaneous sutures, having placed a rod underneath the bowel through the mesenteric window to prevent retraction (Fig. 13-6A &

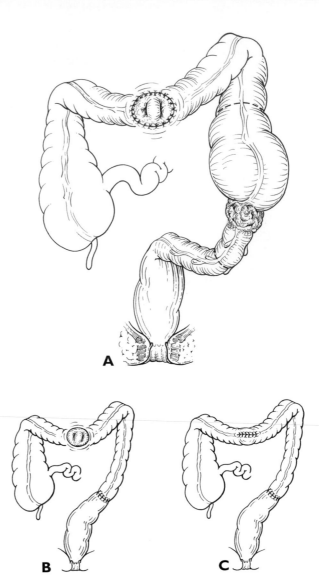

Figure 13-2. ▬▬▬▬▬

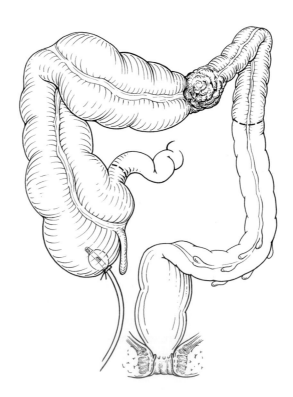

Figure 13-3. ▬▬▬▬▬

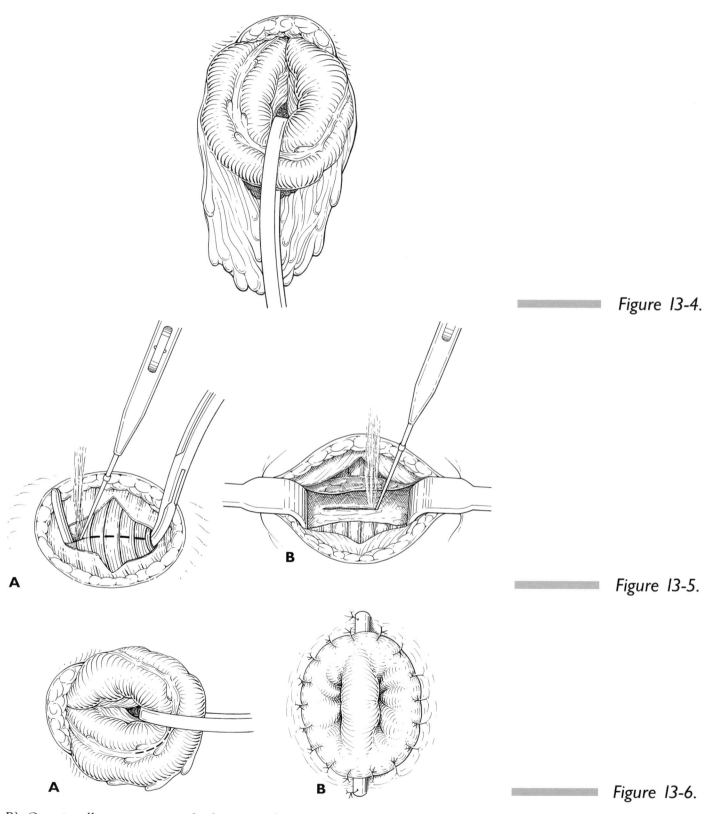

Figure 13-4.

Figure 13-5.

Figure 13-6.

B). Occasionally, in patients with obstructing lesions in the rectum, a loop sigmoid colostomy is more appropriate than a left transverse colostomy. Under these circumstances, a trephine can be made in the left lower quadrant and the sigmoid loop raised in exactly the same manner, preferably leaving a rod through the mesenteric window to avoid retraction in the early postoperative period (Fig. 13-7).

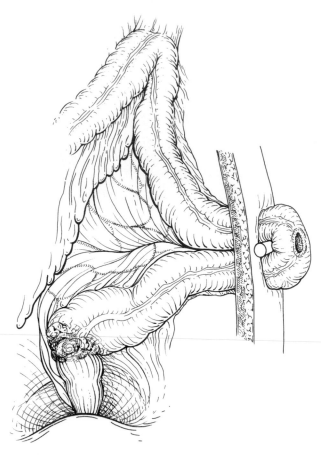

Figure 13-7.

Stage 2: Primary Resection and Anastomosis

The laparotomy wound is reopened and the bowel is resected in the manner described in Chapter 10, the methods of resection depending on the site of the lesion and the anastomosis depending on the surgeon's preference. The loop transverse colostomy should be left undisturbed. In the case of a sigmoid colostomy decompressing a rectal carcinoma, it may be necessary to resect the sigmoid colostomy with the rectal carcinoma and to protect the primary anastomosis by a loop ileostomy (Fig. 13-8).

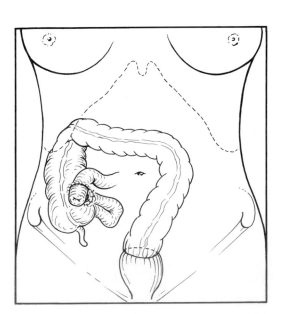

Figure 13-8.

Stage 3: Closure of the Transverse Colostomy

Closure of the transverse colostomy can be performed once the distal anastomosis has completely healed. The stoma is mobilized from the skin, subcutaneous fat, rectus sheath and muscle, and the peritoneum. We prefer a double-stapling technique for closure of a loop colostomy using the linear staple cutter (Fig. 13-9A & B). Alternatively, the colostomy once thoroughly mobilized may be closed by suture (Fig. 13-10). We prefer a Connell technique (Fig. 13-11), but an extramucosal continuous or interrupted closure technique is quite satisfactory and may in fact compromise the lumen of the gut less than the full-thickness inverting technique.

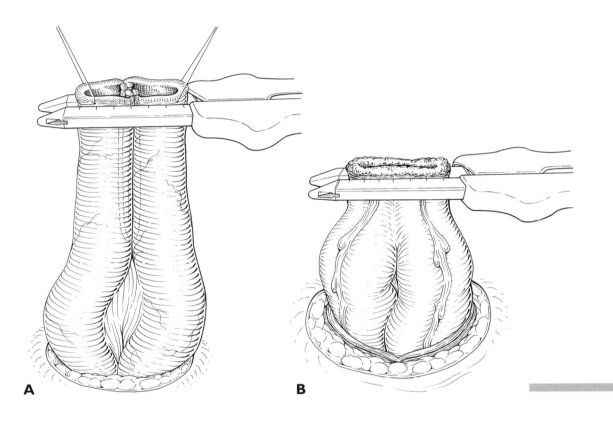

A   B   Figure 13-9.

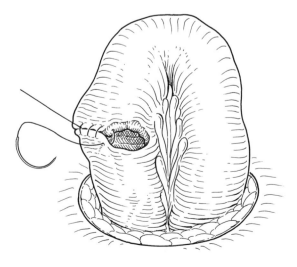

Figure 13-10.

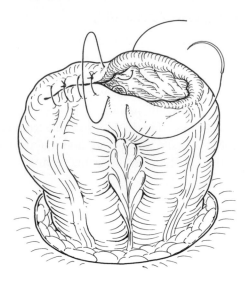

Figure 13-11.

Two-Stage Procedures

Hartmann Resection and Closure

The details of the Hartmann operation as well as restoration of intestinal continuity are described for diverticular disease in Chapter 11. There are, however, certain features of the initial resection specific to the management of large-bowel obstruction. Antibiotic cover and antiembolism prophylaxis with heparin is instituted upon admission. The patient is placed in the modified Trendelenburg Lloyd-Davies position with the feet in Allen stirrups, the bladder is catheterized, and pneumatic leg bags are applied. A midline laparotomy incision is made, the cecum is carefully inspected to ensure that it is not ischemic, and the site of the obstruction is identified. The first major problem is that the large bowel is grossly distended, which makes operative management extremely difficult and potentially hazardous. If a Hartmann resection is to be contemplated as the initial procedure, or indeed, if any primary resection is to be performed without a proximal stoma, it is in our opinion mandatory to decompress the bowel. Fortunately, a large amount of the dilatation is caused by gas, and if a pursestring suture is placed just above the tumor and a sump catheter gently inserted after a tape has been placed around the proximal bowel as a snare (Fig. 13-12), proximal decompression within the segment being resected can often be achieved quite effectively. In order to prevent blockage by solid fecal material, it is important that the assistant keep the end of the suction tube in the gas-filled component and milk the gaseous distension from the right colon into the resected segment. In this way it is possible to establish considerable decompression, which greatly facilitates the subsequent resection.

The obstructing lesion is mobilized in the usual manner by dividing the peritoneum on the lateral aspect of the left colon. The sigmoid is thoroughly mobilized, assuming that the blockage is a carcinoma and that a curative resection is envisaged. A standard left hemicolectomy is thus performed, with high ligation of the inferior mesenteric artery and separate high ligation of the inferior mesenteric vein, taking the descending colon, sigmoid, and upper rectum, as described in Chapter 10. If, on the other hand, there are liver metastases, a local sigmoid resection would be performed. The rectal stump is then closed with a linear stapler (a technique that we prefer) or by a suture technique (Fig. 13-13A & B). If sutures are used, we prefer a two-layer technique, placing the loop on the mucosa with a continuous stitch so that when it is tightened the bowel is inverted and the suture can be completed by returning to the original position. Alternatively, if the rectum is being closed by suture and a crushing clamp has been applied to its end to prevent spillage, we take bites in the first layer from either side to achieve a similar degree of inversion without the risk of contamination.

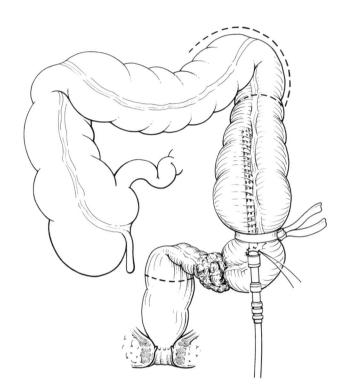

Figure 13-12.

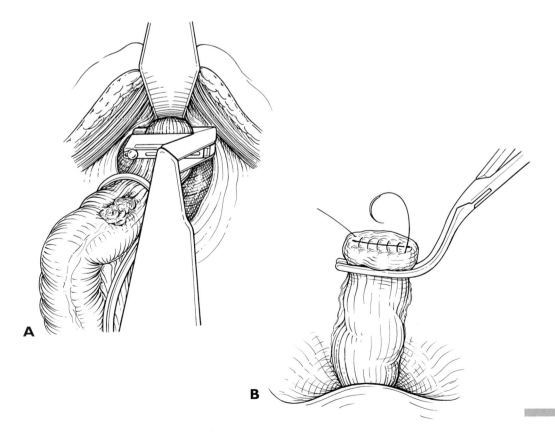

Figure 13-13.

The proximal end of the colon is divided between staples in order to minimize contamination or is covered with a Potts clamp for construction of an end colostomy. It should be noted, however, that if a radical resection for malignant disease is performed as illustrated in Figure 13-12, the splenic flexure will have to be mobilized in order to bring the colon down to a trephine in the left iliac fossa for an end colostomy (Fig. 13-14). Mucocutaneous suture of the stoma completes the colostomy; however, suture of the colostomy should be deferred until the abdomen is closed in order to minimize contamination of the abdominal incision.

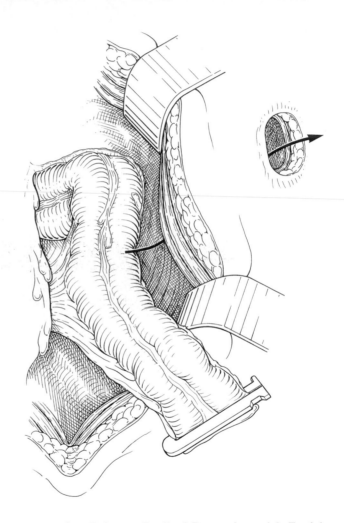

Figure 13-14.

Blind Decompression Prior to Radical Resection with Excision of the Stoma

If there is no clinical evidence of impending perforation of the cecum and no evidence of overt peritonitis, and provided the site of intestinal obstruction has been accurately localized by preoperative water-soluble contrast radiography, it is possible to place a stoma immediately proximal to the obstructing lesion. Hence, for lesions in the rectum or rectosigmoid, a midsigmoid colostomy would be raised; conversely, for lesions in the proximal sigmoid, descending colon, splenic flexure, or left side of the transverse colon, a left transverse colostomy would be raised (Fig. 13-15). Under these circumstances we do not perform a laparotomy unless there is clinical suspicion of cecal perforation, difficulty with identifying the proximal bowel, or problems when raising a stoma. Usually a trephine through the left rectus muscle in the left lower quadrant will facilitate a blind left loop sigmoid colostomy, and a trephine in the left upper quadrant will facilitate the identification and delivery of a proximal loop colostomy in the left transverse colon. If a fairly large trephine needs to be made to accommodate distended proximal obstructed colon, a tape is always placed through the vascular mesenteric window to facilitate delivery of the loop onto the abdominal wall. A piece of intravenous tubing is used as a rod because it can be sutured to the skin and causes minimal trauma to the bowel, yet ensures that the loop does not retract in the early postoperative period (see Fig. 13-6B).

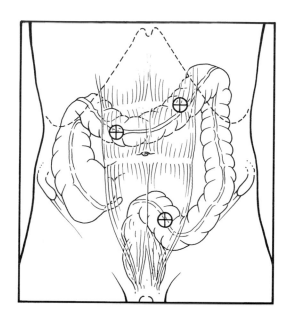

Figure 13-15.

This is an extremely low morbidity procedure but it must be performed by an experienced surgeon, and there must always be a low threshold for performing a laparotomy if there is any difficulty with the construction of the stoma, any doubt about the underlying diagnosis, or any fear that there may be ischemia in the proximal colon or localized sepsis. Nevertheless, if the procedure can be undertaken, decompression occurs immediately and can be achieved while the patient is still anesthetized by placing a flexible sump suction along the proximal colon to evacuate the gas. It also provides an opportunity for resection within 1 to 2 weeks of the initial decompression, preferably during the patient's initial admission, provided there are no medical contraindications to a second anesthetic. Full mechanical bowel preparation can then be performed by standard techniques to clear the proximal colon and by distal colostomy washout and rectal washout to clear the obstructing segment of the colon. At the second operation the tumor and the proximal colostomy are resected in continuity and a primary anastomosis is performed.

The second operation must only be performed when there has been complete decompression of the bowel and when the patient is fully mobile. A preoperative mechanical bowel preparation should have eliminated fecal residue from the proximal colon. The patient is placed in the modified Trendelenburg position with the legs in Allen stirrups. The bladder is catheterized, and a long midline incision is made. Once the abdomen is opened, tapes are placed around both limbs of the loop colostomy in order to prevent any contamination. The loop colostomy is then mobilized from the abdominal wall; this is usually very easy to do because dense adhesions will not yet have formed between the colon and the abdominal wall. When the stoma has been delivered a standard resection of the left colon, sigmoid, and rectum is performed as described in Chapter 10 (Fig. 13-16). After mobilizing the splenic flexure it is usually feasible to perform a primary anastomosis with a circular stapling

336 Atlas of Colorectal Surgery

gun, as described in Chapter 2 (Fig. 13-17). Two closed-suction drains are then placed into the pelvis and the abdomen is closed in the usual way. The patient usually can then be discharged 8 to 10 days later.

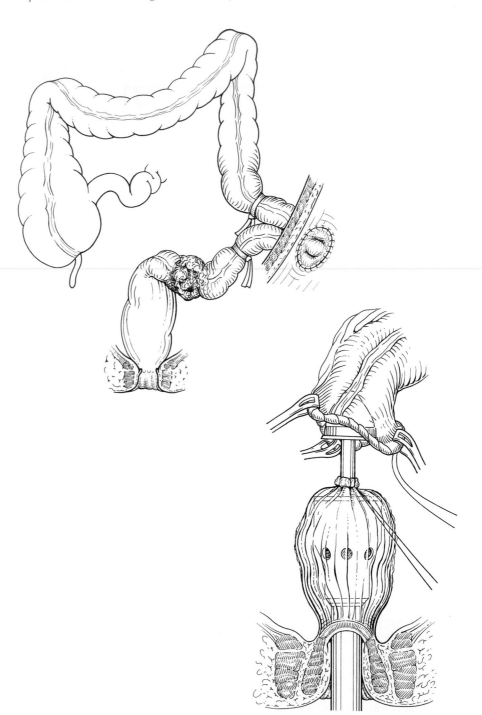

Figure 13-16.

Figure 13-17.

Some patients with an obstructing tumor in the left side of the transverse colon, splenic flexure, or upper descending colon may be managed simply by performing an extended right hemicolectomy, including the transverse and upper left colon, with an ileocolonic anastomosis (Fig. 13-18). This modification is certainly worthy of consideration in patients with adequate anal sphincter function and an obstructing proximal left colonic tumor.

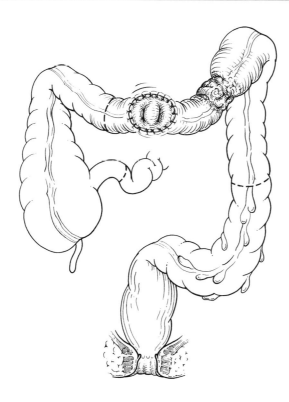

Figure 13-18.

Primary Resection and Double-Barreled Colostomy

There are situations in which primary resection with construction of a double-bar-reled colostomy can be performed as an alternative to the Hartmann procedure. This greatly reduces the complexity of restoring intestinal continuity, which is possibly the greatest argument against using the Hartmann procedure in obstructing colon cancer. The option of resection and double-barreled colostomy is only feasible where after resection there are two mobile bowel segments that can be delivered to the abdominal wall adjacent to one another, thereby facilitating closure. This option is certainly possible for obstructing lesions well above the rectosigmoid junction, but clearly is not an option for malignancy involving the rectum.

The conduct of the initial laparotomy is exactly as that described for the Hartmann procedure, taking care to establish adequate decompression through the resected seg-ment. The bowel ends must be mobilized more widely than for the Hartmann proce-dure and it is wise to resect the obstructing lesion between two separate linear staple cutters in order to minimize contamination and to facilitate the delivery of the two bowel ends through a large trephine in the left rectus muscle. In order to deliver the two bowel ends it is almost always necessary to divide part of the rectus muscle rather than to split it in the line of its fibers. The stapled bowel ends are excised once the abdomen is closed and direct mucocutaneous sutures are applied with a few additional sutures to approximate the two adjacent bowel ends (Fig. 13-19).

Restoration of intestinal continuity is then a relatively easy matter. The bowel ends are mobilized from the abdominal wall by a circumstomal incision. The two forks of a linear staple cutter are advanced between the two adjacent bowel ends once they have been fully mobilized from the abdominal wall; the two ends are then transected beyond the staple line to close the colostomy, thus achieving a functional end-to-end anasto-mosis. A suture technique is just as effective but slightly more time consuming. The defect in the rectus muscle, rectus sheath, and skin is then closed. The defect in the abdominal wall is closed with interrupted Prolene sutures as described in Chapter 4.

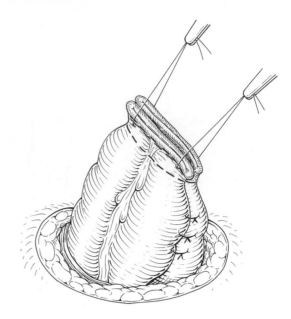

Figure 13-19.

One-Stage Procedures

Primary Resection and Ileosigmoid/Ileorectal Anastomosis

There are certain patients, particularly those with an obstructing lesion in the left side of the transverse colon, splenic flexure, or descending colon, in whom if the patient is sufficiently fit a one-stage primary resection of the proximally dilated colon and a primary colorectal anastomosis or even an ileosigmoid anastomosis may be the best option. Some would even argue that lesions in the lower descending and sigmoid colon should be treated in a similar manner by primary resection and ileorectal anastomosis (Fig. 13-20). On the other hand, elderly patients with compromised sphincter function may suffer from diarrhea and incontinence after such radical ablative surgery. As in all cases of obstruction, each patient must be carefully evaluated and assessed individually to determine the most suitable surgical strategy.

The patient is placed in the modified Trendelenburg position with the legs in Allen stirrups. A urethral catheter is passed. There must be access to the rectum if a

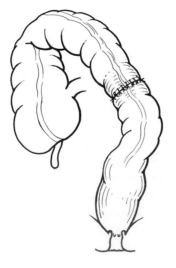
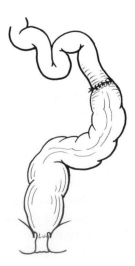

Figure 13-20.

stapled anastomosis is to be performed and tested underwater. A long midline laparotomy incision is made, and a full laparotomy is performed to ensure that there is no evidence of ischemia or sepsis. The surgeon should also assess, stage, and determine the operability of the tumor.

Decompression of the dilated proximal segment through the planned resection site is again desirable in order to minimize contamination and to facilitate a curative resection. For lesions in the left side of the transverse colon and splenic flexure, high ligation of the inferior mesenteric artery may not be necessary; rather high division of the middle colic artery preserving the arcade of Riolan and its supply from the inferior mesenteric artery would be desirable unless the procedure is only palliative. The technique of resection is as described in Chapter 10 and that of primary ileosigmoid or ileorectal anastomosis is as described in Chapter 2. Most ileosigmoid anastomoses will be hand-sewn or stapled using a functional end-to-end anastomotic technique. For ileorectal anastomosis, either a hand-sewn technique will be used or a circular stapler will be passed through the rectal ampulla, as described in Chapter 2. Two drains are placed down to the operation site and the abdomen is closed in the usual manner. If there is any concern whatsoever about the integrity of the ileorectal or ileosigmoid anastomosis, if there is excessive bleeding, or if there is coexisting sepsis or any technical difficulty, a proximal loop ileostomy should always be raised to decompress the anastomosis (Fig. 13-21). Safety should never be compromised in surgery for large bowel obstruction.

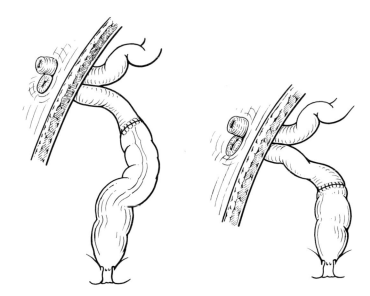

Figure 13-21.

Primary Resection and Anastomosis with On-Table Colonic Lavage

Increasingly, surgeons are attracted by the concept of primary resection and primary anastomosis for obstructing colon cancer. Although this undoubtedly reduces the morbidity of multiple operations, great care should be taken in case selection. Such an option should not be considered unless the patient is fit and can withstand an operation that is likely to take 3 to 4 hours. Furthermore, careful monitoring of pH and fluid-electrolyte balance during the operation is important when colonic lavage is used. There is no doubt that, with staple techniques and the opportunity for early decompression through the ileotomy or the appendicostomy used for irrigation, this method of management is ideally suited for the fit patient and for the patient in whom an obstructing tumor occurs in the presence of coexisting hepatic metastases.

The patient is placed in the Lloyd-Davies position with the feet in Allen stirrups and the buttocks well over the end of the table for easy access to the rectum both to facilitate a circular stapled anastomosis and to test it. The bladder is catheterized, an arterial line should be inserted for regular intraoperative monitoring, and a midline laparotomy incision is made. Careful assessment of the site, nature, and stage of the obstructing lesion is undertaken. It is also important to verify whether there is any evidence of ischemia or sepsis from obstruction. A large Foley catheter (30 Fr) is inserted into the rectal ampulla for subsequent rectal washout. The first move after laparotomy is to insert a flexible saline sump tube into the segment of bowel to be resected to achieve initial decompression, as already described (see Fig. 13-12). Once the gaseous distension is overcome it is much safer and easier to mobilize the splenic flexure and to perform a radical curative resection, as described in Chapter 10. Usually resection of left-sided colonic lesions involves high ligation of the inferior mesenteric artery and separate ligation of the inferior mesenteric vein. At this point a crushing clamp is placed above the saline sump tube and a proximal tape is passed around the colon above the site at which the anesthetic scavenger tubing is to be inserted into the proximal colon. In this way complete control is achieved to allow safe insertion of the anesthetic scavenger tubing. A pursestring suture is placed just above the crushing bowel clamp. The tubing is gently advanced through the pursestring suture and beyond the proximal tape so that it can be secured into position.

A Foley catheter is then inserted into the appendix stump or through the terminal ileum. We prefer the appendix stump, because in our opinion an ileostomy is associated with greater morbidity; furthermore, temporary cecostomy through the appendix stump also provides a method of early postoperative decompression. Hartmann's solution is then used to irrigate fecal material from the proximal colon through the anesthetic scavenger tubing into an attached plastic bag placed on the floor adjacent to the operating table (Fig. 13-22). An irrigation rate of approximately 1 L/10 min

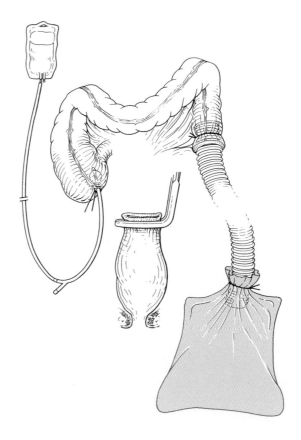

Figure 13-22.

allows rapid elimination of fecal material from the proximal colon. During this maneuver fecal material should be gently milked along the bowel. Sometimes negative pressure may be responsible for collapsing the colon, thus preventing drainage. To overcome this, the receiver bag may have to be elevated in order to allow the colon to empty. Alternatively, a gas vent may be necessary in the scavenger tubing.

Once completely clear fluid is running into the receiver bag, the irrigation can be stopped. At this point it is a good idea to perform a rectal washout while the residual fluid in the proximal colon is syphoning away. The rectum should contain very little material but it is wise to clear it out as effectively as possible prior to the use of the circular stapler. We generally advise resecting the bowel through which the anesthetic scavenger tubing has been passed. The optimum site of transection in the proximal bowel is determined, a crushing clamp is placed on the distal end, and a pursestring suture is placed on the proximal margin after division. To achieve a circular stapled anastomosis, the anvil of the circular stapling gun is inserted through the pursestring suture, the rectum is resected with a linear stapler (TA-55, RL-50, or PIA-58), and double-stapling is done by passing the head of the stapler with its spike through the center of the transected rectal stump. An end-to-end circular anastomosis is thus fashioned. The Foley catheter used for colonic irrigation may be left in situ for decompression; if this is done, the serosa of the adjacent bowel should be sutured to the abdominal wall to minimize contamination when the decompression tube is withdrawn. If testing of the anastomosis underwater raises any doubt about its integrity, the Foley catheter should be withdrawn from the appendix stump and a loop ileostomy raised. The abdomen is then closed in the usual way, placing suction drains to eliminate any hematoma at the operation site. If a loop illeostomy is used, it is everted or sutured to the skin as described in Chapter 4. If the Foley catheter has been left in the cecum for decompression, this too should be secured to the skin with a pursestring suture.

Editorial Commentaries

I agree with Professor Keighley that if surgery for large bowel obstruction is contemplated, the patient should be given a water-soluble contrast enema in order to determine the nature and level of the obstruction.

I agree with Professor Keighley's comments on right-sided obstruction. It is with left-sided obstruction that controversy really lies. Three-stage procedures are rarely necessary today.

I prefer not to perform a loop sigmoid colostomy proximal to an obstructing rectal cancer, as this is the area of bowel used in subsequent anastomoses. If one is going to perform a diverting colostomy, then it should be done in the transverse colon for left-sided disease. Any right-sided obstruction should be treated by resection and primary anastomosis. Hartmann pouches should be stapled closed. I mark the ends of the rectal stump with long Prolene sutures; this facilitates identification of the rectal stump at the time of re-exploration.

With regard to left-sided obstruction, located high in the rectum, in the sigmoid, or higher, my preferred approach is a colectomy and ileorectostomy.

(Continues)

A less optimal option would be an on-table bowel preparation approach, which is described quite adequately by Professor Keighley; I have little to add with the exception that I do use an ileotomy and not an appendicostomy.

Another choice would be resection followed by reanastomosis and proximal diverting ileostomy. Double-barreled colostomy is the next best procedure because it can be done in two stages that are easily performed. The last choice is a Hartmann procedure. Hartmann procedures are often difficult to reanastomose and patients often have to undergo a long procedure again.

On-table bowel preparation, although a very involved procedure, can be an excellent option, and I have used it successfully multiple times. I irrigate with 3 L of saline followed by 3 L of povidone-iodine solution. I would only add that the infusate must be at body temperature; I speak to this based on my own difficult experience in which after infusing room-temperature saline and povidone-iodine, the patient's core temperature dropped dramatically and remained low for a total of 8 hours.

John H. Pemberton

For right-sided colon obstruction a right hemicolectomy and ileocolic anastomosis is usually performed. The exception is that rare entity of unresectable right colon obstruction, in which either an exclusion bypass ileotransverse ostomy or an ileotransverse ostomy in continuity is performed.

For left-sided obstruction, the alternatives available have been well-outlined. Unless the patient is moribund or desperately ill, resective surgery as opposed to colostomy is used. The alternatives are those of the Hartmann resection, with subsequent reanastomosis versus resection anastomosis, and intraoperative irrigation with or without a temporary stoma. The decision between these two is based on the adequacy of the bowel after intraoperative irrigation and how well the patient is doing after the operation. One's bias is toward performing the anastomosis with a temporary ostomy as opposed to a Hartmann procedure, provided there is no associated sepsis.

The other alternative, subtotal colectomy and ileorectal anastomosis for left-sided bowel obstruction, is one that has historically been associated with significant diarrhea and disability, especially in the elderly patient. One would draw the distinction between ileorectal anastomosis and ileosigmoid anastomosis, however. In this latter event, I believe this is a salutary procedure and one in which morbidity is not excessive. This then becomes a procedure of choice for obstructing lesions of the descending colon, for example.

Victor W. Fazio

I do agree with Dr. Keighley's descriptions of the different techniques that can be used in dealing with acute large bowel obstruction. As he mentioned, the management of left-sided large bowel obstruction remains a challenging problem, whereas the treatment of right-sided obstructions has become almost standardized and consists of a one-stage resection with primary anastomosis in the vast majority of cases.

In our opinion, the operative risk and the complexity of emergency surgery for this condition must be minimized. Indeed the first goal is to relieve obstruction without compromising the possibility of further curative resection of the tumor and restoration of bowel continuity when feasible. Acute large bowel obstruction is often encountered at night by little-experienced surgeons in poor-risk patients. Because of the increasing enthusiasm for one-stage procedures with primary anastomosis, the assessment of optimal anatomic conditions allowing such procedures has become crucial. In particular, it is essential to determine whether the wall of the distended bowel is suitable for anastomosis, even after on-table washout. We think only fully skilled surgeons are capable of such a reliable assessment and of performing a safe anastomosis under these circumstances. For this reason we favor loop colostomy for acute left-sided large bowel obstruction.

This quick and safe procedure can be done by trainees and carries a low operative risk. Furthermore, in the absence of perforation with abscess or peritonitis, there is no need for urgent tumor resection, as it has not been shown to improve the long-term prognosis. As Dr. Keighley wrote, we think this colostomy must be performed "blind." This technique induces minimal peritoneal adhesions and allows tumor resection with anastomosis 2 to 3 weeks later. In the interoperative period, the patient and the bowel are prepared, and a careful workup of the disease is made. Prior to the operation, the site of the obstruction has to be clearly defined by water-soluble contrast radiography. A midline incision is mandatory in the presence of small bowel distension, which may be attributable to peritoneal carcinoma, if the viability of the cecal wall is doubtful, or if peritonitis or abscess is suspected. The colostomy is made as close as possible to the tumor, both being resected during the second stage. Because the site of the obstruction is frequently on the sigmoid or rectosigmoid junction, a horizontal incision is made in the left iliac fossa and the rectus muscle is crossed. Sometimes the colon has to be freed from the peritoneum to allow it to be brought to the skin surface without tension. For this, a silicone tube is passed through the mesentery beside the colon, and is used to pull up the colon to the skin through the rectus muscle. The incision, which often must be made large so as to accommodate a distended bowel, sometimes has to be repaired carefully around the colon. The tube is then replaced above the skin by a plastic rod. The colon is opened and sutured to the skin by interrupted Vicryl Dec. 1.5 sutures. In obstructing rectal tumors the colostomy does not compromise the mobility of the splenic flexure and can be maintained during the second stage to protect a low colorectal anastomosis. It has the disadvantage, however, of excluding a large bowel segment above the tumor, which cannot be properly cleaned and implies a third procedure.

When urgent tumor resection is required, the Hartmann procedure is often the only option, allowing both treatment of perforation and complete tumor resection. Indeed, the latter, due to its width, does not allow a double-barreled stoma. However, this technique may be advisable in aged patients

(Continues)

with obstructing advanced tumors in a mobile segment of the colon. After wrapping the tumor and washing out the cavity, tumor resection is completed without the splenic flexure needing to be mobilized. The bowel is divided after stapling. The distal stump staple line is reinforced by a continuous one-layer Vicryl suture. Due to the high risk of leakage from the stump in these conditions, we advocate its drainage by a Mikulicz sack with two to three gauze meshes. The device goes through the inferior part of the midline incision. A small silicone tube is placed at the bottom of the sack, allowing daily washouts after day 9 in order to facilitate mesh retrieval (one mesh per day and the sack the day after). This safe method allows complete drainage of the pouch of Douglas and prevents the peritoneal spillage from the rectal suture line. Once the sack is taken out, a small tube (Ch 10) is placed in its track to enable daily irrigation (usually saline plus povidone-iodine 250 cc/day) until its closure.

As far as one-stage procedures are concerned, we agree with Dr. Keighley's statements. However, when choosing these options, particularly the colorectal anastomosis after on-table lavage, we think that loop colostomy to protect the anastomosis must be avoided, otherwise the method has no advantage over blind loop colostomy. On the other hand, this stoma does not prevent anastomotic leaks, only reduces their gravity. The suture technique by itself does not differ from our so-called unique technique: continuous one-layer full-thickness suture. When choosing total colectomy with ileorectal anastomosis, it may be advisable to close the distal ileum with a stapler and to perform a side-to-end anastomosis because of the discrepancy in luminal diameters of the two segments.

Rolland Parc

14

Colorectal Trauma

Susan Galandiuk

The mortality rate for victims of colonic trauma was more than 90 percent during the American Civil War, and dropped to 60 percent with the advent of regular laparotomy during World War I. The routine use of fecal diversion and blood replacement during World War II was associated with a further reduction in mortality to 30 percent. During the Korean and Vietnam conflicts, improved patient transportation and use of broad-spectrum antibiotics resulted in a 10 to 12 percent mortality rate. This rate has continued to improve and is now approximately 3 percent among the civilian population. Treatment of colorectal trauma must, however, be individualized. The presence of shock and associated injuries, the degree of contamination, the nature of the injury, and preexisting medical conditions determine the way colonic or rectal injuries are treated. Options in the management of colon injury include primary repair with or without proximal diversion, exteriorization, and resection and primary anastomosis or diversion.

Principles

Like any trauma victim, the patient with suspected intra-abdominal injury is further evaluated after the airway, breathing, and circulation have been evaluated and secured. If during the subsequent survey a stab wound is found to have penetrated the fascia, intra-abdominal exploration or diagnostic laparoscopy is indicated. In the event of blunt trauma or a bullet wound of uncertain trajectory, diagnostic peritoneal lavage should be performed. Following the insertion of a nasogastric tube and Foley catheter, a small incision is made below the level of the umbilicus (Fig. 14-1A), and a lavage catheter is inserted into the peritoneal cavity under direct vision (Fig. 14-1B & C). In patients with a pelvic fracture and suspected retroperitoneal hematoma, and in pregnant patients, the incision for diagnostic peritoneal lavage should be made supraumbilically. If no blood can be aspirated through the catheter, 1 L of normal saline is infused into the peritoneal cavity and then allowed to return by gravity flow (Fig. 14-1D). Gross and microscopic analysis of this fluid may demonstrate a red blood cell count > 100,000/mm³, a white blood cell count > 500/mm³, or amylase, bile, bacteria, or vegetable matter, any of which indicates intra-abdominal injury. In patients with a pelvic fracture and in those with gunshot wounds or bullets in the pelvis or buttocks or gunshot injuries in which the bullet trajectory is uncertain,

may become a nidus of infection. There is little valid data regarding the use of intra-operative colonic lavage in the trauma patient, most probably because the prerequisite of a stable patient and time are often lacking. Normal saline irrigation should be used to remove contaminants after a colon injury has been repaired. Additional irrigation with an antibiotic-containing solution is also an option. The rate of postoperative wound infection is quite high in the presence of significant intraoperative contamination, particularly when a colostomy must be constructed. In these cases, the wound should be left open or closed over a drain and antibiotic wound irrigation continued postoperatively.

Surgical Management

Injuries to the Right Colon

Because of the relatively liquid consistency of right colon feces, contamination is likely to be more extensive in right colon injury than in left colon or rectal injury. However, bacterial content is lower in the right colon than in the left colon and rectum. In the presence of hypotension, significant contamination, significant associated injuries (i.e., duodenal or pancreatic trauma), or a significant elapse of time from injury to operation, primary anastomosis is not undertaken. With high-velocity missile injury, there is generally a greater degree of tissue injury and devascularization. In such cases, resection is usually performed with construction of an ileostomy and a mucous fistula (Fig. 14-2). In the stable patient with little contamination and no other serious associated injuries, resection with primary anastomosis (see Ch. 2) may be performed (Fig. 14-3). Interestingly, given good intraoperative judgment regarding all these factors, there is little reproducible difference between primary repairs and diversion in the management of right colon trauma. For lesser injuries, the edges of the defect should be trimmed to remove nonvascularized or injured tis-

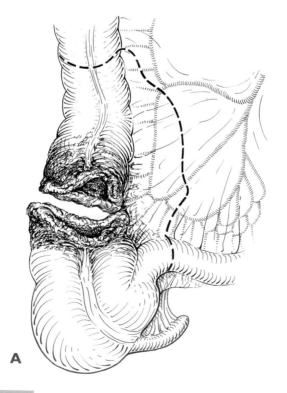

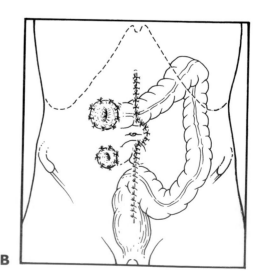

A

B

Figure 14-2.

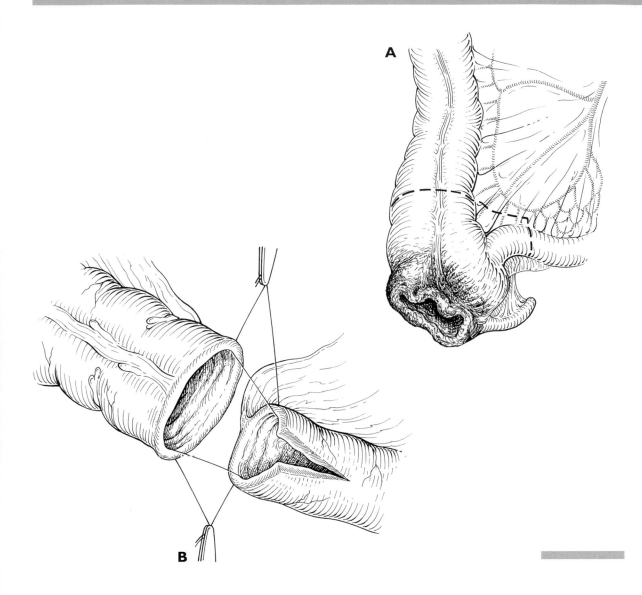

Figure 14-3.

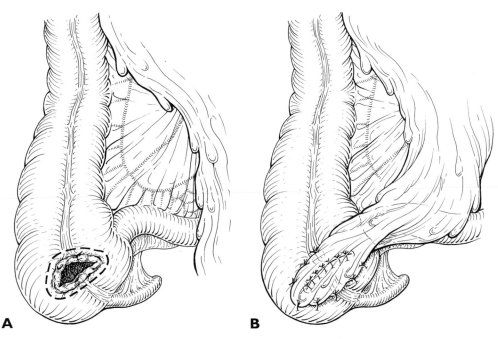

Figure 14-4.

sue and, most important, to ensure that there is adequate bleeding from the wound edges (Fig. 14-4A). A double- or single-layer transverse closure is performed and the omentum, if present, is used to buttress the repair (Fig. 14-4B). Injuries of the cecum and right colon are usually not exteriorized as loop colostomies because of the very large diameter of the bowel at this location.

Injuries of the transverse colon may be managed by primary closure if there is little contamination and the injury involves the antimesenteric border. Alternatively, because of the length of the transverse colon mesentery, larger injuries can be exteriorized as a loop transverse colostomy, which in many cases dose not require laparotomy for closure. A muscle-splitting stoma aperture is made through the lateral portion of the rectus muscle (see Ch. 4). To limit contamination, these injuries are temporarily closed with a running suture (Fig. 14-5A & B). The colon is brought through the stoma aperture and tacked to the subcutaneous fat with interrupted 3-0 chromic catgut sutures. This keeps the bowel in place during closure of the abdomen and also permits the stoma to be constructed without a rod. After the laparotomy wound is closed, the area of the temporarily closed defect is excised longitudinally in the direction of the tenia, and the stoma matured using chromic catgut (Fig. 14-5C). Many colorectal trauma patients present in shock and there is no opportunity for preoperative stoma marking. Stoma place-

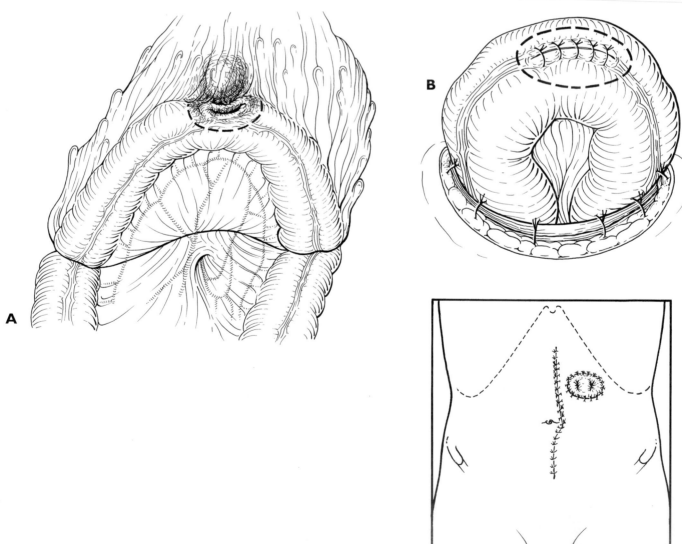

Figure 14-5.

ment in overtly bad locations, such as the waistline or directly adjacent to the iliac crest, must be avoided. There is more danger of wound contamination from a poorly fitting appliance than there is from a properly located stoma closer to the wound.

Injuries to the Left Colon

Many reviews have established that limited injuries of the left colon can be safely managed by primary closure. Although left colon resection with primary anastomosis has been successfully performed in many stable trauma patients, this should not be done without careful patient selection. In the unstable patient or the patient with significant associated injuries, and when there has been a significant delay between injury and operation and/or significant contamination, a primary resection with construction of an end colostomy and mucous fistula is preferred (Fig. 14-6A & B). The colostomy aperture should be made in the lateral portion of the rectus muscle. A longitudinal incision is made in the anterior fascia, and the rectus muscle is separated using a clamp (Fig. 14-6C & D). Following division of the posterior rectus sheath, the colon is brought through the aperture and tacked to the subcutaneous fat using absorbable interrupted sutures, and the stoma site matured following closure of the laparotomy incision (Fig. 14-6E & F). A mucous fistula should be formed whenever there is a long distal bowel stump and a proximal colostomy has been constructed. Because preoperative mechanical bowel preparation is impossible, luminal obstruction by retained fecal contents may occur later. Continued secretion of mucous may also lead to leakage from the distal colon stump. At the time of colostomy closure, preparation of the distal colon by irrigation is facilitated through the mucous fistula. Sizable sigmoid injuries can be exteriorized easily as a loop sigmoid colostomy. As for other colon injuries, associated significant trauma in the vicinity of the colon injury should create a low threshold for colostomy construction. If the injured segment of bowel has a particularly short mesentery, a proximal diverting colostomy may be constructed following primary repair or primary resection and anastomosis. The entire circumference of the injured segment should always be

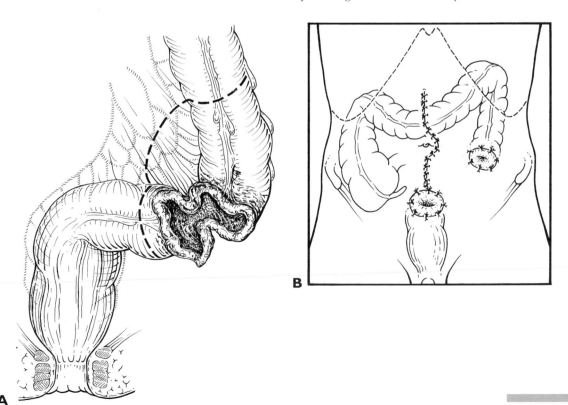

A   B

Figure 14-6.

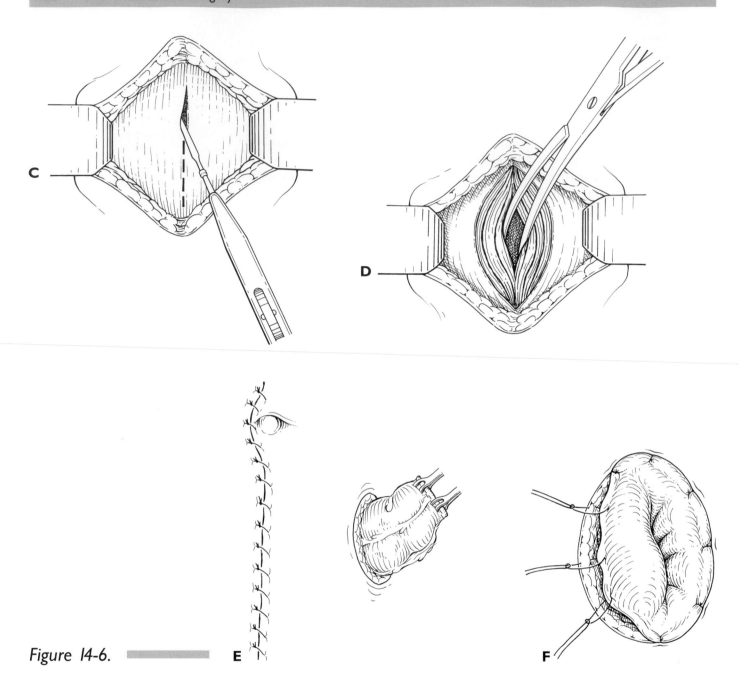

Figure 14-6.

examined. This involves complete mobilization of the injured segment to ensure that injury to the retroperitoneal posterior colon wall has not been missed.

Injuries to the Rectum

Management of injuries to the intraperitoneal rectum is similar to that of the sigmoid colon (Fig. 14-7). Due to the fact that the rectum is fixed in the pelvis, exteriorization as a colostomy cannot be performed. A proximal sigmoid loop colostomy, or alternatively an end sigmoid colostomy and mucous fistula or a Hartmann pouch, can be constructed. Loop sigmoid colostomies are completely diverting if properly constructed. Nevertheless, a pursestring suture of 3-0 chromic can be placed in the efferent limb, if desired (Fig. 14-8A). It will resorb by the time the colostomy is closed. A loop colostomy can also be made to provide complete diversion by applying a linear stapler across the efferent limb prior to stoma maturation (Fig. 14-8B).

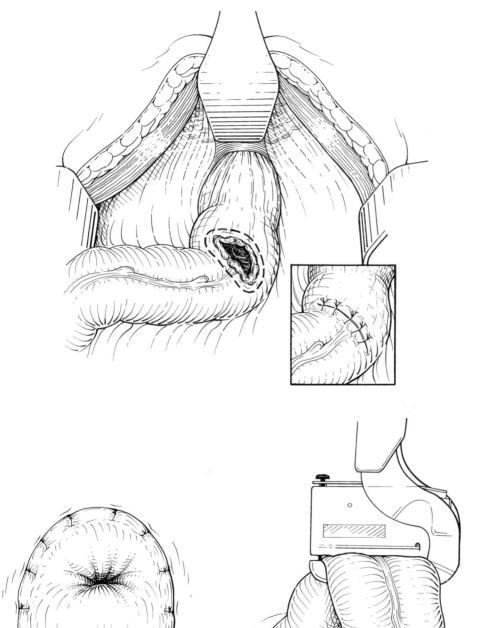

Figure 14-7.

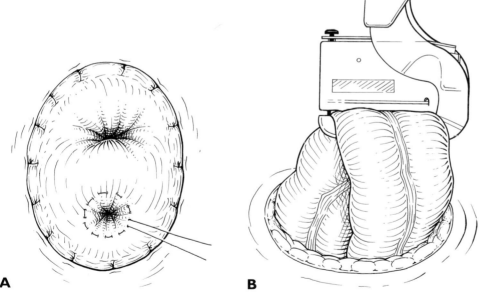

A   **B**

Figure 14-8.

With rectal injuries requiring fecal diversion, rectal washout should be performed. Rectal washout has been shown to result in both reduced morbidity and mortality. This can be done by irrigating the distal limb of bowel with 2 to 3 L of normal saline or dilute povidone-iodine solution with simultaneous anal canal dilatation. If there is a retrorectal injury, the presacral space should be drained. This can be done through the perineum or through the abdomen (Fig. 14-9). Military experience with high-velocity missiles has demonstrated that presacral drainage combined with diversion and rectal washout effectively reduces morbidity and mortality. However, in blunt injury, in the absence of posterior rectal injury, insertion of presacral drains either transperitoneally or transabdominally may act to open virgin tissue planes to potential contamination. Delayed operative management also escalates morbidity and mortality in such injuries. In addition to rectal trauma, severe crush injuries of the pelvis may also be associated with genitourinary injury as well as potentially life-threatening bleeding from the fracture site or injured internal or external iliac vessels.

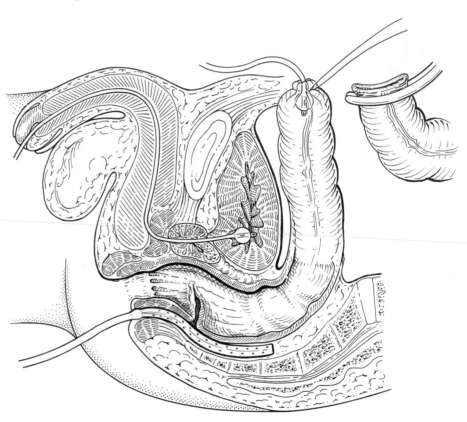

Figure 14-9.

Anal Trauma

Traumatic injury to the anal sphincters may occur in a variety of ways, the most devastating being in association with an open pelvic fracture, as seen in industrial crush injuries and pedestrian–motor vehicle accidents. In addition, trauma to the anal sphincters may be iatrogenic, such as occurs during episiotomy, or related to foreign bodies such as vibrators or unusual sexual activity. In the severely injured trauma patient, management of life-threatening injuries always takes precedence over sphincter reconstruction. Rectal washout, proximal colostomy, and local wound care, including cleansing of perineal wounds, should be undertaken. Care should be taken in debridement, because significant portions of anal sphincter can be removed by overzealous debridement. Pulsatile irrigation is often useful if there is severe contamination of a perineal laceration. After the patient has been stabilized, examination under anesthesia may permit adequate assessment of sphincteric injury and may even permit primary sphincteroplasty. The technique of repair is similar to that for repairs following obstetric injury: an overlapping repair of muscle (Fig. 14-10). In the recent trauma patient, there is very little scar tissue. The ends of the muscle may hold sutures better if they are first buttressed with a running 2-0 suture of nonabsorbable suture material. In crush- or blast-injured patients with a large defect in the area, later coverage with a myocutaneous flap may be useful. If a large wound is allowed to heal by secondary intention alone, formation of scar tissue and fibrosis of sphincter

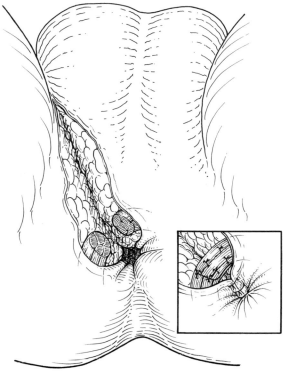

Figure 14-10.

ends may result in poor function if sphincteroplasty is subsequently undertaken. For smaller, less severe injuries, fecal diversion may not be required, especially if there is no full-thickness injury of the lower rectum.

Conclusion

In managing patients with colorectal trauma, there are no universal guidelines. Treatment of each patient must be individualized depending on the nature of the injury, velocity of the projectile, degree of contamination, severity and number of associated injuries, stability of the patients, and interval between injury and operation. Careful attention to these factors will result in acceptably low post-operative morbidity and mortality.

Editorial Commentaries

There may be a place for laparostomy in the assessment of potentially traumatic injuries to the colon.

Michael R. B. Keighley

I make the following few comments only to detail our approach to colonic trauma.

(Continues)

The clinical indications for exploration of patients with abdominal stab wounds are (1) hemodynamic instability; (2) blood from an orifice (such as a nasogastric tube, the rectum, or the genitourinary tract); (3) evisceration; (4) radiographic evidence of pneumoperitoneum; and (5) peritonitis. Patients who meet none of these criteria may undergo the following management options: (1) observation; (2) exploration of the stab wound to determine presence of the fascial penetration; (3) diagnostic peritoneal lavage; and (4) mandatory exploration.

Of all stab wounds to the anterior abdominal wall, 50 percent penetrate the abdominal wall fascia, and 50 percent of these are associated with intraperitoneal injury. Dr. Galandiuk's policy is mandatory exploration of the abdominal cavity by means of either laparotomy or laparoscopy if the wound has penetrated the fascia. This recommendation is appropriate. Some institutions, however, still utilize diagnostic peritoneal lavage to avoid nontherapeutic laparotomy, the rate for which is reported in the literature to vary between 50 and 75 percent. On the other hand, all patients with gunshot wounds that traverse the peritoneal cavity should undergo exploration; the incidence of intraperitoneal injury is fully 95 percent.

Blunt trauma to the colon is extremely rare, occurring in fewer than 10 percent of patients who have incurred blunt trauma. In the hemodynamically stable patient, computed tomography is safe and has a higher degree of diagnostic accuracy than even diagnostic peritoneal lavage. The rate of nontherapeutic celiotomy will also be lower if hemodynamically stable patients are scanned rather than lavaged.

The only patients who require urgent mandatory operation after blunt trauma are those with pelvic fractures; these patients need emergency colon diversion. Diagnostic laparoscopy is only mentioned in passing in the chapter, and rightly so; it is important to point out that there are no data to suggest diagnostic laparoscopy is efficacious in the evaluation of abdominal trauma.

I am grateful to Dr. Michael P. Bannon, our traumatologist at the Mayo Clinic, for his review of this chapter.

John H. Pemberton

Dr. Galandiuk has provided an excellent overview here. There are no significant areas in which I differ from her recommended treatment.

Victor W. Fazio

15

Colorectal Bleeding

Michael R. B. Keighley

Principles

Lower gastrointestinal bleeding may be massive or chronic. Chronic bleeding requires detailed investigation, particularly to exclude conditions such as carcinoma, polyps, arteriovenous malformations, Crohn's disease, ulcerative colitis, hereditary disorders affecting the small or large intestine, and a variety of other disorders posing diagnostic difficulties. This chapter describes the management of massive lower gastrointestinal bleeding, which is likely due to angiodysplasia, diverticular disease, Meckel's diverticulum, or colorectal varices, or to conditions such as Crohn's disease, malignancy, polyps, or aortoenteric fistula.

It must be remembered that the color of the blood lost does not signify the site of bleeding, merely the speed of blood loss, because blood in the bowel acts as a cathartic. It is also essential to exclude an upper gastrointestinal source of the bleeding and generalized bleeding disorders, and to ensure that the patient has had no previous vascular surgery, as this might indicate an aortoenteric fistula.

The process of resuscitation and investigation must proceed simultaneously in the patient with massive gastrointestinal bleeding. Fortunately, in many patients the bleeding episode stops spontaneously, allowing the clinician the opportunity to investigate the source of the bleeding before a second episode occurs.

Diagnosis

A quick general examination should help to exclude possible hereditary hemorrhagic telangectasia. The next step is to perform a gentle rectal examination and careful proctoscopy, because anorectal varices might only be detected by this means. A sigmoidoscopy is then performed, preferably after the patient has used a disposable enema to remove clotted blood from the rectum. Investigation next involves upper gastrointestinal endoscopy. If no source of the bleeding is found, an aggressive mechanical bowel preparation is started in order to clean all blood from the colon. Colonoscopy is then performed, with diathermy available to treat angiodysplastic lesions should any be found. If bleeding continues despite these measures, a red cell scan might identify an area of interest for subsequent angiography. Angiography should be performed with facilities for embolization if it is deemed appropriate. If laparotomy is to be performed subsequent to angiography, the angiogram catheter should be left in the feeding vessel so that if a bleeding lesion is demonstrated, on-table angiography can be undertaken; otherwise angiographic access to the site of bleeding will have to be obtained through cannulation of the mesenteric vessels feeding the suspected lesion. These measures are diagnostic in 80 percent of patients, but there always remains a group of patients in whom the source of blood loss cannot be identified.

Surgical treatment will be indicated if there have been repeated episodes of blood loss from an identifiable lesion or if massive blood loss continues. In the latter situation an identifiable lesion may not have been apparent during preoperative investigation.

Surgical Management

Laparotomy should be performed with the patient in the modified Lloyd-Davies position with the legs in Allen stirrups. The bladder should be catheterized. Antibiotic prophylaxis is given. Subcutaneous heparin is administered because, despite the fact that an underlying bleeding disorder might be responsible for the intestinal bleeding, there is still a risk of thromboembolism. The operating table should be equipped with radiographic facilities in case on-table angiography is necessary. It is also essential that there be facilities for panendoscopy with transillumination, and on-table colonic lavage.

The strategy should be to perform a limited resection where it is deemed safe and appropriate rather than to perform a subtotal colectomy; hence if there are clear clues as to the source of bleeding, or if the bleeding lesion can be positively identified, a segmental resection is preferred to a blind subtotal colectomy. Once the patient has been prepared, a Park's anal retractor should be inserted and the anorectum examined before commencing laparotomy, just in case a lesion in the anorectum has been missed. It is also wise at this point to repeat the sigmoidoscopy. A midline laparotomy is then performed and the bowel is carefully inspected after thorough mobilization of the hepatic splenic flexure and left colon. It is important that the stomach and duodenum, as well as the small bowel and Meckel's diverticulum, be checked for the presence of blood. Blood in the colon should be noted, particularly whether it lies on the left or the right side.

If the source of blood is still not obvious, the next step is to perform on-table colonic lavage followed by panendoscopy. An appendicostomy is performed and a Foley catheter is inserted into the cecum (Fig. 15-1A). Anesthetic scavenger tubing is then placed into the rectum and tied into position with a pursestring suture around the anus (Fig. 15-1B). The colon is irrigated with 10 to 12 L of Hartmann's solution until the material passing through the scavenger tubing is completely free of altered blood. Once the colon is completely clear, it is then possible to perform panendoscopy. This is a very quick procedure: the colonoscope is passed and threaded by the surgeon through to the cecum so that the colon can be inspected carefully as the scope is withdrawn. Using transillumination, it is usually easy to demonstrate a lesion in the wall of the colon that may be the source of bleeding. If no abnormality is identified, the colonoscope is passed back into the cecum and threaded through the ileocecal valve and along the terminal ileum so that as much of the distal small intestine as possible can be inspected using transillumination. If a lesion still is not found, a second endoscope is passed from above through the duodenojejunal flexure to inspect the upper jejunum (Fig. 15-2). In this manner it is nearly always possible to identify the source of blood loss. If a bleeding lesion is identified in the right colon, a

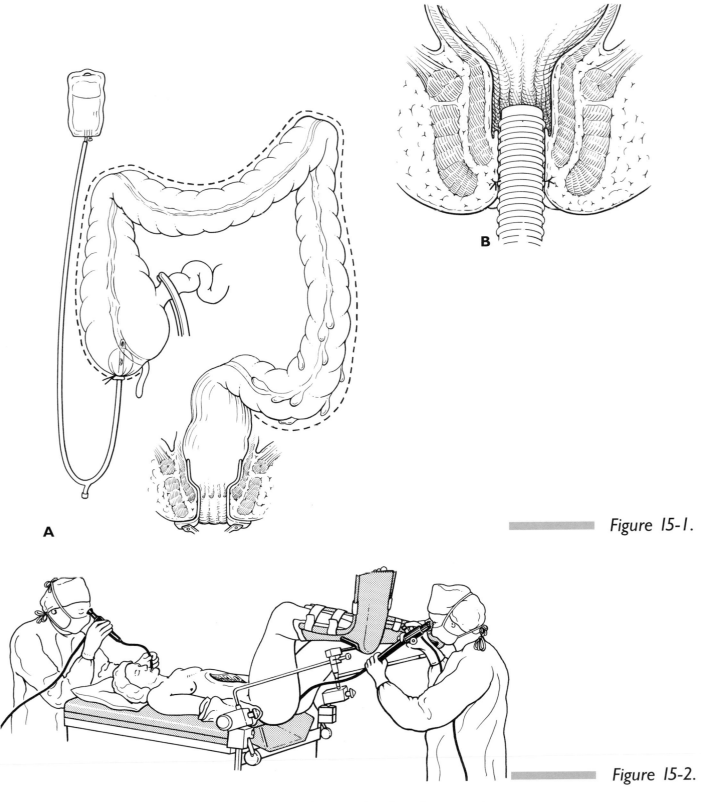

A

B

Figure 15-1.

Figure 15-2.

limited resection should be performed; similarly, if a lesion is found in the sigmoid colon, a sigmoidectomy alone would be advised (Fig. 15-3). If, on the other hand, no bleeding source can be identified and there is no lesion in the small intestine, a subtotal colectomy and an ileorectal anastomosis might be appropriate (Fig. 15-4). The method of resection and anastomosis is as described in Chapters 2 and 10.

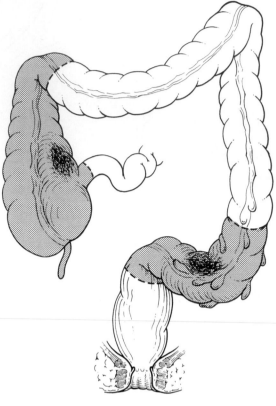

Figure 15-3.

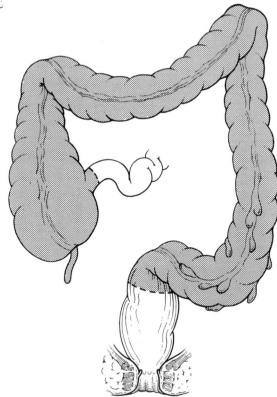

Figure 15-4.

The resected specimen is examined by a pathologist. The main artery is identified and a cannula placed within it; a larger cannula is placed into the draining vein. Heparinized saline is infused through the specimen and the bowel is sent to pathology for injection studies (Fig. 15-5). The abdomen is closed in the usual manner, with closed suction drains placed if necessary.

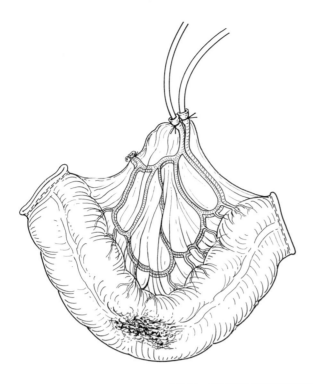

Figure 15-5.

Editorial Commentaries

I have little to add except my generally negative feelings about preoperative colonoscopy. Acute massive gastrointestinal bleeding almost always ceases within a short time, allowing the patient to be completely prepared and a complete evaluation to be undertaken. The futility of performing emergency colonoscopy without adequate preparation in the presence of active bleeding makes this a little-appreciated procedure. It really gains nothing. Another procedure that yields very little is radiolabeled blood imaging for bleeding.

The general approach provided by Professor Keighley is excellent, especially his intraoperative management techniques. These techniques are used at the Mayo Clinic and nearly always result in the successful location of the source of the bleeding. However, as these patients often have multiple angiodysplastic lesions, bleeding nearly always recurs. Blind subtotal colectomy and ileorectostomy are almost never performed anymore for this problem.

John H. Pemberton

The general approach to the management of colorectal bleeding is well-outlined in this chapter. In general, we do not perform upper gastrointestinal endoscopy quite as early in the course of the investigation as outlined here; rather, we pass a nasogastric tube to ascertain if the bleeding is from the stomach or duodenum. Clear bile-stained material is presumptive of a source of bleeding other than the stomach or duodenum. We agree with the generalization that tagged red cell scanning should be done early in the workup

(Continues)

and as a prelude to angiography. We have been somewhat aggressive in performing colonoscopy early in the case, when the patient is still stable. Unlike Dr. Keighley, we do not use embolization, as we feel it is too hazardous in terms of its likelihood to induce ischemia to the colon. Rather, we use the angiogram catheter to administer vasopressin.

Surgery is indicated, then, in patients who have had significant blood loss in whom there has been evidence of continued bleeding despite measures to stop the bleeding. These measures include transfusion, correction of any coagulopathy, and the use of intra-arterial vasopressin where a bleeding point has been demonstrated. Where the bleeding point has not been demonstrated and where the stomach and small bowel have been excluded as the source, surgery is recommended. I would agree with Dr. Keighley's recommendation that segmental resection is ideal, but should only be used if a clear point of bleeding can be identified. If vascular ectasia can be recognized angiographically or endoscopically, and the bleeding point is demonstrated as coming from the right colon, then a right colectomy is performed even if diverticular disease is found in the left side.

In the patient in whom the bleeding point cannot be identified, subtotal colectomy, ileostomy, and oversewing of the rectal stump is the preferred procedure.

Victor W. Fazio

16

Intestinal Fistulas

Victor W. Fazio

A *fistula* is an abnormal communication or tract connecting two epithelial surfaces. Factors promoting persistence of a fistula include distal obstruction, specific infection, the presence of a foreign body, malignancy, and radiation injury. In this chapter, we will deal with the most common types of enteric fistulas. These include (1) enterocutaneous, (2) enteroenteric, (3) enterovesical, and (4) enterovaginal types. The approaches to management of these fistulas will be outlined in turn.

Enterocutaneous Fistulas

Enterocutaneous fistulas are abnormal communications between the intestinal tract and skin. Prior to the modern era of nutritional support with parenteral hyperalimentation, mortality rates of 20 to 40 percent were common. This section will deal primarily with small bowel cutaneous fistulas, although reference is made to other varieties. The more common causes of such fistulas are postoperative anastomotic breakdown; intraoperative or postoperative trauma (e.g., abdominal wall closure with transfixion of an underlying bowel loop, drain erosion, abscess erosion into an adjacent intestinal loop or anastomosis); and Crohn's disease, radiation enteritis, or malignancy ("spontaneous" fistulas). Fistulas are commonly classified as high or low output, *high output* generally denoting a fistula draining in excess of 200 ml/day for at least 48 hours. These fistulas may also be categorized by anatomic location.

Principles of Management

Resuscitation. Fluid, electrolyte, and acid-base deficiencies are corrected. Use of nasogastric suction is a controversial issue, with disadvantages probably outweighing advantages. For long-term control of a problematic high-output fistula, gastrostomy is a better alternative to tube suction aspiration via the nasogastric route.

Sepsis. Abscesses are identified by computed tomography (CT) or ultrasonography and drained. If cellulitis, phlegmon, or undrainable sepsis is present, systemic antibiotics effective against enteric organisms are used after first obtaining material for culture where possible.

Fistula Output Collection. Erosion of the skin around the fistula is prevented or minimized by appropriate application of a skin barrier and a drainable collecting system. An enterostomal therapist is invaluable, as in some complex fistulas it may take up to 1 1/2 hours to provide a good seal to a drainage system.

Identifying the Cause and Site of the Fistula. This is done by the usual methods of history, physical examination, and special studies, including sinography and contrast roentgenography. As well, one will note the natural history of specific diseases (e.g., malignancy and inflammatory bowel disease) for which nonoperative measures are likely to be futile in the definitive management of such fistulas. Coexisting disease is attended to. The main purpose of investigation is to identify specific disease and to exclude obstruction of the bowel distal to the fistula. Obstruction is commonly present at or just beyond the site of the fistula.

Response to Therapy. Unless the patient is to be taken to the operating room urgently, total parenteral nutrition (TPN) is instituted. Patients who fail to improve (as shown by reduced volume of fistula output) on TPN within 3 to 5 days are unlikely to respond adequately without surgery.

Timing and Indications for Surgery. In the postoperative patient with small bowel cutaneous fistula resulting from iatrogenic injury or anastomotic dehiscence, management is largely dependent on when the fistula occurs and whether or not it is high output.

Early-Appearing Fistulas (0 to 10 Days Postoperatively). If output is low, TPN is used and the management is expectant. If the output is high—and in this context, even 100 ml/day may qualify—laparotomy is performed. One must keep in mind that the circumstances encountered at this reentry into the abdomen can *never* be as favorable as those encountered at the prior operation that led to the development of the enterocutaneous fistula. Except in rare circumstances, the urge to do a simple suture repair of the fistula must be resisted in favor of exteriorizing the fistula site or repairing the defect (with or without resection) with proximal ileostomy. Neither in early- nor in late-appearing fistulas is "patch grafting" an alternative.

Intermediate-Appearing Fistulas (10 Days to 8 Weeks Postoperatively). This is a "hands off" interval during which the only justifications for operative intervention are intestinal ischemia, hemorrhage unresponsive to medical treatment, and intra-abdominal abscess not amenable to CT guided drainage. The patient is otherwise managed with home TPN and—if this fails to heal the fistula—deferring of surgery for at least 3 months if not longer.

Late-Appearing Fistulas (2 to 3 Months or Later). These are usually managed by operative means when prognosis and risk-benefit analysis favors surgery.

The timing of surgery in all cases relates to the phenomenon of adhesion formation. The "obligatory" fusion of intestine with other loops and the parietes seems to reach its zenith at about 3 weeks after surgery, after which there is a refractory period ranging from a few weeks to several months before these formidable adhesions soften and allow easier separation of the bowel loops. The more complicated and/or septic the situation was at the last laparotomy, the longer the "recovery" period should be before reentry into the abdomen. In fact, even with these guidelines, the task of reentry may be too hazardous and the experienced surgeon will back out early in the course of reoperation if no reasonable headway is being made—or if iatrogenic enterotomies occur. The surgery of enterocutaneous fistula would in fact be a relatively simple undertaking were it not for the "cementlike" adhesions and bowel obstruction that is so often encountered with an obliterated peritoneal cavity.

Principles of Surgery

Prevention of Continued Contamination of the Peritoneal Cavity. Ideally this is done by resection of the fistulized segment and bowel anastomosis. If this is not possible—and sepsis is not otherwise controllable—then a proximal diverting stoma is performed. If necessary, this may be a "high" stoma or jejunostomy. At operation—through an epigastric or even left subcostal incision—the duodenojejunal junction is identified and the distalmost segment of bowel that can be traced from the duodeno-jejunal flexure is brought out as a loop stoma proximal to the source of the intestinal defect. However, except in the occasional intermediate-appearing fistula, this is rarely needed.

Incision Planning. Incisions are planned with a view to preserving potential ostomy sites, which are marked preoperatively. Avoidance of incisions that closely parallel old incisions will minimize ischemic incision skin bridges. Commonly the previous midline incision is used while the lower abdominal fistulous opening is excised (Fig. 16-1).

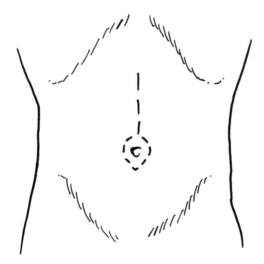

Figure 16-1.

Mobilization of the Small Bowel. The abdomen is entered, usually in the epigastrium through the upper part of the previous midline incision. Adhesions here are usually less formidable and there is a lesser likelihood of starting off with an enterotomy. The underlying bowel loops are identified and teased or dissected away from the posterior aspect of the wound and lateral abdominal wall. Where possible, the matted loops of small bowel are exteriorized onto the anterior abdominal wall to allow easier loop separation. Usually this is not entirely possible. The entire small bowel needs to be mobilized to evaluate possible obstructed sites or other bowel defects. Adherent loops of small intestine are then separated; usually this becomes more difficult as one approaches the fistula source. The muscular coats of adjacent loops may appear to have fused or even be absent. Separation of these loops may be almost impossible without producing an enterotomy. This may be facilitated by tracing the fusion planes of the mesentery proximal and distal to the site of maximal mucosal fixation. Gentle finger compression/dissection may further clarify a plane, especially where the loop of intestine is abutting the lateral abdominal wall. One maneuver I find occasionally helpful is to inject normal saline (using a 10-ml syringe and a 23-gauge needle) into the site of fusion of these loops (Fig. 16-2). Creating an edematous layer between the loops lessens the risk of enterotomy with sharp scissor dissection in this fabricated plane (Fig. 16-3).

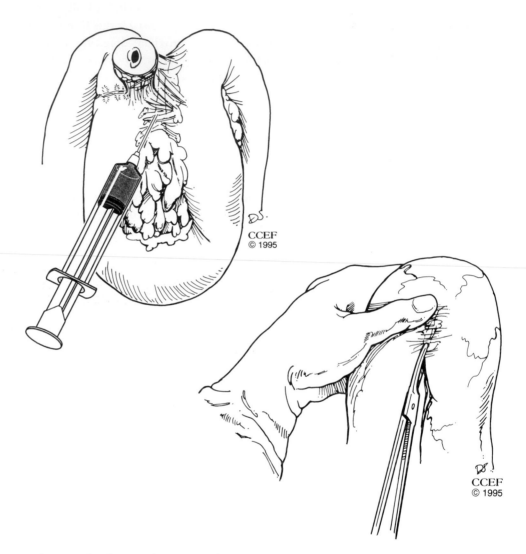

Figure 16-2.

Figure 16-3.

A general rule is to dissect out the easy segments first, as this will often help facilitate the approach to the difficult, fixed fused segment. This is especially true when a problematic loop is densely adherent deep in the pelvis. By retrieving the easier loops first, and by tracing the entrance and exit loops of the fused segment, the safety of the bold scissor dissection of the apex of this loop is enhanced. In cases where reoperative pelvic surgery is likely, preoperative passage of ureteric stents is often helpful.

In particularly difficult cases, where bowel serosa is intimately fused to the abdominal wall, a permissible and sometimes useful technique is to incise the abdominal fascia from the peritoneal aspect, dissect in the extrafascial plane, and reenter the peritoneal cavity several centimeters away at a point where serosal separation is easy or already has been achieved.

Specific Fistula Procedures

There are certain procedures that are *not* done. Serosal patch surgery is of historic interest only. Nothing less than a mucosa-mucosa closure is acceptable. Suture closure of the unprepared defect is associated with a high leakage rate—similar to closure of an ostomy without preparing the bowel opening. In most cases, there will be associated fibrinous thickening of the wound edge, or a septic membrane that will mandate resection of the fistula-bearing segment.

Resection of the Fistula-Bearing Bowel Segment. This is the usual procedure of choice. In cases of established fistulas in which the adjacent bowel is reasonably soft, supple, and free of disease, where there is no adjacent abscess, and where distal bowel obstruction has been ruled out, end-to-end anastomosis is done following the principles outlined in Chapter 2. A two-layer anastomosis of absorbable suture is preferred. The cutaneous fistula opening and its tract, including fat and fascia, is mobilized to the enteric communication and resected (Fig. 16-4A–C).

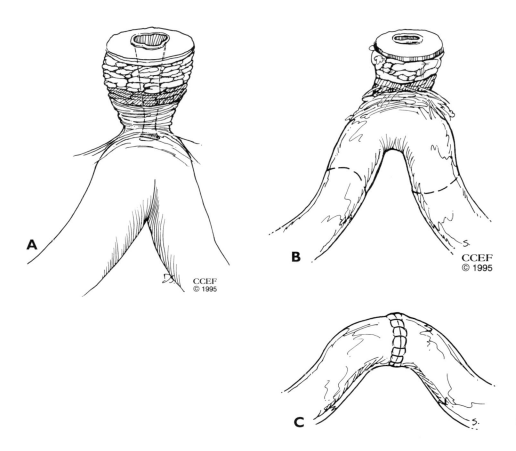

Figure 16-4.

If several enterotomies in adjacent segments are made in the course of identifying the fistula, it may be appropriate to make two or more resections and anastomoses. In such cases, I will commonly use stapling techniques to expedite the procedure.

Resection with No Anastomosis. This is done for patients with an established stoma (e.g., ileostomy patients) in whom an ileostomy fistula or fistula arising from the nearby ileum is found. A peri-ileostomy fistula is a difficult problem to handle, occurring as it usually does from the abdominal wall component of the ileostomy and at a time when reentry into the abdomen is quite difficult (i.e., 7 to 14 days postoperatively) (Fig. 16-5). Indeed, there is little or no alternative to reoperating, as pouching of a skin level parastomal fistula is particularly difficult because leakage from the appliance seal and the accompanying painful skin excoriation mandate intervention. The ileostomy and terminal ileum are so adherent at this stage that "simple" delivery of a few more inches of bowel out of the abdominal wall aperture (by local surgery) is often impossible. Thus a midline laparotomy—with all the attendant risks of enterotomy to the underlying intestinal loops—is usually required to aid in the delivery of the ileostomy and fistula. If the ostomy site is quite septic, relocation of the stoma may be needed. When enough length has been delivered, the ileum is transsected below the fistula and matured (Fig. 16-6).

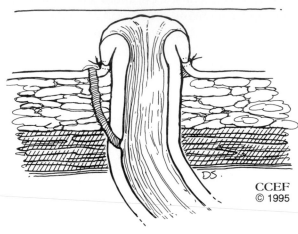

Figure 16-5.

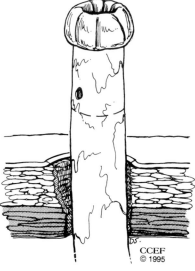

Figure 16-6.

In the scenario in which the fistula arises several inches to a foot or so from the ileostomy, the surgeon will make a judgment about the risks and benefits of performing a limited resection and anastomosis versus a much longer resection of bowel including the ileostomy with construction of a neo-end ileostomy. Where the patient is vulnerable to developing short-bowel syndrome, anastomosis with preservation of as much small bowel as possible is performed.

Ileostomy. Ostomy may be used as a definitive procedure in conjunction with resection or may be used alone in cases where reentry into the abdomen is especially problematic and yet intra-abdominal sepsis continues. This will be temporizing until reentry is feasible, and may be used proximal to a bowel anastomosis where there is a high chance of leakage. In very unusual cases in which multiple fistulas are present (Fig. 16-7) or there is extensive pyogenic membrane remaining, a series of mucous fistulas may be constructed distal to the diverting ostomy (Fig. 16-8).

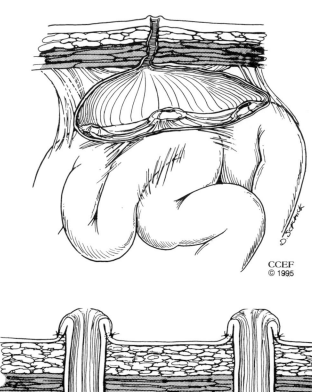

CCEF
© 1995

Figure 16-7.

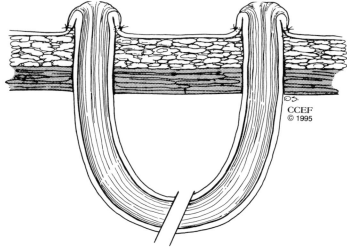

CCEF
© 1995

Figure 16-8.

Bilateral Exclusion Bypass (Thiry-Vella Loop). Bilateral exclusion bypass (Fig. 16-9) is rarely used, but is appropriate when the hazards of removing a bowel segment are considered excessive (e.g., in certain radiation- or malignancy-related fistulas, and especially in those small bowel fistulas arising in the pelvis that discharge onto the perineum or into the vagina). The bowel segments proximal and distal to the isolated loop are anastomosed. Ideally, one or more limbs of the isolated loop are exteriorized as a mucous fistula, so that in the event of a later obstruction at the fistula source, stump blow-out will be avoided.

Other Considerations. *Anastomotic Quarantine.* Where feasible, anastomoses are wrapped or quarantined from raw surfaces or "beds" where a phlegmon resided using omentum or even small bowel mesentery itself. One useful "trick" is to leave most or all of the mesentery of a resected small bowel loop, from which a small pedicle may be created that will quarantine the anastomosis.

Repair of Damaged Serosal Surfaces. Inevitably, serosal injury or myotomies or enterostomies will be made in many or most operations for enterocutaneous fistulas. These are all repaired carefully using 3-0 polyglycolic acid sutures. Care is taken not to narrow the lumen and the repair is oriented so that the closure is made as nearly

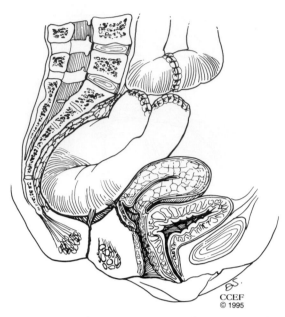

CCEF
© 1995

Figure 16-9.

transversely as possible. With long myotomized segments, the surgeon will have to choose between sacrifice (resection) and "chancing it" (i.e., leaving the affected segment in situ). The latter is reasonable, especially if part of the intestinal muscle wall remains.

Checking for Occult Enterotomy. At the end of the procedure, one that is usually prolonged and has involved extensive repair work, it is tempting to close as quickly as possible. If there is one thing worse than surgery for enterocutaneous fistula, it is reoperative surgery for recurrent fistula. The enterotomy repairs done at this time may be incomplete and some enterotomies may be inadequate or missed. This is best checked by irrigating the last-recognized enterotomy with saline, allowing distension of the bowel upstream and downstream to check for leaks. Alternatively, the bowel may be insufflated with air or carbon dioxide as it is held under a saline abdominal fill to check for bubbles.

Management of the Cutaneous Abdominal Wall Component of the Fistulous Tract. In many cases, especially midline wound fistulas, the abdominal wall component of the fistulous tract is excised. In lateral fistulas, the tract is debrided and curetted. This approach may also be applied to the midline wound, as there is commonly a long cutaneous, fascial or subfascial component, with an inflammatory rind of granulation tissue extending for several inches. If left, there is pronounced thickening of the abdominal wall at that point. Suture closure of the abdomen at this point will cause a slow "cut through" of the sutures. Thus, this inflamed, thickened part of the fascia and enterocutaneous tissue should be excised—my preference being with cutting cautery. Figure 16-10A shows a duodenal repair for duodenocutaneous fistula. The fistula tract may suppurate unless curetted (Fig. 16-10B).

For lateral fistulas, especially where the tract is long and tortuous, I use a subfascial Penrose drain to traverse the tract and quarantine small bowel from the deep aspect. This drain is removed after 10 to 14 days, in the outpatient department (Fig. 16-10C).

Abdominal Closure. The fascia is closed with interrupted No. 1 Prolene. The abdominal cavity and wound are copiously irrigated with saline solution. The skin is

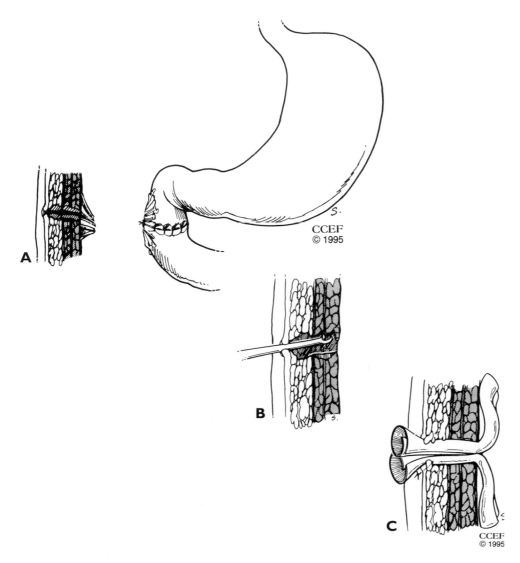

CCEF
© 1995

A

B

C

CCEF
© 1995

Figure 16-10.

left (almost) entirely open; the skin opposite stoma sites is closed only for an inch or so to allow for a good skin barrier seal. Above and below this, the skin is approximated with two or three sutures to allow for wide wound drainage. Delayed primary closure is carried out after about 7 days. If the fascia is deficient, I will avoid using nonabsorbable mesh at this time. The skin and subcutaneous fat is closed over dental rolls to spread the suture tension evenly.

Enteroenteric Fistula

Enterocolic fistula may arise from the same conditions that cause enterocutaneous fistulas. Ileocoloduodenal fistulas were discussed above. The principles of surgery here are to resect the source of the fistula and to wedge out the secondarily affected bowel segment. Thus with Crohn's disease of the ileum and a localized perforation that has eroded into either an adjacent proximal small bowel loop or sigmoid colon, a terminal ileal resection is done. The secondary organ (i.e., proximal small bowel or sigmoid colon), is treated by taking a small margin of bowel just outside of the fistula orifice (i.e., a wedge excision) with primary suture closure of the defect (Fig. 16-11A & B).

In the case of the primary disease in the sigmoid colon (e.g., diverticulitis or carcinoma of the sigmoid), the ileosigmoid fistula is treated by formal sigmoidectomy and

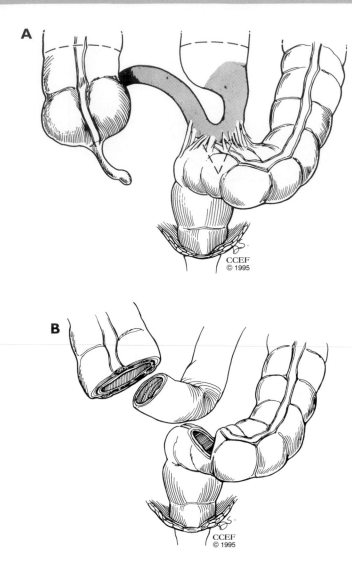

Figure 16-11.

wedge excision of the small bowel fistulous component, and primary closure of the defect (Fig. 16-12). An exception exists in certain cases of Crohn's-induced ileosigmoid fistula in which the sigmoid colon is affected by phlegmonous inflammation or is part of an abscess cavity wall. In such cases, I prefer to do a limited sigmoid segmental resection. The ileum to ascending colon and sigmoid to sigmoid anastomoses are then carried out (Fig. 16-13).

Gastrojejunal cutaneous fistula usually arises secondary to recurrent peptic ulceration and may involve the transverse colon as well. Figure 16-14A–C shows the principles of resection. Duodenal defects remaining after excision of ileoduodenal or coloduodenal fistulas may be remedied by a side-to-side duodenojejunostomy (Fig. 16-15).

Enterovesical Fistula

There are numerous causes of enterovesical fistula, but the most common include Crohn's disease (ileovesical, colovesical fistulas), carcinoma of the rectosigmoid, diverticulitis, and radiation injury. The principles of fistula surgery hold true, namely resection of the disease-bearing segment, detachment or wedge excision of the aperture pertaining to the fistula defect on the secondarily involved organ, with bowel anastomosis and primary closure. In fact, for benign causes, such as diverticulitis and

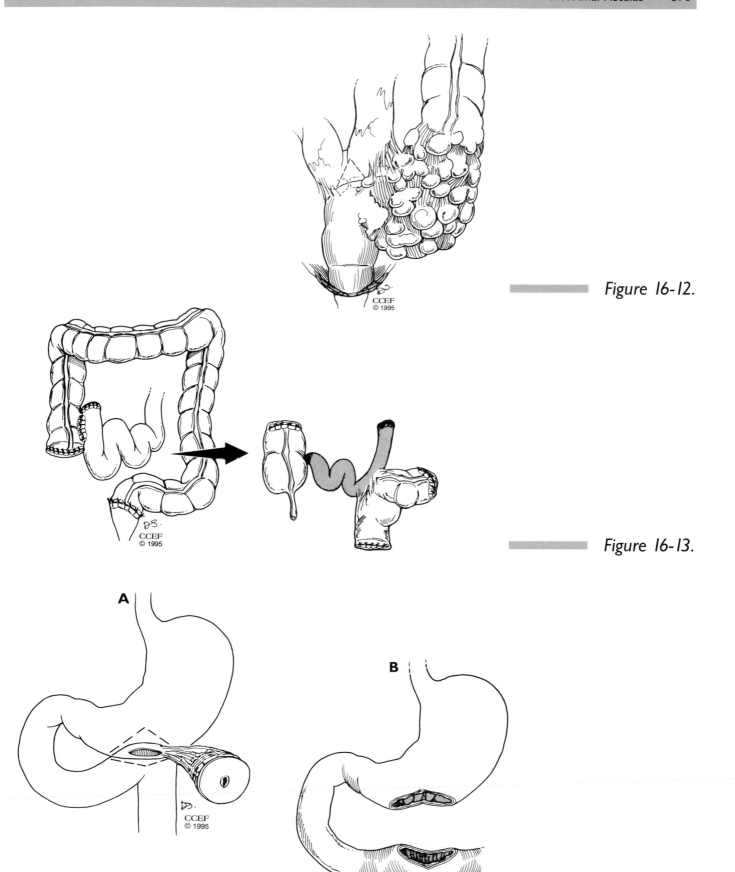

Figure 16-12.

Figure 16-13.

Figure 16-14.

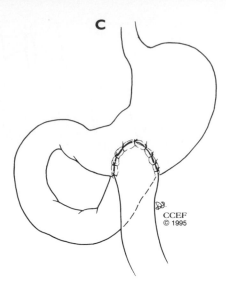

Figure 16-14.

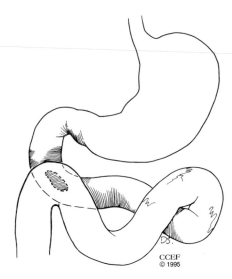

Figure 16-15.

Crohn's disease, no resection of the secondary fistulous orifice is done (Fig. 16-16A–B). The bowel is separated from the bladder in these cases by the pinch/fracture technique. However, it is important to exclude underlying colonic malignancy by sigmoidoscopy and biopsy, if necessary, at the time of surgery. Should malignant enterovesical fistula be present, then a 2-cm-wide margin of the bladder peripheral to the fistulous orifice is required. After bowel resection, a primary anastomosis is almost always done, with interposition of omentum between the anastomosis and bladder defect. The bladder defect is often difficult to see. The granulation tissue on the back of the bladder is curetted and trimmed to freshen the edges. Any overt defect is sutured closed; a urinary catheter is left in place for 7 to 10 days. Any capsule of inflammatory phlegmon remaining at the bladder base is drained by latex rubber drains for 10 days.

It is important to be sure that ureteric obstruction or injury is not sustained when dealing with the bladder defect after resection of a malignant colovesical fistula. Should the defect encroach on the trigone, J-stents should be placed into the ureters. A two- or three-layer closure of the bladder should then be performed with 0-0 and 2-0 polyglycolic acid sutures. Again a urinary catheter is left in place for 7 to 10 days. Cystography is usually done prior to catheter removal to confirm healing.

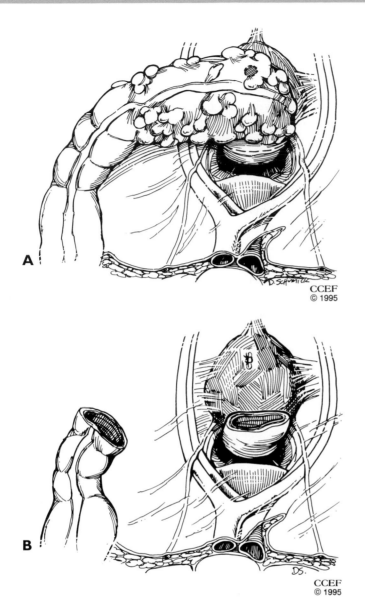

Figure 16-16.

Enterovaginal Fistula

The identical principles of fistula surgery hold for this rather common type of fistula as well, namely resection of the primary diseased segment. Most cases occur when the uterus has been previously removed. Colovaginal fistulas are commonly due to diverticulitis or occur postoperatively after colonic resection; typically a colorectal anastomotic defect is the source of the problem. Ileovaginal fistula is a complication of Crohn's disease or radiation enteritis.

Editorial Commentaries

Like Dr. Fazio, we tend to avoid early intervention in early low-output intestinal fistulas. We find that even when a fistula becomes manifest within

(Continues)

the first week of operation, reoperation is generally difficult, and that many of these fistulas will close spontaneously provided local sepsis is controlled, there is no abscess between the intestinal defect and the abdominal wall, there is no distal obstruction, and there is no evidence of persistent intestinal disease (undetected Crohn's disease or radiation enteritis).

We would not necessarily immediately operate on all late fistulas. Certainly patients with Crohn's disease and severe coexisting malnutrition may require TPN prior to surgical intervention. Similarly, established fistulas arising from radiation damage may not always justify further surgery, because the dangers of reoperation may outweigh their benefits.

We agree with Dr. Fazio that it is wise to try to enter the peritoneal cavity of a patient with a postoperative enterocutaneous fistula well away from the site of previous sepsis and fibrosis. We like to isolate segments of bowel that are at risk of "springing a leak" by tying tapes around these at-risk segments. We also tend to use sharp dissection, and this is one of the situations in which a scalpel blade often provides the only method of separating densely fibrinous loops of bowel from one another and particularly from the abdominal wall.

Special mention should be made of postirradiation enterocutaneous, enterovesical, and enterovaginal fistulas. These fistulas are the most difficult ones to manage because there is a high risk of repeated fistulation unless nonirradiated bowel is used for subsequent reconstruction. Postirradiation fistulas in our experience are almost always diverted after resection. Coloanal sleeve resections tend to be used for sigmoid and rectal fistulas, and exclusion bypass may have to be used for ileal fistulas deep in the pelvis.

Finally, mention should be made of the place of laparostomy in the management of severe recurrent postoperative enterocutaneous fistulas. There are certain situations in which it may be unsafe to close the abdominal wall. This is particularly so if there is a risk of bleeding, sepsis, or recurrent fistulas. Patients with a laparostomy often require ventilation, and they may require repeat abdominal wound toilet. However, many of these patients, even if they develop a subsequent fistula, can be managed successfully without the risk of fatal sepsis.

We tend to use single-layer extramucosal techniques for intestinal anastomosis and for closure of intestinal defects, because this causes less risk of narrowing the lumen of the bowel. Generally, we do not advise delayed closure of skin wounds. If skin wounds are to be left open because of the risk of infection, by the time they are ready for secondary closure, healthy granulation tissue has formed and the process of secondary healing is rapidly progressing.

Michael R. B. Keighley

Dr. Fazio's principles of managing intestinal fistulas are excellent. I agree entirely that gastrostomy tubes are better than nasogastric tubes for long-term control, and that consideration to early gastrostomy is imperative. I agree completely with the "hands-off" policy regarding fistulas that present between 10 days and 2 months postoperatively. This is the worst possible time to be back in the abdomen, and the patient can only be made worse by attempts to "rummage around." In addition, if the patient has fibrous scarring, going into the abdomen even in less than 10 days can be a daunting adventure.

Ureteral stents should be placed with little hesitation when reoperating for intestinal fistulas. The old belief that stents help because they allow one to know when one has cut across the ureter is really not true. I find them extremely helpful in difficult situations.

When closing after enterocutaneous fistula surgery, I usually close the skin of the midline incision. I agree that mesh is rarely indicated after the first reoperation.

With regard to Dr. Fazio's approach to the sigmoid colon, I agree that when the ileum has "kissed it" with Crohn's disease, a limited, even wedge, resection of the sigmoid is indicated. Sometimes it is difficult to know if there is concomitant sigmoid disease, but flexible sigmoidoscopy often helps to identify its presence.

With regard to the approach to the bladder after removing an enterovesical fistula, I agree completely with "pinching off" the fibrous fistula between the bowel and the bladder, but one can almost never put a stitch in the resultant opening, as the reaction is so firm. Placement of a suction drain in the cul-de-sac, however, will control any leakage that may occur from a tiny bladder opening that cannot be closed. I have actually never seen urine come out of such a drain postoperatively.

I have not used a laparoscopic approach in patients with severe postoperative adhesions and enterovesical cutaneous or enteroenteral fistulas.

John H. Pemberton

17

Rectovaginal Fistulas

Victor W. Fazio

Although the term *rectovaginal fistula* applies to any communication between the rectum and vagina, the entity discussed here is more properly termed *anovaginal fistula*. Most fistulas arise at or just above the dentate line and traverse the rectovaginal septum, with their exit between the fourchette and the posterior vaginal fornix. The more common acquired rectovaginal fistulas result from trauma (e.g., childbirth, surgery), cryptoglandular sepsis, inflammatory bowel disease, irradiation, and specific infectious disease.

Principles

The patient should be worked up for the specific cause of the rectovaginal fistula, and that cause treated appropriately where indicated (e.g., drain the specific infection or treat the underlying Crohn's disease).

The operation must be timed appropriately (e.g., a traumatic childbirth injury would lend itself to repair at that time). However, if *that* repair fails, the edema, induration, and possible sepsis will need to resolve (e.g., after 2 to 3 months) so that the definitive repair may be done on supple tissues. The bowel should be prepared so that it is empty and broad-spectrum antibiotic coverage provided (e.g., cephalosporin and metronidazole). A Foley catheter is placed in the bladder.

Certain disease processes may require different strategies: radiation fistulas will usually require rectal resection and coloanal anastomosis; rectovaginal fistulas due to Crohn's disease may require treatments as varied as advancement flaps, sleeves, or proctectomy, depending on the specific fistula and patient.

Fecal diversion must be considered in certain cases. Although there is no rule about this, commonly used guidelines include the use of a diverting colostomy where the risk of nonhealing of the repair is higher than usual. Such circumstances include the following:

Multiple previous repairs.
Associated major sphincter injury (e.g., cloaca).
Inflammatory bowel disease, especially where, for example,
  Crohn's disease is producing systemic symptoms, or if rectal/anal inflammation is such that an advancement sleeve operation is under consideration.

Operative Choices

Repair of rectovaginal fistulas may be approached transanally, transvaginally, or perineally. The choice of operation is usually dictated by one's training and experience. Success with all of the above approaches has been reported. My own preference has been for the transanal repair, as this would have theoretical advantages over both of the other alternatives:

1. By repairing a defect on the bowel side, this would obviate the risk of stool accumulating (producing sepsis) below a transvaginal repair.
2. By avoiding division of the internal and part of the external sphincter—as occurs with perineal body division for the perineal, transsphincteric approach—future sphincter continence is not jeopardized. If sepsis complicates a perineal repair, the muscle repair may very well break down. On the other hand, this repair is the preferred approach when a significant sphincter injury accompanies a rectovaginal fistula.

Transanal Technique

The recto(ano)vaginal fistula can have varying presentations and "morphology." The opening may be at or below the dentate line, or extend 2 to 5 cm above the dentate line. (For very difficult fistulas at the level of 6 to 7 cm from the anal verge, alternatives such as coloanal anastomosis, or even the York-Mason posterior transsphincteric approach, to "get at" the fistula may be necessary.) The fistula may vary from 1 to 2 mm to a large opening that easily admits the index finger. Herein I will describe three approaches that I commonly use for specific sets of circumstances.

Advancement Rectal Flap. The patient is given a general anesthetic (others prefer regional anesthesia) and placed in the prone jackknife position. The patient has already been given washout enemas (in addition to the bowel preparation). The vagina and perineum are prepared with povidone-iodine.

Effacement sutures (four to six in number) are placed on the anal verge. By placing the sutures at the verge—*not* near the dentate line—and suturing to the perineal skin about 7 cm distant from the verge, the fistula is "lowered" to the operator; this is a very cost-effective alternative to commercially available self-retaining retractors (Fig. 17-1). Because a patient may strain or cough during the procedure, a gauze

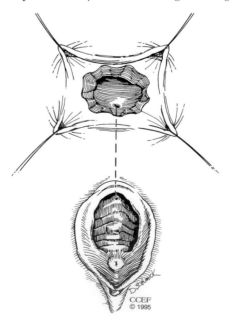

Figure 17-1.

dressing (tied to a stout silk ligature) is placed in the mid- to upper rectum to absorb any mucus or rectal content that could grossly contaminate the operative field.

The anterior mucosa of the anal canal is infiltrated with 1:100,000 epinephrine in saline solution to provide hemostasis as well as help to clarify the plane of anterior dissection. Further injection to clarify the plane is done with injectable saline (thus minimizing the cardiovascular effects of too much epinephrine). Using the cutting cautery, a curvilinear incision is made just caudad to the fistula extending to the right and left to about one-third to one-half circumference (Fig. 17-2). By avoiding the rectangular flap, the concern about ischemia of the edges is nullified.

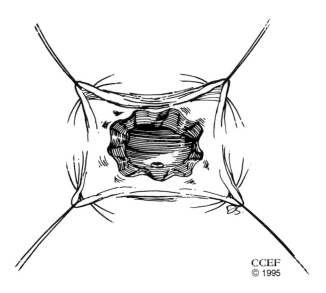

Figure 17-2.

At the start, the flap consists of mucosa and submucosa only. As the dissection is carried cephalad, a flap of increasing bulk is obtained, incorporating portions of circular muscle of the rectum (Fig. 17-3). The edges, right and left, are vulnerable to attenuation, and, therefore, continued saline injection is used to "thicken" the flap. In fact, this ensures a good blood supply to the distal flap.

The dissection is carried as far superiorly as is deemed necessary—given that the distal edge of the flap needs to be excised and a tension-free advancement of the flap

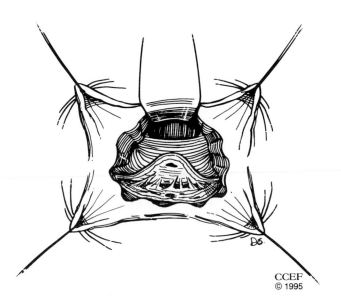

Figure 17-3.

to the dentate line has to be done. If needed, the dissection can be (and for rectal sleeve advancement, has to be) carried out to the anterior peritoneal reflection, exposing the entire septum.

Attention is now turned to the fistula tract through to the vagina. Excision of this tract is not easily done, as the tissue is friable. Furthermore, the defect resulting from excision is alarming. However, unless complete curettage is carried out and the surgeon satisfied with its conduct, excision is best—as this assures "healthy" tissue with a good blood supply.

The defect is now closed. Depending on the local situation, one or more layers of muscle (sphincter) closure over the defect can be done. Figure 17-4 illustrates a vertical repair of interrupted 20-polyglycolic acid. A UR6 needle is particularly helpful. In certain cases, a transverse closure may be more appropriate. The principle is that of obtaining a well-vascularized repair. The vaginal mucosal defect is left open.

At this point, hemostasis of the rectovaginal septum is obtained. Beware of creating a bed of charcoal with excessive diathermy. During the dissection, continuous lavage with saline or dilute tetracycline solution is performed.

The flap is drawn caudad and the fistula component is excised (Fig. 17-5). I use scissors so I can appreciate bleeding from the cut edge. At this point an assessment is

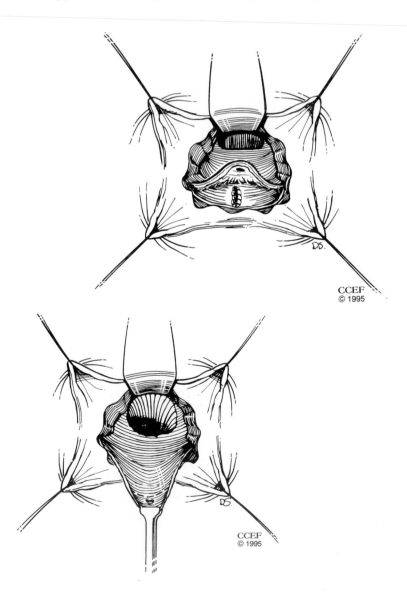

Figure 17-4.

Figure 17-5.

made regarding the extent to which any tension will be present in the mucosa to dentate line closure. If the flap is thick enough, sutures between the deep aspect of the flap (*not* full thickness) and the underlying muscle will help take off the tension (Fig. 17-6A). Figure 17-6B shows this in profile. The mucosal/submucosal flap is then sutured to the dentate line with interrupted 3-0 polyglycolic acid (Fig. 17-7).

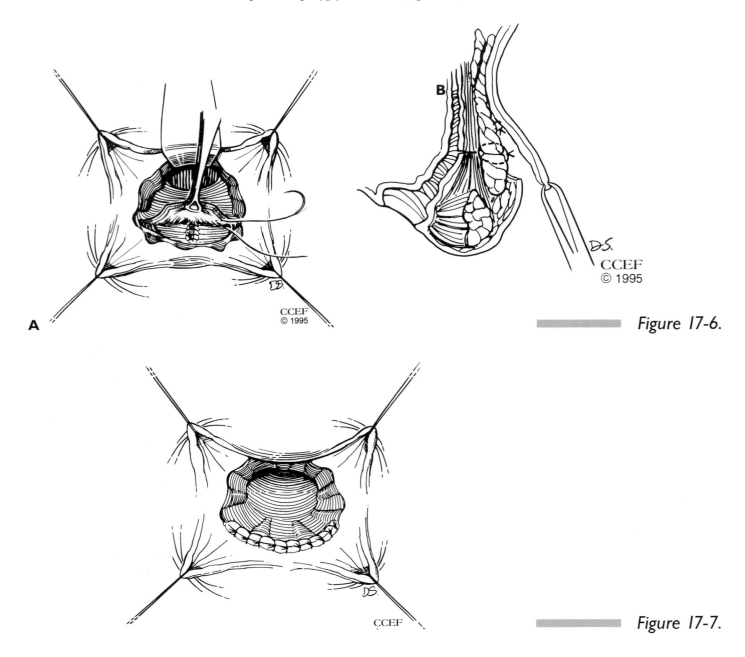

Figure 17-6.

Figure 17-7.

Side to Side Flap.   This procedure is used when the rectal defect is at a distance from the dentate line (e.g., 2 to 5 cm above the dentate line). Raising a curvilinear or rectangular flap has obvious limitations in terms of cephalad extent of mobilization. Although not as "scientific" a procedure as the advancement—because both the defect in the muscle as well as the mucosa are in apposition after repair is made—still the relative ease of the procedure makes it attractive as an alternative (Fig. 17-8).

Figure 17-9 shows a vertically oriented repair, used when the defect is disposed in this direction.

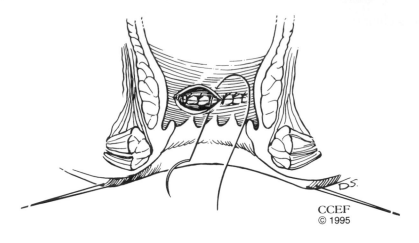

Figure 17-8.

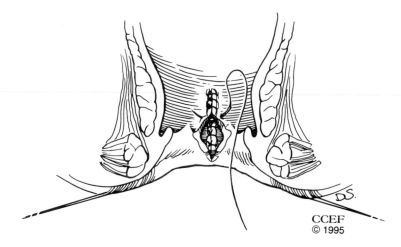

Figure 17-9.

Advancement Rectal Sleeve. This is a complex procedure, as it involves complete or near complete (i.e., 90 percent) detachment of the mucosa of anal canal from the dentate line, distal to the fistula source. The entire anal canal is mobilized up to the anorectal ring, above the level of the levators. The extrarectal (supralevator) space is entered and the lower rectum is circumferentially mobilized. This involves dissection through the cephalad extent of the internal sphincter (middle coat of the rectum) as well as the longitudinal muscles. This procedure is really best reserved for patients in whom the anal canal mucosa is severely diseased (i.e., ulcerated, as in some cases of Crohn's disease) or if there is too much tension in a regular curvilinear flap. Although more demanding technically, the advancement sleeve enables excellent rectal mobilization, similar to an Altemeier procedure for rectal procidentia. A temporary ileostomy is usually added. Figure 17-10 shows the entry into the supralevator space as well as the excision of anal canal mucosa *above* the dentate line.

The medial aspect of the internal sphincter is exposed (Fig. 17-11). After delivery of the mobilized rectum through the anus, the segment of rectum incorporating the fistula opening is trimmed (Fig. 17-12). The cut end is then sutured to the dentate line, as per the regular advancement flap (Fig. 17-13).

Transvaginal Technique

With this approach, the patient is placed in the lithotomy position. The fistula is cored out from the vaginal side and the edges of the vaginal wound are mobilized for 2 to 4 cm (Fig. 17-14). The rectal defect and an adjacent margin of rectal wall are exposed (Fig. 17-15). Alternatives of rectal closure include a pursestring suture (2-0 polyglycolic acid) versus conventional one- or two-layer interrupted sutures. If any of the septum can be imbricated over the rectal repair, then this is done. The vaginal defect is closed with the same type of suture (Fig. 17-16).

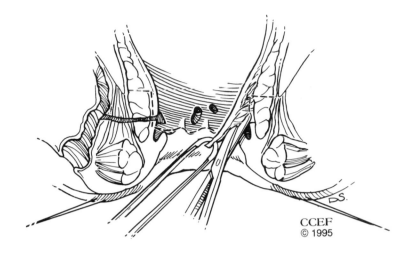

Figure 17-10.

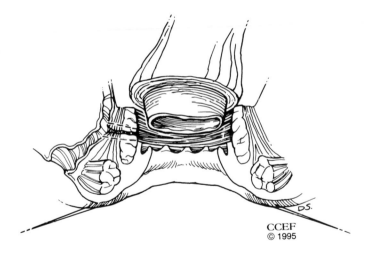

Figure 17-11.

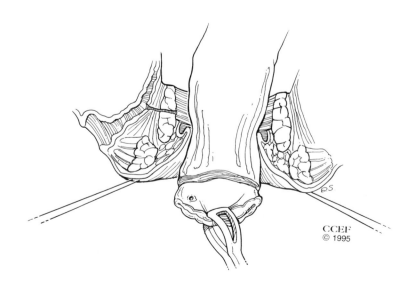

Figure 17-12.

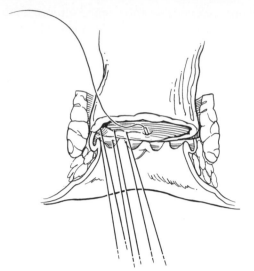

Figure 17-13. ▬▬▬

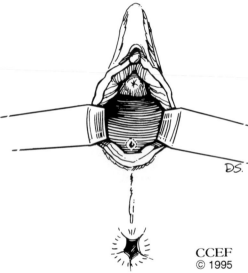

Figure 17-14. ▬▬▬

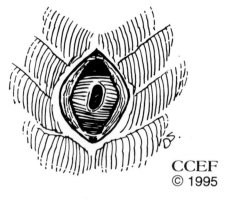

Figure 17-15. ▬▬▬

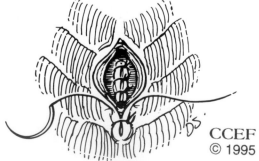

Figure 17-16. ▬▬▬

Transperineal Technique

The transperineal technique is valuable when dealing with a rectovaginal fistula associated with sphincter injury and incontinence. The fistula tract is incised (Fig. 17-17) and then the edges are excised to eliminate granulation tissue (Fig. 17-18). A layered repair is then made, using an overlapping technique for the internal and external sphincter (Fig. 17-19). A suture of 0-0 polyglycolic acid is used to "rebuild" the perineal body. The vaginal and rectal mucosa is then closed (Fig. 17-20).

Postoperative Care

Postoperative care of the rectovaginal fistula patient is controversial. Issues of controversy include the following:

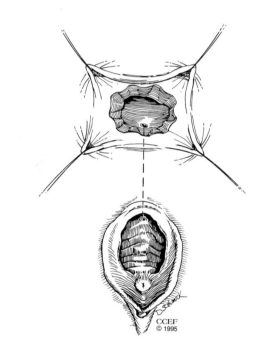

Figure 17-17.

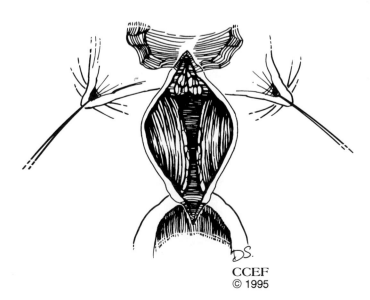

Figure 17-18

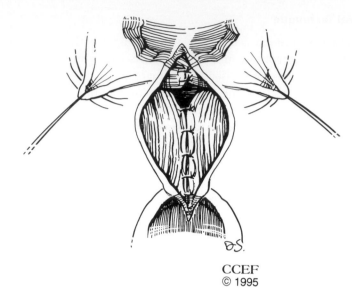

Figure 17-19.

CCEF
© 1995

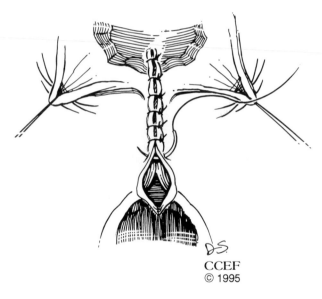

Figure 17-20.

CCEF
© 1995

To confine the bowel or not?
Antibiotics: type, duration, and method of delivery?
Allow the patient to ambulate or not?
Diet: nothing by mouth to ad lib diet?

In practice, I give the patient intravenous antibiotics for 4 to 5 days, usually a third-generation cephalosporin and metronidazole. Following discharge, the patient is prescribed antibiotics by mouth for a further 10 days. The bowels are confined with antidiarrheals for 2 days or so, at which point the urinary catheter is removed. The patient is given liquids only by mouth for 2 days before being given a low-residue diet. Patients are encouraged to walk from the first postoperative day, but to avoid vigorous exercise for 3 months.

If an ostomy is used, it is reversed after 3 months upon demonstration of a healed fistula repair.

Editorial Commentaries

I entirely agree with the approach described by Dr. Fazio for rectovaginal fistula. Where possible, we use a transanal approach, but like him, reserve a perineal approach for patients in whom there is a sphincter injury. We tend to defunction difficult repairs and, provided there has been a full mechanical bowel preparation, prefer loop ileostomy to colostomy.

Michael R. B. Keighley

Dr. Fazio's approach in general is an excellent one. I tend to use the transperineal approach more commonly and reconstruct the pelvic floor anteriorly, including the levators, puborectal muscle, and sphincters, as most rectovaginal fistulas that are not caused by Crohn's disease involve destruction of the perineal body and the anterior sphincter apparatus secondary to obstetric injury.

The management of Crohn's rectovaginal fistula is extremely complex and controversial. In the past I have treated such fistulas using the same approach as described above but added diversion of the fecal stream to the management technique. I have been successful using this approach, although I know that failure may occur any time!

John H. Pemberton

Index

Page numbers followed by f indicate figures